Radioimmunoassay
and related techniques
METHODOLOGY AND CLINICAL APPLICATIONS

Radioimmunoassay and related techniques

METHODOLOGY AND CLINICAL APPLICATIONS

JAN I. THORELL, M.D.

Associate Professor of Clinical Chemistry,
University of Lund; Head Physician,
Department of Nuclear Medicine,
Malmö General Hospital,
Malmö, Sweden

STEVEN M. LARSON, M.D.

Chief, Radioimmunoassay Section, Laboratory Service,
Assistant Chief, Nuclear Medicine Section, Medical Service,
Seattle Veterans Administration Hospital;
Associate Professor of Medicine,
Laboratory Medicine and Radiology,
University of Washington,
Seattle, Washington

with 132 illustrations

The C. V. Mosby Company

Saint Louis   1978

Printed in the United States of America

Distributed in Great Britain by Henry Kimpton, London

The C. V. Mosby Company
11830 Westline Industrial Drive, St. Louis, Missouri 63141

Library of Congress Cataloging in Publication Data

Thorell, Jan I   1934-
   Radioimmunoassay and related techniques.

   Bibliography: p.
   Includes index.
   1.   Radioimmunoassay.   2.   Radioisotopes in medical
diagnosis.   I.   Larson, Steven M., 1941-   joint author.
II.   Title.   [DNLM: 1.   Radioimmunoassay.
2.   Radioligand assay.   QY250 T488r]
RB42.T48   616.07′56   77-23927
ISBN 0-8016-4944-7

GW/CB/B   9   8   7   6   5   4   3   2   1

To our families

PREFACE

During the last few years we have often been asked to recommend an introductory text on radioimmunoassay. This request has been made in many different situations: in elementary courses for medical students or medical technologists; in more advanced courses for scientists and practicing physicians; and in consultation with scientists, research trainees, and laboratory supervisors who were about to start immunoassay work for the first time. Frequently, the radioimmunoassay literature available has been too specialized. Multiauthor books and symposia, by experts writing for experts, are difficult for the beginner to utilize. On the other hand, "beginner oriented" writings, such as journal survey articles, are often too short and superficial for the serious student. Accordingly, we have written this text as both a general survey of the field and as a source of information that is detailed enough to be used as a basis for actual performance of important assays.

As we prepared this text on radioimmunoassay and related methods, we were struck by the diversity of the field. Applications of this methodology impinge on many aspects of biologic, chemical, and physical sciences. With such great diversity it is a practical impossibility to encompass all of the relevant scientific knowledge that relates to this discipline. For this reason, we have restricted the scope of this book to include the more practical aspects of this methodology that will enable practitioners in the field and interested students to obtain a thorough grounding in the basic principles of these techniques. In addition, the combination of a methodology and clinical applications in the same volume is an attempt to bridge the gap between the laboratory and the clinical.

The abundance of different methodologic variants, despite the common principles used in most methods, has made this condensation necessary. This overview does not intend to cover all possible variants reported. However, the principle of the main procedures given in the boxes is that we have performed the method in our own laboratories and, for most methods, in heavy clinical practice over a long period. This at least implies that they have worked well in our hands and should not involve unanticipated problems in actual performance.

The impact of methodologic advances on progress in medicine should not be underestimated. Radioimmunoassay serves as an important example of what a new methodology with a greatly improved sensitivity can mean in terms of advancing scientific knowledge. What of the future for this technology? We believe that the clinical utilization of radioimmunoassay is only at the threshold of an era of many new applications and developments of importance both for everyday clinical medicine and advanced biomedical research. The recent rapid advances of biochemistry are likely to help us to achieve even better binding reagents, in particular more specific and highly avid antisera. Newer labels may be employed that will improve the sensitivity of this test still further. Simpler methodologies and more rapid separation techniques will undoubtedly appear. For some clinical assays, the baton has already been passed from the researcher to the industrialist, and more practical applications to clinical medicine can be anticipated in the future.

This text would not have been possible without the expertise and experience of our collaborators in the laboratory. Thanks to the keen interest of Mr. Ingvar Larsson, M.S., and Mr.

Åke Forsberg, B.A., all boxes and appendixes have been put together from our current laboratory manuals. The extensive typing was done by Mrs. Britta Thelander and Mrs. Ina Blair. During the course of our collaboration we have received valuable advice and support from Henry N. Wagner, Jr., M.D., Johns Hopkins Medical Institutions, Baltimore, Maryland; Tyra T. Hutchens, M.D., University of Oregon Health Sciences Center, Portland, Oregon; and Bertil Nosslin, M.D., Malmö General Hospital, Malmö, Sweden. We extend our gratitude to them and all the other capable workers who have contributed to this volume.

Jan I. Thorell
Steven M. Larson

CONTENTS

PART I

Methodology

1 INTRODUCTION

Radioimmunoassay (RIA) and related competitive protein-binding methods began a little over 20 years ago as a cumbersome research methodology in a few specialized laboratories. Since that time there has been a phenomenal proliferation of these techniques to the measurement of hormones and other substances present in minute quantities in biologic fluids. It is almost impossible to exaggerate the diversity of applications for this methodology. Virtually every branch of medical and biologic research has been affected by these techniques. In particular, endocrinology has been greatly enriched by the new knowledge that has come as a direct result of RIA methods. These methodologies are being introduced into clinical medicine at a rapid rate, and the growing commercial availability of radioassay kits promises to revolutionize the routine practice of hospital laboratories.

TERMINOLOGY

The term radioimmunoassay was coined by Berson and Yalow in describing their original methodology. This term is adequate when radioassays are described in which antibodies are used as specific binding reagents; but because many assays utilize binding reagents other than antibodies, a more general term is required. Several different terms have been proposed, including saturation analysis, competitive radioassay, competitive binding assay, displacement analysis, radiostereoassay, and competitive protein-binding procedures. Each of these terms has deficiencies when used to describe the whole class or technique. Two examples serve to indicate the deficiencies: no assay works at saturation conditions in the sense that all receptor sites are occupied; an increasing number of radioassays are not competitive.

We have adhered to the term radioligand assay for the following reasons. The word ligand emerges from the Latin word "ligare," which means "to bind." The term ligand is a common denominator for compounds participating in interactions between macromolecules and smaller molecules. All radioassay methods of the type discussed here involve the binding of a compound to some sort of specific receptor. Accordingly, the term ligand assay need not be confined to any special type of interaction occurring in the assay or to any particular type of components participating in this reaction. Also, this nomenclature will conform to that currently used in chemistry and biochemistry to describe the interaction between big and small molecules. The prefix "radio" in radioligand assay indicates that radioactive nuclides are used as the indicator for the purpose of quantitation. Radionuclides are by no means the only indicator that may be used for this purpose. Assays in which an enzyme or a fluorescent substance is used may be called enzymatic ligand assay or fluorescent ligand assay, respectively. Explanations of other terms that may be encountered during a discussion of in vitro radionuclide methodology are given in the glossary of radioligand assay terms below.

GLOSSARY OF TERMS USED IN RADIOLIGAND ASSAY

accuracy (of assay) Closeness to "true" or real value.

affinity Property of substance bound. Strength (energy) of binding to the receptor.

analyte Substance to be measured by an assay system.

antibody A protein formed as part of an immunologic response to a foreign substance. The antibody specifically combines with the foreign substance and to a variable extent with substances of similar structure.

antibody, first Term used in double-antibody assays to indicate the antibody binding the substance to be assayed.

antibody, second Term used in double-antibody assays to indicate a precipitating antibody, which binds the first antibody, in order to separate "bound" from "free" ligand.

antigen A substance that is capable of inducing formation of antibodies and that reacts specifically to the antibodies so produced.

antiserum Serum from an immune animal, contains various antibodies.

autologous Term of immunologic relationship, from same individual.

avidity Property of binder, strength (energy) of binding of ligand.

competitive inhibition Describes inhibition of binding of radioligand to receptor by ligand.

competitive protein binding Synonym for radioligand (assay), emphasizing importance of protein receptors in in vitro assays that utilize competitive inhibition.

competitive radioassay Synonym for radioligand assay, emphasizing competition between radioligand and ligand for a specific receptor binding site as the basis for in vitro radioassay.

damage Jargon term used to indicate denaturation of the radioligand. This may occur during the process of radiolabeling—"labeling damage" (in the case of labeling by means of radioiodination, "iodination damage"). If it happens during the incubation period of an assay, it is often referred to as "incubation damage" or during storage of the radioligand as "storage damage."

displacement analysis Synonym for radioligand assay, emphasizing the principle of displacement of radioligand by stable ligand as the basis for in vitro radioassay.

hapten A substance that is not immunogenic in itself, but becomes immunogenic when complexed to another compound. The antibody produced will bind the noncomplexed hapten also; for example, steroids and digoxin.

heterologous Xenogeneic, from an individual of another species.

homologous From another individual of same species: *syngeneic* if genetically identical, *allogeneic* if genetically different.

immunogen A substance capable of inducing an immune response when introduced into an immunologically competent host.

immunoglobulins A group of serum proteins of which the following classes are known: IgG, IgM, IgA, IgD, IgE. They emerge as the effect of an immunoresponse and have the property in common to specifically bind the antigen. IgG is quantitatively dominant and is the usual binding antibody in RIAs.

immunoradiometric assay Ligand to be measured is assayed directly by combination with specific labeled antibodies rather than in competition with a labeled derivative for a limited amount of antibody.

incubation damage Alteration in binding characteristics of a ligand during the incubation period of an assay (usually applied to radioligand). This may result, for example, from aggregation of molecules, enzymatic degradation, radiation damage, or deiodination.

incubation period, first Ambiguous term used to describe (1) period of preincubation of ligand and binding agent before addition of radioligand (disequilibrium assays) or (2) period of incubation between ligand, radioligand, and binding agent before addition of precipitating (second) antibody (double-antibody assays).

incubation period, second Ambiguous term used to describe (1) period of incubation after addition of radioligand (disequilibrium assays) or (2) period of incubation with precipitating (second) antibody (double-antibody assays).

iodination damage *See* damage.

ligand The substance that is bound. In radioassays usually the hormone or other moiety that is to be assayed.

precision (of assay) Degree of agreement of repeated measurements of a quantity. Usually expressed as the coefficient of variation for repeated measurements of the same sample: intraassay if it refers to precision within an individual assay run, interassay if it refers to results from different sets of assays.

quality control In general terms, the analytical and other steps that must be taken to ensure that results of assays are reliable and representative for the true concentration of the material to be assayed.

radioimmunoassay Radioligand assay in which the receptor is an antibody.

radioligand Radioactive form of ligand.

radioligand assay General term for in vitro radioassay based on receptor-ligand binding.

radioreceptor assay Term usually used when a cell-associated receptor (membrane, cytoplasm, nucleus) is used as the binder for a radioligand assay. May also be used less commonly as a general term for in vitro radioassay based on receptor-ligand binding.

radiostereoassay Synonym for radioligand assay, emphasizing the importance of tertiary protein structure and specific complementary orientation of ligand and receptor in in vitro radioassay.

receptor A substance (a protein) that specifically binds a certain compound (ligand). In radioligand assays most commonly an antibody but includes other binders such as plasma transporting proteins, enzymes, or cell-associated binding substances (membrane receptor, intracellular receptor).

saturation analysis Synonym for radioligand assay, emphasizing the progressive saturation of available receptor-binding sites with ligand, and the subsequent nonavailability of receptor sites for binding of radioligand, as the basis for in vitro radioassay.

sensitivity Minimum quantity detectable. Depends in part on assay precision.

specificity Ability to assay a single substance in heterogeneous mixtures. For RIA, the capacity to discriminate antigens of similar structure.

standard A substance, usually chemically identical to the substance to be assayed, that is added to certain reference tubes in an assay series to serve as a yardstick for quantitation of the contents in the samples. It is not necessarily of maximum purity. An International Standard is a particular preparation of a substance that has been adopted by the World Health Organization as a common reference for quantity of this substance.

titer Measurement of antibody concentration. For RIA, the titer is frequently defined in terms of the dilution of antiserum that will bind 50% of added radioligand.

CHARACTERISTICS OF RADIOLIGAND ASSAY

Receptors that bind radioactive substances were first used to assess the binding capacities of proteins such as thyroxine-binding proteins and transferrin. Competition between radioligand and ligand in the unknown sample for a specific receptor-binding site was first used from 1956 to 1960 as a means of measuring ligand concentration by Berson and Yalow and associates. This concept has been called the principle of competitive inhibition. These investigators deserve much of the credit for developing the basic techniques for radioligand assays in general. Their initial studies were of insulin metabolism in diabetes. They were able to achieve ^{131}I labeling of insulin in specific activities high enough to permit adequate assay

Table 1-1. Ligand-receptor combination in radioligand assays

Antibodies		Plasma transporting proteins		Tissue receptors	
Ligand	Antibody to	Ligand	Receptor	Ligand	Receptor
Protein hormones	Protein hormone (sometimes conjugated)	Thyroxine	TBG	Vitamin B$_{12}$ Nucleotides	Intrinsic factor Nucleotide binding
Steroid hormones	Steroid-protein complex	Vitamin B$_{12}$	Transcobalamin	Estrogen	Uterus cytosol receptor
Enzymes	Enzyme	Testosterone	Testosterone-binding globulin	ACTH	Adrenal cortex Cell membrane receptor
Nucleotides	Nucleotide-protein complex	Cortisol	Corticosteroid-binding globulin	Insulin	Liver, placenta Cell membrane receptor
Virus	Virus, in animal or human				
Drugs	Drug-protein conjugate				

sensitivity. They also devised methods for separation of the unbound radioligand from that bound to specific antibody. This work resulted in the first RIA, which was for serum insulin, in 1960. The use of a nonimmune serum-binding protein for a competitive assay was independently developed by Ekins, who devised a method for measurement of thyroxine using the thyroxine-binding properties of specific binding globulins in human plasma. The subsequent development of a series of RIAs for other hormones and biologically important substances was greatly facilitated by the work of Hunter and Greenwood in 1962, who developed the chloramine-T method for readily labeling proteins with high specific activities of ^{131}I.

Radioligand assay methods have in common a binding reagent (receptor) that selectively binds the substance to be measured (ligand). Antibodies have been the most extensively used type of receptor (RIA), but the specific binding properties of other proteins have also been used (Table 1-1).

The revolution in the measurement of biologic substances created by radioligand assays was primarily an effect of a dramatic increase in *sensitivity* in comparison with other chemical methodologies. This sensitivity is related to the

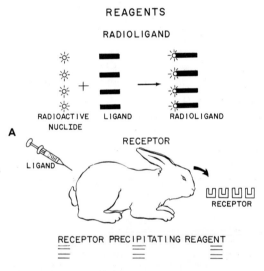

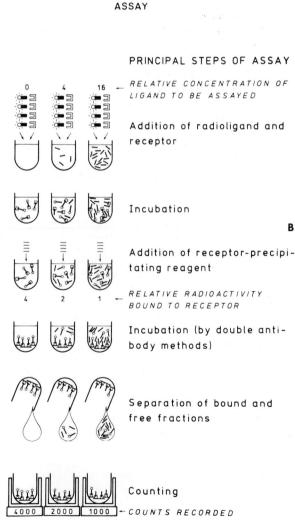

Fig. 1-1. Diagram of principles of a competitive type of radioligand assay. **A,** Reagents used for competitive type of radioligand assay. The ligand is labeled with a radionuclide to form the radioligand. Ligand is injected (as immunogen) into an animal to produce specific antibodies as receptor. **B,** Assay performance for radioligand assay of competitive type. Radioligand and receptor are added to the incubation mixture. During the incubation step, the reactants come to equilibrium, and there is competition between the ligand and radioligand for a specific receptor site. After equilibrium has been achieved, relatively little radioligand is bound in the tubes that originally contained a high relative concentration of ligand (16). A receptor-precipitating reagent is added, and the bound and free fractions of radioligand are separated and counted. The lowest counts (1,000) occur in the tube with the highest original relative concentration of radioligand (16).

extremely sensitive methods for the detection of radioactivity. For example, it is possible to measure the radioactive isotope ^{125}I in quantities as small as 10^{-14} g (or approximately 10^{-12} M) with good precision. Since the serum concentration of most hormones is on the order of 10^9 to 10^{10} M, detection of hormone levels at the lowest physiologic concentration is now possible. The radioactive tracer used in these assays is called the radioligand.

The other main feature of this methodology is *specificity*. Most biologically active compounds are built up by the common elements C, O, H, and a few others. The uniqueness of these compounds is therefore determined not so much by their overall composition but by the order in which the elements are put together. It is the architecture of the compounds that determines their function. A unique structure will give the molecule a unique external configuration. This is also the basis for the assay specificity. The ligand is bound by the receptor at a specific receptor-binding site. This binding site has a configuration that is complementary to a particular area on the surface of the ligand. The binding between ligand and receptor can be viewed as the fitting of a key into a lock. The ability of a receptor to recognize the external configuration is therefore the basis for identification of the particular compound in a biologic fluid. Antibodies have been produced that have such high specificity that they can distinguish between two peptides that differ by as little as

one atom, for example, thyroxine and triiodothyronine. The fit between receptor and ligand also influences the strength of the bond, a factor that along with the specific activity of the radioligand determines the sensitivity of the assay.

In addition, radioassays have been refined to the point that they are relatively easy to perform on a mass scale with a high degree of precision. These techniques lend themselves relatively well to automation. In this regard we are already beginning to see in the clinical laboratory the fruit of a decade or more of rapid commercial development.

PRINCIPLES OF RADIOLIGAND ASSAY

In order to establish a radioligand assay, three prerequisites must be met: (1) a receptor must be available that specifically binds the substance (ligand) to be measured; (2) the ligand must be labeled with a radioactive nuclide (radioligand); and (3) separation must be achievable between the ligand bound to the receptor and the ligand that is unbound. The radioligand assay may be divided into two general categories: competitive and noncompetitive radioligand assay.

Competitive assays

The competitive assay is still the most common type. The principles of such methods are shown in Fig. 1-1. In this case, the specific

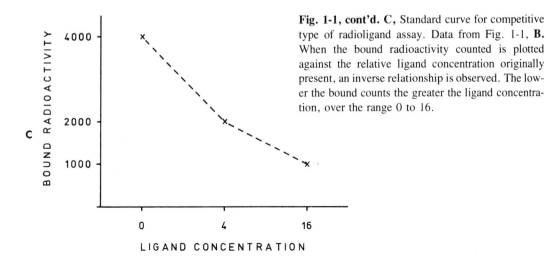

Fig. 1-1, cont'd. C, Standard curve for competitive type of radioligand assay. Data from Fig. 1-1, **B.** When the bound radioactivity counted is plotted against the relative ligand concentration originally present, an inverse relationship is observed. The lower the bound counts the greater the ligand concentration, over the range 0 to 16.

receptor is an antibody directed against the ligand to be measured. The ligand is injected into a species of animal that sees this substance as foreign and produces a specific antibody against the ligand. The radioligand is produced by coupling of radioactive nuclide to the ligand as a marker for the ligand substance to be measured (Fig. 1-1, *A*). The principal steps of assay are illustrated in Fig. 1-1, *B*. The amount of antibody used (in this simplified example) has

a binding capacity that approximately corresponds to the amount of radioligand present. If there is any native (unlabeled or "cold") ligand present, it will compete with the radioligand molecules for the limited number of binding sites. As the concentration of native ligand increases, less and less radioactive material will be bound to the receptor. Thus the greater the concentration of native ligand in the biologic specimen, the lower the amount of ra-

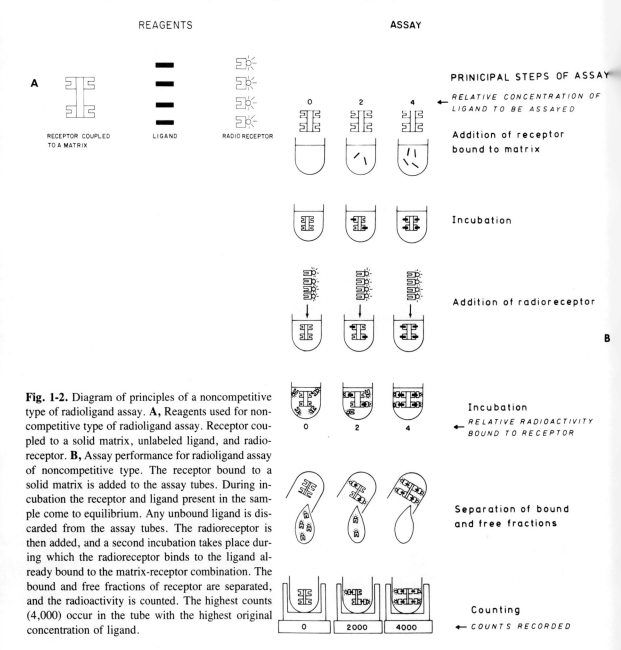

Fig. 1-2. Diagram of principles of a noncompetitive type of radioligand assay. **A,** Reagents used for noncompetitive type of radioligand assay. Receptor coupled to a solid matrix, unlabeled ligand, and radioreceptor. **B,** Assay performance for radioligand assay of noncompetitive type. The receptor bound to a solid matrix is added to the assay tubes. During incubation the receptor and ligand present in the sample come to equilibrium. Any unbound ligand is discarded from the assay tubes. The radioreceptor is then added, and a second incubation takes place during which the radioreceptor binds to the ligand already bound to the matrix-receptor combination. The bound and free fractions of receptor are separated, and the radioactivity is counted. The highest counts (4,000) occur in the tube with the highest original concentration of ligand.

dioligand bound to the receptor. This can be considered as a progressive dilution of radioligand bound to the receptor, or as a progressive dilution of radioactive material with nonradioactive material, thereby reducing the specific activity of the ligand bound to the receptor. In this way, radioligand assay may be considered an application of the general principle of isotope dilution, in which the receptor serves to remove an aliquot of the tracer for subsequent measurement of its specific activity.

There is usually an incubation period for most assays, during which time the binding reaction between receptor and ligand comes close to equilibrium. For most assays the molar concentration of the receptor is chosen to be about the same order of magnitude as the expected concentration of the ligand in the unknown samples. In general, the more dilute the receptor is, the more sensitive the assay will be. At these low concentrations of reactants, longer incubation times will be necessary in order to achieve a sufficient binding of ligand to receptor.

After the binding reaction is completed, the receptors must be separated from the rest of the mixture in order to determine the amount of radioactivity that is bound. A variety of different techniques have been employed for this purpose. In some circumstances, a second period of incubation may be required, as with the double-antibody techniques. The receptor-bound radioactivity is then separated from the free radioactivity, and the amount of bound radioactivity is determined. As can be seen from inspection of Fig. 1-1, *B,* there is an inverse correlation between the amount of radioactivity bound and the concentration of native ligand present in samples. This relationship is usually not linear (Fig. 1-1, *C*). In order to be able to measure the amount of ligand in an unknown biologic sample, such as plasma or urine, a series of assay tubes must include a standard series of tubes that contain known amounts in sequential increment of the substance to be assayed. Based on the radioactivity bound to the receptor in these standard tubes, a standard curve is drawn (Fig. 1-1, *C*). From this standard curve, the amount of ligand in an unknown sample can be estimated.

Noncompetitive assays

In these techniques the antibody is usually labeled instead of the ligand. These methods are particularly useful when the ligand cannot be labeled easily, as in the case of hepatitis-associated antigen or other viruses. This procedure is illustrated diagrammatically in Fig. 1-2.

In this technique the receptor is coupled to an insoluble, solid phase matrix. This matrix may be either a powder or disc, or the inside of the test tube. An additional set of receptors is labeled with radioactivity. In the initial phase of the assay (Fig. 1-2, *A*), the receptor preparation is incubated with the sample containing the ligand to be assayed until all ligand present is bound to the receptor. In step two, a second set of receptors is added, which are soluble but have a radioactive tracer labeled to their

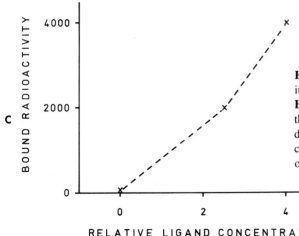

Fig. 1-2, cont'd. C, Standard curve for noncompetitive type of radioligand assay. Data from Fig. 1-2, **B.** When the bound radioactivity is plotted against the relative concentration of ligand to be assayed, a direct relationship is observed. The greater the bound counts, the greater the relative ligand concentration, over the range 0 to 4.

outer end. This radioreceptor adheres to any bound ligand present in the sample (Fig. 1-2, *B*). This methodology requires that the ligand be sufficiently large to have two or more molecular regions that can act as combining sites (divalent or polyvalent). Following the incubation with radioactive receptor, the matrix is washed and all nonbound radioactivity is removed. The radioactivity remaining bound to the matrix is measured. The activity bound to the solid phase is proportional to the amount of nonradioactive ligand present. A standard curve is constructed by including within the assay run a series of tubes that contain incremental amounts of known standard. The standard curve in this type of assay is directly proportional to the concentration of standard; that is, the larger the amount of ligand present, the larger the amount of radioactivity bound to the receptor (Fig. 1-2, *C*).

SUMMARY

1. RIA and related clinical methods (radioligand assay) derive their unique usefulness from their very great sensitivity. These methods permit measurement of biologically important substances down to concentrations of 10^{-12} mol/liter.

2. These methods are all based on binding interaction between large and small molecules, the receptor and the ligand, respectively, hence the general term for this class of radioassay: radioligand assay. This binding can be visualized as a "key in lock" interaction of molecules with complementary surface structures.

3. Radioligand assay is a method that is applicable to the measurement of many biologically important substances of diverse types, including hormones, drugs, and proteins. Development of such methods depends principally on the availability of a relatively pure preparation of the compound to be measured and a specific binder for this compound.

In subsequent chapters, each of the reagent components of the radioligand assay, as well as the kinetics of the interaction, is discussed. The initial half of the book relates to technical aspects of assay performance. The second half of the book contains discussions of the many important clinical applications of RIA and related clinical methods.

2 RECEPTORS FOR RADIOLIGAND ASSAYS

The properties of the binding reagent (the receptor) of radioligand assays are among the major factors that determine the quality of the assay. As discussed in detail in the section on quality control, the quality of any assay is determined by four factors: *sensitivity, specificity, precision,* and *accuracy.* Of these, specificity is predominantly a property depending on the receptor, whereas sensitivity is limited by two factors; the avidity of the receptor and the specific activity of the radioligand (see Chapter 3). In essence, the specificity denotes the uniqueness of the binding, and the avidity denotes the strength of binding. The way in which the receptor properties influence specificity and avidity is illustrated in Fig. 2-1. Precision and accuracy are mainly determined by the design and performance of the assay.

The *specificity* is the ability of the assay to measure one specific compound and no other. The specificity or rather lack of specificity is a major problem in some assays but not in others. If a compound to be assayed in plasma is the only one of its type present and there exists no other with structural similarities in plasma, then there is no need to anticipate interference from any other material. However, for many biologically important compounds, a number of compounds exist with similar chemical structures. Usually we do not want to include these substances in the assay, because they have different biologic effects. Steroid hormone assays are one example of assays with serious problems of this type; there are many steroid derivatives with small differences in structure but with marked differences in physiologic effects. In this situation, production and selection of adequate receptors (antisera) may require significant effort. Sometimes it is not possible to achieve a receptor with specificity adequate to measure a particular compound in the presence of other similar compounds. The situation can be improved sometimes by chemical separation to isolate the compound to be measured from those causing undesired cross-reactions; solvent extraction and washing procedure or various types of chromatography are the purification procedures most often used (see Chapter 5).

The *avidity* of the receptor reflects the energy in the binding between the ligand and the receptor or, in simple terms, the firmness of the

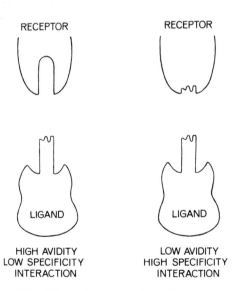

RECEPTOR   RECEPTOR

LIGAND   LIGAND

HIGH AVIDITY   LOW AVIDITY
LOW SPECIFICITY   HIGH SPECIFICITY
INTERACTION   INTERACTION

Fig. 2-1. Schematic presentation of the concepts avidity and specificity. At high avidity the "strong" high-energy binding is indicated by the large contact areas between receptor and ligand; however, this does not necessarily imply a unique fit (high specificity) between them. The high-specificity binding, on the other hand, indicates a unique fit; but this does not in itself make it a "strong" high-avidity binding.

binding. To be able to measure the minute amounts of hormones and other biologic reactive compounds with sufficient sensitivity, the energy of the binding has to be very high. Antisera optimal in this respect are sometimes quite rare, so the avidity of the antibodies is usually the limiting factor for the sensitivity of an RIA.

IMMUNE RECEPTORS (ANTIBODIES)
General properties

It has long been known that higher animals have the ability to react to foreign material in their bodies and that these reactions, which are part of the defense mechanisms against invasive organisms such as bacteria and viruses, are quite specific. Immunity against measles virus does not help against German measles. It has been shown that these responses to foreign material are mediated by the immunologic system and that many of the reactions are caused by humoral principles circulating in the blood plasma. These principles have been identified as antibodies; they have the property of binding to and thereby neutralizing foreign material.

The ability of antibodies to recognize such foreign material is related to two general properties of antibodies: the binding of this material is highly specific to the chemical structure of the reacting material, and it occurs only to material foreign to the individual in which the antibodies circulate. The latter phenomenon depends on an ability of the system that produces antibodies to recognize "self" from "nonself" material. Altered material from the individual's own body may acquire nonself properties. In this way antibodies may act as a sewage removal system. The ability of antibodies to recognize one particular material as distinct from any other is highly developed, and it is this particular characteristic that is the basis for the use of antibodies as an analytical tool in all immunologic methods. We will see how extremely small alterations in the structure of a molecule sometimes will drastically change its binding to antibodies but also that there are limitations in the ability of the antibodies to discriminate between similar structures. Antibodies are usually not preformed in the individual but are produced in response to the entry of the foreign material into the body. Material that induces an immunoresponse is called an *immunogen*. The substance that is bound by *antibodies* is called *antigen*. Most substances are both immunogen and antigen, but these two properties are distinct and not all antigens have the ability to initiate the formation of antibodies.

Antibodies are a group of related proteins in blood plasma and certain other extracellular fluids. They are collectively called immunoglobulins (Ig). Previously the term γ-globulin was used because of the electrophoretic mobility of the main body of the immunoglobulins. There are five known types or classes of immunoglobulins: IgG, IgM, IgA, IgD, and IgE.

The basic structure of all immunoglobulins is similar with a pair of large polypetide chains (heavy chains, H), that consist of 446 amino acids, each associated with a smaller chain (light chain, L) 214 amino acids long. The chains are arranged as shown in Fig. 2-2, joined by disulfide bonds. Each immunoglobulin molecule has the ability to bind two antigen molecules, one at each of the two binding sites, which are located at the outer open end of each pair of H-L chains. Differences in the chemical composition of these two ends of the molecules (the so-called variable portions of the chains) are the structural basis for the differences in the binding characteristics of different antibod-

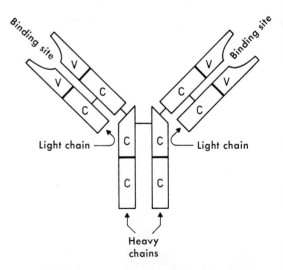

Fig. 2-2. Schematic presentation of immunoglobulin G (IgG) structure. *C* denotes regions with a constant structure and *V* the variable regions that constitute the binding sites, in which the variability is the basis for the configuration of the binding site to fit to its corresponding antigen.

ies. The configuration of this binding site can therefore assume such a variety of forms that it very specifically fits to the surface of any antigenic material. The various types of immunoglobulins have somewhat different biologic functions. IgG is the quantitatively dominant immunoglobulin in plasma. It has a molecular weight of about 160,000 daltons. It is the class of immunoglobulin usually utilized as binder in RIA. Its concentration in plasma is about 10 g/liter (1%).

The immunoglobulins are produced by B-lymphocytes. The process of their maturation and development to antibody-producing cells is complex and only partly known, as is the effect of interaction with the other type of lymphocyte, the T-lymphocytes. The following description is a highly simplified view of the events. After administration of the immunogen, it is believed to be bound to receptors on the surface of certain lymphocytes. This binding induces the production of an immunoglobulin with a structure of the variable portion that can bind this particular antigen. Then the lymphocytes carrying this information start multiplying, and all the new lymphocytes so produced carry with them the ability to produce antibodies against this particular immunogen.

The production of immunoglobulin in response to stimulation with an immunogen follows a certain time course. The antibody produced initially is of the IgM type, which is a large molecule consisting of 5 units of IgG-type antibody and accordingly has 10 antigen-binding sites. The induction of the IgM response is very rapid, and IgM antibodies may appear in plasma as early as 12 hours after immunization. The production of IgM antibodies continues to increase exponentially for about 1 week. Then the cells producing the IgM antibodies switch to synthesis of IgG antibodies; the IgM level in plasma declines, and the level of IgG begins to rise. The IgG production after a single stimulus usually reaches a peak after 1 or 2 months; then it declines slowly. Production may continue for extended periods, sometimes many months or even years. If the same stimulus is repeated with a new injection of the same immunogen (the "booster injection"), there follows a rapid IgG response without any previous IgM induction.

Not every substance foreign to the body will induce an immunoresponse. Small molecules usually do not; the approximate lower limit for immunogenicity is a molecular weight of 1,000 to 10,000 daltons. Certain types of compounds are more immunogenic than others. Most large proteins and carbohydrates are immunogenic. However, the antibodies developed to the substance will bind only to a very small portion of the antigen molecule. For proteins it is a section comprised of only a few amino acid residues that participate in the binding to the binding site (receptor) of the antibody. This implies that the binding to antibody may occur with any compound that has the structure of this antigenic combining site. Such a molecule may be too small to induce the production of antibodies and is for this reason called an incomplete antigen, or hapten. If a hapten is chemically coupled to a large molecule, the combination of the hapten and the large molecule may act as a complete antigen or an immunogen. This phenomenon has been extensively utilized for the production of antisera against small molecules in RIAs (such as steroid hormones and thyroid hormones). The small molecules are coupled with large protein molecules, such as serum albumin or thyroglobulin. This complex is administered to an animal that produces antibodies against this complex and in which some of the antibodies are directed against the hapten. These antibodies may then be used in an assay for this particular small molecule, where its property of binding with the antibody even when not coupled to the serum albumin is employed.

The antibodies produced in response to an immunogenic stimulus constitute only a very small fraction of the total antibody population occurring in plasma of that animal. In most assays there is, however, no need for isolation of this particular fraction from the other antibodies present, since the assay system only measures the binding of one particular radioactive antigen. Other antibodies present will not interfere in this binding between the labeled antigen and its particular antibody. These mutually associated antigens and antibodies are called homologous antigen and antibody. In certain assay systems, one may utilize antibody that is raised against a different immunogen;

in this case the antigen and antibody are called heterologous.

Kinetics of antigen-antibody binding

The reaction between antigen and antibody is a reversible reaction and involves noncovalent bonds (electrostatic, hydrogen bonding, and van der Waals interactions). In many antigen-antibody systems, the primary reaction is followed by secondary reactions. For example, the primary antigen-antibody complexes join together and form aggregates. The complexes build up large lattices with reduced solubility in water, which cause them to precipitate. Other secondary effects induced by the binding between antigen and antibody are agglutinations and cell toxic reactions.

In RIAs, it is believed that only the primary antigen-antibody reaction occurs (except in separation with double-antibody precipitation). However, the data available in this respect are quite limited, and the long incubation time needed in some assay systems indicates that secondary reactions, which usually take much longer than the primary reactions to develop, may be involved. The kinetics of binding reactions between ligand and receptor in nonimmune radioligand assays is essentially the same as that of the primary antigen-antibody reactions; this discussion applies to all such receptor-ligand systems.

The reversible primary reaction between antigen and antibody obeys the law of mass action, assuming that the two antibody-binding sites of each antibody molecule are reacting independently with the same energy. Accordingly, this reaction can be characterized in common thermodynamic terms. From the law of mass action:

$$L + R \underset{k_{-1}}{\overset{k_1}{\rightleftarrows}} LR \tag{1}$$

where L denotes the ligand (antigen), R the receptor (antibody), and LR the complex of ligand bound to the receptor (antigen-antibody complex). In the following discussion, we assume that the ligand and radioligand behave identically in the reaction, so we do not need to treat them separately. L, therefore, applies to either unlabeled or labeled material or any combination thereof, and k_1 and k_{-1} are the rate constants for the association and dissociation reactions, respectively. The quantitative reaction between the reactants when the reaction has reached equilibrium is characterized by the following formula:

$$[L] \times [R] \times K_a = [LR] \tag{2}$$

where the brackets denote the molar concentrations of L, R, and LR. K_a is a constant for the overall bind-

ing reaction (association constant). The overall reaction is the combined effect of the association and dissociation rates:

$$K_a = \frac{k_1}{k_{-1}} \tag{3}$$

Formula (2) can be rearranged to:

$$K_a = \frac{[LR]}{[L] \times [R]} \tag{4}$$

K_a is the factor that at equilibrium governs the quantitative relation between the concentration of free ligand [L], bound ligand [LR], and unoccupied receptor sites [R]. K_a is expressed in liters per mole. Sometimes the dissociation constant, K_d, or the Michaelis-Menten constant, K_m, is used to express these relationships. The two constants are the inverse of K_a. K_a is an expression for the avidity of the binding between ligand and receptor. The higher the avidity, the higher will be the proportion of the reagents in the bound form. At low concentration of the reactants (as in the case in radioligand assays) K_a must be very high to give sufficient binding.

The following interpretation of this equation in connection with RIA may explain the importance of the constant K_a in particular to the sensitivity of the assay. It is applied to the simplified example given in Chapter 1 (Fig. 1-1).

In this case, it is evident that if these assays are to work as a "saturation analysis" system, the binding capacity of the receptor should be about equal to (or less than) the amount of radioligand added to the system. It is only in this situation that added unlabeled ligand will compete with the radioligand for the binding sites, and the bound radioactivity will decrease. This decrease must reach a certain magnitude to be recorded as a real (significant) decrease. The overall imprecision of assays usually implies that the decrease in the bound activity has to be about 10% of the total activity to be significant. Thus the smallest amount of the unlabeled ligand that will significantly inhibit or compete with the binding of the radioligand is on the order of one-tenth the amount of radioligand. (The influence of the quantitative relation between ligand and radioligand on the sensitivity of assay is highly dependent on assay precision, which is discussed at length on p. 79.) Most protein hormones occur in plasma in a concentration of about 10^{-9} mol/liter. According to the discussion above, the concentration of radioligand should at the most be $10 \times 10^{-9} = 10^{-8}$ mol/liter. At saturation the molar concentration of the binder should be the same. The total concentration of receptor is [LR] + [R]. In this case [LR] + [R] should be about $10 \times 10^{-9} = 10^{-8}$. At saturation, the number of receptor sites still unoccupied (R) is approaching 0. Assume that 90% of the receptor sites are occupied. Thus, $[LR] = 0.9 \times 10^{-8}$ and $[R] = 0.1 \times 10^{-8}$ (or the ratio $[LR]/[R] = 9$).

Substituting this in (4) gives:

$$K_a = \frac{0.9 \times 10^{-8}}{[L] \times 0.1 \times 10^{-8}}$$

or

$$K_a = \frac{9}{[L]}$$

or

$$\frac{1}{K_a} = \frac{[L]}{9}$$

The inverse of K_a is accordingly 1/9 of the concentration of free ligand. In our example, the free ligand present $[L]$ corresponds to the amount of ligand we want to measure (10^9), since this was the amount that was added in excess of the binding capacity. Accordingly,

$$\frac{1}{K_a} = \frac{10^{-9}}{9} = 1.1 \times 10^{-10}$$

Thus, $K_a \approx 10^{10}$, or the inverse of K_a is approximately one tenth of the amount we want to measure.

What would be the effect if K_a were markedly smaller? Assume $K_a = 10^9$. Still, to be able to achieve a competitive situation, the receptor must be close to saturation as before. This implies that the amount of radioligand is equal to or larger than the binding capacity. As in the previous case, a 90% occupancy of the receptor would make $[LR]/[R] = 9$. Substituting these figures in (4) we find:

$$10^9 = \frac{9}{[L]}$$

or

$$[L] = 1.1 \times 10^{-8}$$

Thus to be able to achieve a 90% saturation of the receptor, as much as 10^{-8} mol/liter of the ligand must be in the free form. This implies that we must add about two times more of the radioligand to saturate the receptors than in the previous example with a K_a of 10^{10}. The effect of this is that before any cold ligand is added, 50% of the total radioactivity is in the free form; the 10^{-9} mol/liter of the ligand we want to measure constitutes only 5% of the amount of radioligand. According to the initial discussion of this example, the addition of 5% unlabeled ligand would not be detectable. The smallest detectable concentration in this example would be 2×10^{-9} mol/liter. A further decrease of K_a will make the relation between the amount of radioligand and

ligand even more unfavorable and decrease sensitivity further. As will be evident in later sections, many radioligand assays suffer from borderline low-avidity antisera that make it necessary to work with correspondingly high amounts of radioligand and low bound fractions even when no unlabeled ligand is present (for example, on the order of 30% to 50%).

In conclusion, a low K_a may be compensated for to an extent by increasing the amount of radioligand, but it will reduce the working range of the assay. In practical terms, $1/K_a$ should be at least two to ten times the molar concentration K_a we want to measure. The influence of K_a on the assay sensitivity is illustrated in Fig. 2-3.

If $1/K_a$ is very much larger, for example, 100-fold the concentration to be measured, then the receptors are almost completely saturated by addition of radioligand in the same amount as the binding capacity. That is, about 99% of the added radioactivity is bound (as in the example in Fig. 1-1). This implies that the assay works almost as an ideal isotope dilution method, which gives the highest possible theoretical sensitivity to an equilibrium type of assay. At this condition, a doubling of the total concentration of ligand will always cause a reduction of bound activity by 50%. A steeper slope of the dose-effect relation (the standard curve) cannot be achieved in a competitive type of assay permitted to react approximately to equilibrium and with identical behavior of ligand and radioligand. In such an assay the specific activity of the radioligand will be the sensitivity-limiting factor. The reason for this is that as long as the factor $1/K_a$ is much higher than the concentration of the ligand to be assayed, the amount of receptor can be further diminished (antibody-diluted) and still maintain saturation condition. This scaling down of the amounts of reagents will improve sensitivity in proportion to the decrease in the amount of receptor, providing that the radioligand still can be detected at this low concentration. Fig. 2-3 also shows that a low avidity cannot be appropriately compensated for by increasing the specific activity. But with a very high avidity of the receptor, an increased specific activity of the radioligand will increase the sensitivity of the assay proportionately.

The most common approach for characterization of the binding reaction follows the Scatchard presentation of the law of mass action (Fig. 2-4):

$$\frac{r}{c} = nK_a - rK_a \tag{5}$$

where n is the valence of the antibody, r the ratio of bound antigen to total antibody, and c the concentration of free antigen. In this connection, it is most

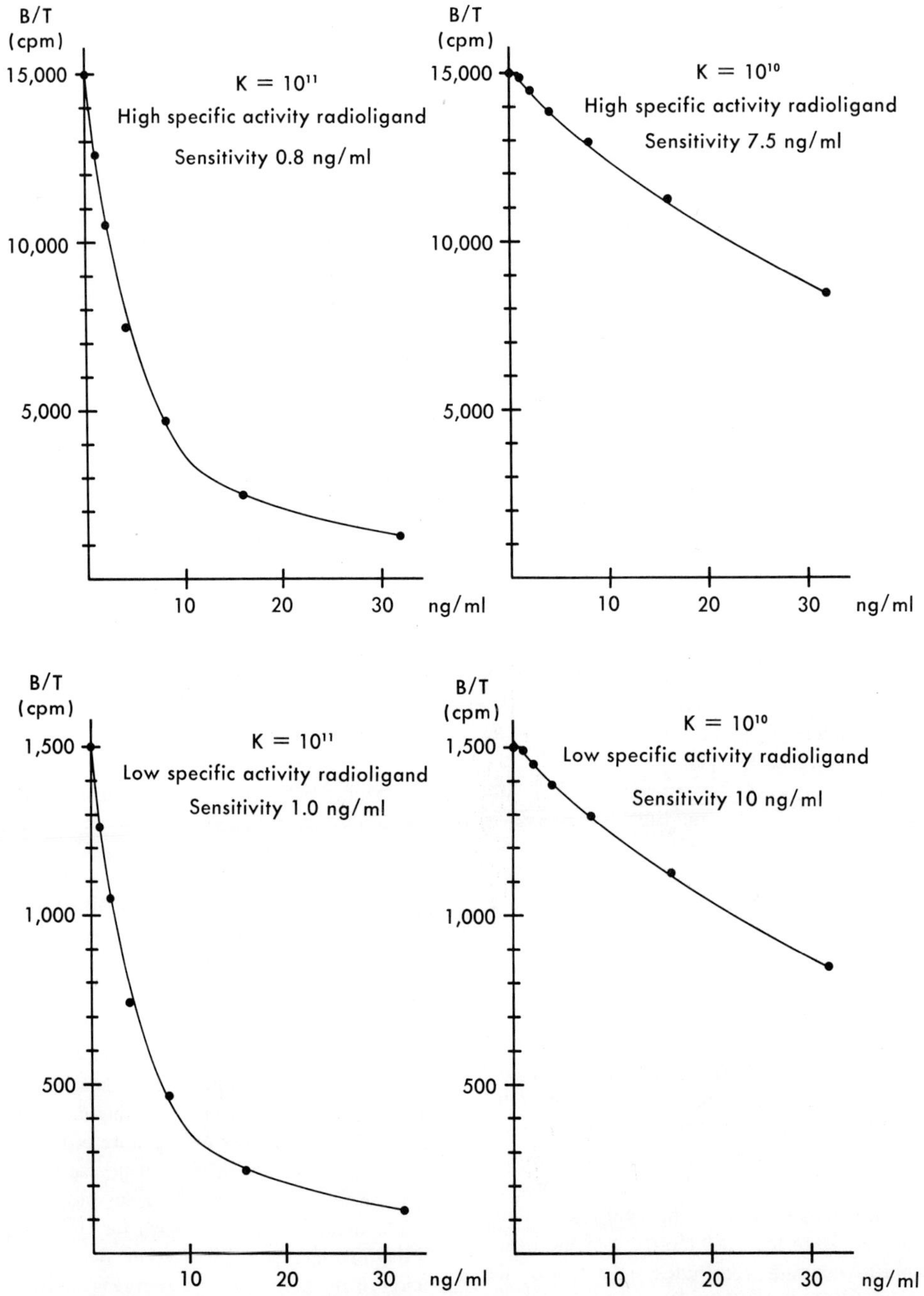

Fig. 2-3. The effects of antibody avidity and specific activity of radioligand on the sensitivity of a radioimmunoassay. Comparisons between the two pairs of standard curves located beside each other illustrate the marked influences of a 10-fold difference in K_a-value. Comparisons between the upper and lower set of curves shows the relatively small effects of a 10-fold difference in specific activity (high and low specific activity radioligands, respectively).

often used in a form applicable to the actual assay data:

$$\frac{B}{F} = K_a \, (R_{tot} - LR) \tag{6}$$

where B and F stand for bound and free activity, respectively, R_{tot} for the total molar binding capacity of the antibody, and LR for the molar amount of ligand bound to the antibody. The left side of this equation can be replaced by the actual assay data and listed just as a number of counts recorded, since the units cancel out. R_{tot} is always constant in a particular assay, since the amount of total antibody added is the same in all assay tubes. Therefore $K_a \times R_{tot}$ is a constant, and the equation is actually a form of a common straight line equation *(y = kx + b)* and shows how B/F varies with the amount of ligand bound (Fig. 2-4). Accordingly, K_a is the slope of this line *(k)*. If B/F = 0 (that is, *y* = 0, the point at which no radioactivity is bound, which can be achieved by saturating the receptor with a large excess of unlabeled ligand), the equation becomes R_{tot} = LR. Accordingly, the intersection with the *x*-axis is the total receptor-binding capacity. Intersection with the *y*-axis occurs when the bound ligand approaches 0 or, in practical terms, when no cold ligand is added and the amount of radioligand is kept as small as possible. The slope of the line (K_a) then is the ratio between the *y* and *x* intercepts at these points. By this method K_a can easily be calculated from any experimental assay data (Fig. 2-4).

We have shown previously that K_a for the binding between ligand and receptor is the factor that characterizes the potential sensitivity of the assay. Thus K_a is a term frequently used for describing the properties of an antiserum. B/F is readily available in any assay, and LR is easily calculated from the data (fraction bound (B/T) × total concentration of ligand) at any point. It must be noted that the total concentration of ligand includes both labeled and unlabeled ligand and that it should be expressed in moles per liter.

For most RIA systems, the Scatchard plot does not give a straight but a curvilinear relationship. This is believed to be due to heterogeneity of antibody sites. Various approaches have been used to measure the heterogeneity of K. One is the Sips distribution function, and another has been described by Karush. However, the reactions between ligand and receptor in an assay are probably considerably more complex than what we have assumed here. There is a multitude of different interactions that make up the overall binding rate. As will be discussed in later sections, there are heterogeneities not only in the avidity of the antibody site, but also in antibody specificity, radioligand quality, and ligand purity. Accordingly, any experimentally estimated value of K_a must be regarded as an average association constant for the sum of all these reactions under the particular experimental conditions of measurement. This variety of factors that affects the apparent K_a of any assay situation explains why different investigators may calculate differently the K_a for any one particular antiserum. Even within

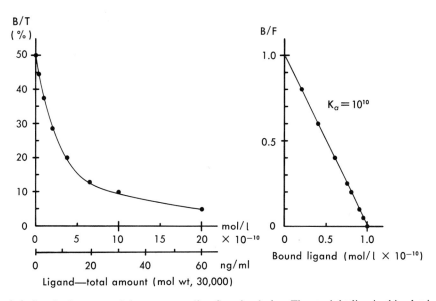

Fig. 2-4. Standard curve and the corresponding Scatchard plot. The straight line in this plot indicates one order of antibody affinity only.

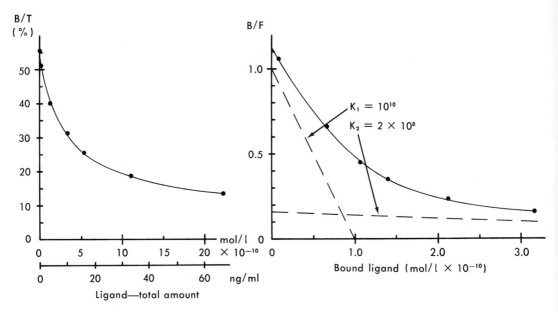

Fig. 2-5. Standard curve and the corresponding Scatchard plot. The curved line here indicates two populations of antibodies. The line is resolved in two components: one *(K₁)* with high avidity and low capacity, the other *(K₂)* with a lower avidity but a high capacity component. It is evident that the sensitivity is determined by the high avidity component *(K₁)*.

the laboratory, the results may vary from assay to assay.

Despite its curvilinearity, the Scatchard plot may be used for calculation of K_a, since the approximations involved in the calculations as such are probably not greater than all others involved. The curved line can usually be resolved into two straight lines (Fig. 2-5). When the assay has a relatively wide working range (for example, with $B_0/T > 50\%$), the slope of the upper, steeper straight line will be relatively little influenced by the slope of the lower, shallow line. The slope of the upper line is the important slope, since that defines the most avid receptor and gives the best indication of the sensitivity of the assay.

An alternative method for estimation of K_a is to measure the free antigen concentration for half-saturation of the antibody. This is based on the Michaelis-Menten presentation of the law of mass action, where the K_a is numerically equal to the inverse of the substrate concentration that half-saturates the enzyme. This is illustrated in Fig. 2-11, *B*.

NONIMMUNE RECEPTORS
Cellular receptors

All hormone actions on target organs in the body are believed to be initiated by the coupling of the hormones to cell receptors that initiate some metabolic events when activated by the hormone. One of the main functions of these receptors is to identify the incoming signals, that is, to ascertain that the effect caused by one hormone is not induced by any other. Many hormones have rather similar structures, for example, the gonadotropins luteinizing hormone (LH) and follicle-stimulating hormone (FSH), and many of the steroid hormones, so these receptors must have a high specificity. Despite exposure of the target cells to all the different hormones within the body fluids, only one (or a few) particular hormonal molecule or molecules will exert a certain biologic action. The specificity of cellular receptors in binding the hormones is accordingly of the same magnitude as discussed for antibodies previously. However, a principal difference is that the cellular receptors actually participate in the biologic specificity discrimination, the mechanism by which the cells dinstinguish between hormones with different biologic effects. This is achieved when the receptor binds the biologically active part of the hormone molecule (often called the ''biologically active site''). The binding sites of antibodies, on the other hand, are not necessarily directed toward the biologically active site of the molecule, since the antibody response against a foreign molecule is not related to the biologic function of that molecule. Accordingly, binding of a hormone to a cell receptor reflects the biologic activity of the hormone, whereas binding of antibody to antigenic binding site frequently does not. Particularly when dealing with hormones with large structural similarities, such a dissociation between antigenic and biologic activity may cause considerable differences in the specificity of binding to antibodies and to cell receptors.

Principally, there are two types of cell receptors. Those binding large polypeptide hormones are located on the outside of the cell wall (the plasma membrane) since these large hormones are excluded from penetrating into the cell. Steroids that are lipophilic penetrate the lipids of the plasma membrane into the cells and have their receptors located in the cytoplasm. The receptors located in the plasma membrane are relatively firmly bound to the lipid structure of the cell wall. The receptors may be extracted from the membrane by the use of detergents, but such an extraction has been reported to alter the binding characteristics of the receptors. For this reason, assays based on cell membrane receptors have so far employed homogenized cell membranes. In this way the receptors are kept in a nonsoluble state, analogous to the solid phase coupled antibodies used in several RIAs. (See Chapter 5.)

Transporting proteins

Another group of substances with binding (receptor) properties consists of certain plasma proteins that serve as carriers for small hormones of low molecular weight and other small molecules. The diffusion of such small molecules through the extracellular space is prevented by binding to the large proteins, and in this way even freely diffusible hormones stay in the circulation for long periods. This group includes such proteins as thyroid-binding globulin (TBG), transcortin, and sex hormone–binding globulin. These proteins were commonly used as binding proteins in earlier assays but recently have to a large extent been substituted

by specific antibodies when they become generally available. Other transporting proteins have a transfer function through structures that the unbound substance cannot penetrate. An example of this is intrinsic factor from the gastric mucosa, the function of which is to translocate vitamin B_{12} from the intestinal tract into the circulation.

PRODUCTION OF ANTISERA

One of the early difficulties that had to be overcome before RIA could be applied to direct measurement of hormone levels in biologic fluid, without extensive initial purification of the samples, was the production of antisera with sufficient sensitivity (avidity) and specificity. Over the past 15 years experience has shown that proper consideration of a few general principles will make the production of specific antisera more certain.

Choice of animals for immunization

In most instances rabbits are quite suitable, since they are easily handled and are large enough to permit the easy collection of relatively large quantities of serum over extended periods. Large quantities of immunogen are not required; this is particularly valuable in the case of expensive or otherwise rare material. Sometimes the immunogenic response is affected by variation in the species specificity of the immunogen. For example, most large proteins show such species variation in the structure of the proteins that they are immunogenic in almost any vertebrate species. Others, such as some polypeptide hormones and other smaller molecules, show so little species variation that they may not be recognized by the immunized animal as foreign and, therefore, will not produce any immunologic response. In such cases, a careful selection of the animal may improve the situation. For example, guinea pig insulin varies more from human insulin than does rabbit insulin, and guinea pigs have usually been found to produce better insulin antisera more consistently than rabbits. In some cases, even the injection of immunogens believed to have a structure identical to the corresponding proteins in the animal to be immunized may result in antibody production (for example, immunization of cows with bovine insulin). Such results indicate that the immunogens may have become modified during their extraction or purification or in the coupling procedures involved in the production of the immunogen. Certain genetic differences in immunoresponsiveness may also influence the results. For this reason, immunization of less common animals, such as turkeys or monkeys, is sometimes attempted when immunization of rabbits or guinea pigs fail. Another factor that affects the responsiveness to an immunogen is the presence of systems in the immunized animals that neutralize the injected immunogen. It is believed, for example, that it is easier to produce antisera against estrogens in goats than in rabbits because of the low affinity of the goat sex hormone–binding proteins. For most RIA applications even small animals may be used to produce antisera, because the antisera are used in very high dilution. For example, it is not uncommon that a good antiserum may be used at a final dilution of 1 : 1,000,000; 1 ml of the antiserum will suffice for 2,000,000 assay tubes. For certain applications, such as the production of the precipitation antibody in double-antibody assays, the antiserum must be used at relatively high concentration to produce an adequate precipitate. The consumption of this antiserum may then be significant, and in this case it is preferable to use large animals (goats, monkeys) that are able to produce many liters of good antiserum.

The immunogen

The prerequisite for immunogenicity of any foreign material is that it must come into contact with the immunologic defense system. Large molecules, such as proteins and large carbohydrate compounds, are broken down to smaller components before reaching the circulation if entering via the digestive tract. For this reason, immunogens must be administered parenterally.

The purity of the immunogen is at times critical although not always. Impurities induce antibodies too, and their influence in the assay depends on how they are related to the compound (ligand) to be measured. If the impurities are structurally unrelated to the ligand and the radioligand is not contaminated with them, they do not interfere in the assay. If the radioligand contains a significant amount of the contaminant in a radioactive form, it will bind to the antibodies if these occur in sufficiently high concentration (high titer). This may reduce the working range of the assay. If the contaminant also is contained in the standards, which is more difficult to reveal, it may affect assay accuracy and cause nonparallel inhibition curves of samples and standards. The influence of contaminants also depends on their occurrence or concentration in plasma. If it is very high as in the case of albumin, which is a common contaminant in many biologic materials, the antibodies are likely to be completely saturated by the addition of plasma to the sample test tube. These antibodies will not interact in the assay any longer, but if the radioligand contains a significant fraction of labeled albumin, it will appear as a nonimmunoreactive radioactivity. If the radioligand contains no trace of the contaminant, the contaminant-antibody will not influence the assay, which is the case in assays with antibodies produced against haptens coupled to bovine serum albumin (BSA) or human serum albumin (HSA) if the radioligand contains no radioactive BSA or HSA.

Of much greater importance—or nuisance—is the occurrence of contaminants that are structurally related to the primary immunogen (and the ligand). One area in which this has caused many complications is assay for pituitary glycoprotein hormones (see Chapter 10 for details). Antibodies against such related contaminants may partially cross-react with the primary antigen at the same time as the primary antigen reacts to a much higher degree with the contaminant. If now the standard and the plasma samples contain different proportions of contaminants and of the primary antigen, their sum effect will be different in standards and plasma samples. The net effect of this is that the results of the assay will not reflect the amount of the primary antigen in the sample but a combination of this and the amount of contaminants, where the contribution from each of these components cannot be predicted. For example, if the contaminating agent is a precursor of the primary antigen and such precursors occur in plasma, the result of the assay may be highly influenced by the variation in the concentrations of the precursors rather than by the concentration of the primary antigen.

Antibodies to contaminants are also prone to cause difficulties in relation to the purity (or potency) of the standards used. Two standards, of which one is pure while the other contains substantial amounts of contaminants, will give different results (potency estimates) with such antisera, even if both standards contain the same amount of the primary antigen. For example, such effects are frequently found with some of the current standard preparations for pituitary hormones, which contain as little as a few percent of the active compound.

It has been proposed that the occurrence of contaminants with related structures, for example, degradation products arising during the purification or production of the immunogens, may increase the immunogenicity of the preparation. Results with more recently produced antisera against highly purified pituitary glyco-

protein hormones tend to disprove this theory and indicate that the best antiserum is produced with the purest immunogen.

Haptens

As described in the antibody introduction, haptens are not active as immunogens, because of their small size. Such compounds are made immunogenic by coupling to a larger molecule. Albumins from different species (ovalbumin, BSA, or HSA) have been most extensively used as carrier proteins for hapten. In recent years, other macromolecules have been used as well, for example, poly-L-lysine (a synthetic polyamine), thyroglobulin (cow), and hemocyanin (a large protein, molecular weight above 2 million daltons, from the keyhole limpet, which is highly immunogenic). The two latter macromolecules have been successfully applied to many different haptens.

When the hapten is a polypeptide, the cou-

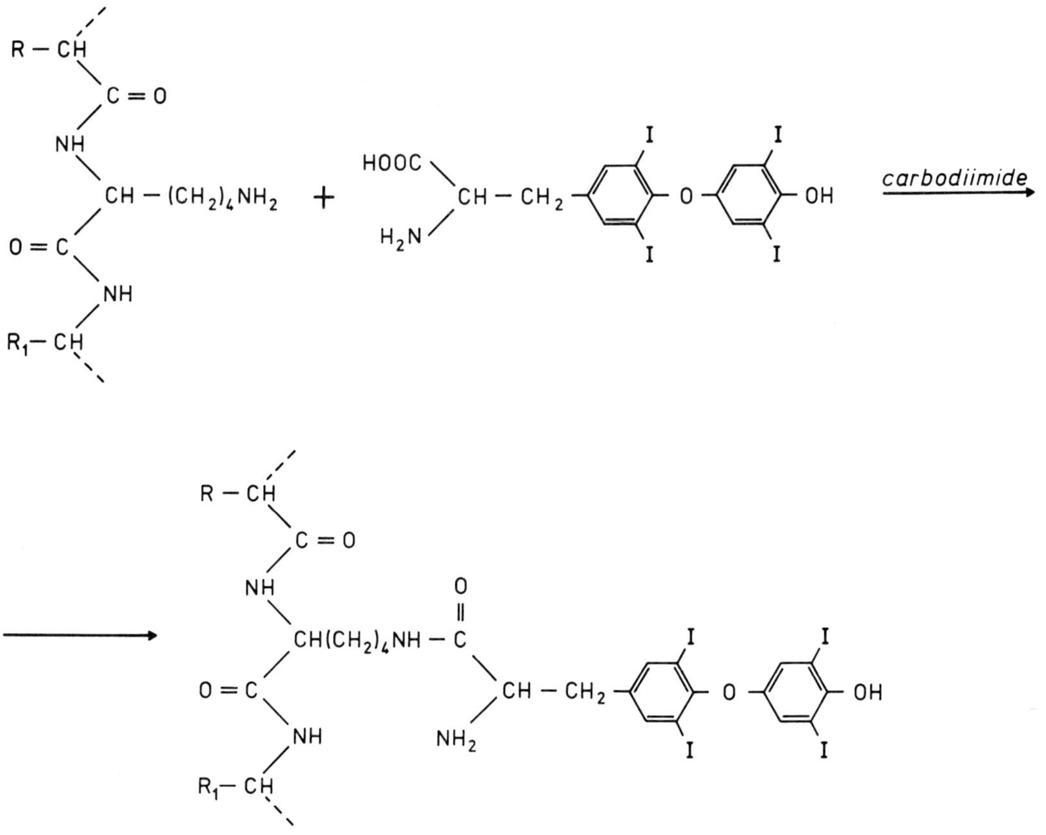

Fig. 2-6. Principle for coupling a dipeptide (thyroxine) to a lysine residue of BSA by means of carbodiimide.

Table 2-1. Methods for coupling haptens (R_1) to carrier proteins (R_2)

Reagent	Type of bond	Reactive group in hapten utilized for coupling
Carbodiimides	R_1—CONH—R_2	—NH_2 or —COOH
Isobutyl chloroformate	R_1—CONH—R_2	—NH_2 or —COOH
Isoxazolium	R_1—CONH—R_2	—NH_2 or —COOH
Glutaraldehyde	R_1—NH—CH(OH)(CH$_2$)$_3$CH(OH)NH—R_2	—NH_2
Diisocyanates (Toluene-2-4-diisocyanate)		—NH_2
Diazotized benzidine	R_1—N=N——N=N—R_2	Tyrosine, histidine, or lysine

Table 2-2. Methods to introduce an active group in haptens for coupling to other compounds

Group to which active species is coupled	Reagent	Compound produced	
Hydroxyl	Succinic anhydride	Hemisuccinates	$R—O—\overset{\displaystyle O}{\overset{\|}{C}}—(CH_2)_2\overset{\displaystyle O}{\overset{\|}{C}}—OH$
Hydroxyl	Phosgene	Chlorocarbonates	$R—O—\overset{\displaystyle O}{\overset{\|}{C}}—Cl$
Vicinal hydroxyl groups	Br CN	Imidocarbonate	$\begin{array}{c}—O\\ \\ —O\end{array}\!\!\!>\!C{=}NH$
Keto or aldehyde	O-(carboxy methyl) hydroxylamine	O-(carboxymethyl) oxime	$R—CH=N—O—CH_2COOH$

pling is usually achieved by means of a peptide bonding at amino or carboxyl groups. A number of reactions are described to achieve this (Table 2-1). Some reagents, such as carbodiimide, couple both to amino and carboxyl groups, so the bonds may occur via any free amino or carboxyl group of the hapten and the carrier protein. Thus carrier proteins also may be coupled to carrier proteins, and hapten to hapten, rather than just hapten to carrier protein. This may make the final product inhomogeneous, con-taining many different types of immunogens. With reagents such as glutaraldehyde, which couples only to amino groups, the conjugates have a more specific structure, with all haptens bound via the *N*-terminal or other free amino ends. This method is described in Appendix 2.

With haptens other than polypeptides, the hapten must first be chemically modified so that it acquires a group that permits conjugation via a peptide bond. Various methods to produce such reactive groups are given in Table 2-2

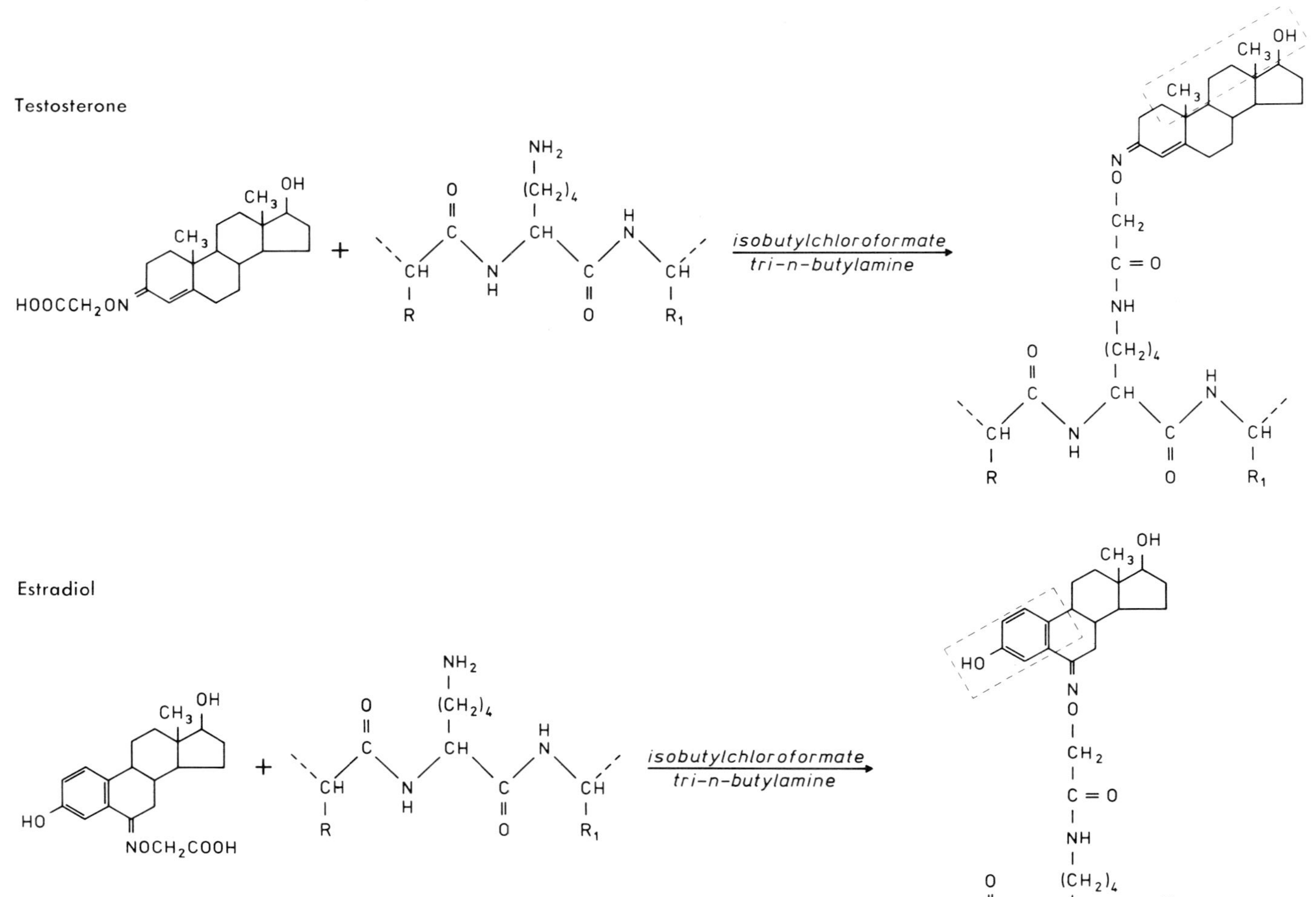

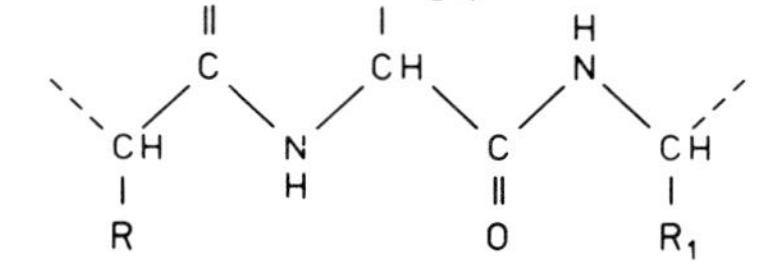

Fig. 2-7. Two examples of reactions used for coupling steroids to BSA via different carbons of the steroid structure. In both cases hydroxyl groups have been activated to form a carboxymethyloxime. The coupling is performed to carbons distant from the part of the steroid structure, which is characteristic for the particular biologic activity (region surrounded by broken lines).

and Appendixes 3 and 4. For example, the use of such procedures is necessary in the conjugation of steroids to proteins.

For haptens such as the steroids, where there is a family of chemically related compounds with highly different biologic activity, the conjugation must be done to a specific part of the steroid to achieve sufficient specificity. The goal is that the immunogen induces antibodies that bind to a part of the hapten (antigenic determinant) that coincides with the part of the molecule that constitutes the biologically active site. Antibodies formed to a hapten conjugate are more likely to be directed to parts of the hapten that project out from the carrier. For this reason the opposite part of the hapten is chosen for the conjugation. This is illustrated for some steroids in Fig. 2-7, and the procedures are given in Appendixes 5 to 7.

The ratio between hapten and carrier protein (the average number of hapten molecules coupled to each protein molecule) in the immunogen is important, since it influences the immune response to the hapten. With the largest type of carrier proteins it is possible to cover the surface with 20 to 100 hapten molecules.

After the conjugation, unreacted hapten and other reagents are removed.

The result of the conjugation procedure can be tested in different ways. By including a small portion of the hapten in radioactive form, the yield of the reaction is easily estimated. In some instances the yield can be measured by spectrophotometric determination of the amount of hapten present before and after conjugation. The purity of the conjugate may be tested by gel chromatography. Such testing of conjugate hapten is described in Appendixes 5 to 7.

The conjugated hapten is then used for immunization in the same way as the complete antigen, that is, injected in an adjuvant mixture.

Adjuvants

The immunoresponse to the foreign substance is often relatively weak. One method used to enhance the response is to administer the immunogen together with an adjuvant. The adjuvant acts as a nonspecific stimulator to the lymphoid system, causing a foreign-body reaction with granuloma formation. Another adjuvant effect is to prolong the adsorption of the immunogen, thereby extending the phase during which the lymphocytes of the host are exposed to the immunogen. The adjuvant may contain inorganic or organic material (such as killed bacteria); many different types of adjuvant have been described. The most commonly used technique in later years has been to emulsify the immunogen in an oil phase, with or without addition of killed mycobacteria (Freund's adjuvant). This simultaneous injection of killed virus material has also been suggested as a general stimulus of the immune system. The preparation of an immunogen in Freund's adjuvant is described in Appendix 1.

Amount of immunogen

The amount of immunogen injected has varied, but lately there has been a tendency toward progressively lower doses. Previously, 1 mg/kg body weight was a common dose, but such amounts, particularly if given repeatedly, may induce immunologic tolerance rather than an immunoresponse. Doses of immunogen on the order of $10\mu g$ to $100\mu g$/kg can induce very high titers. The tendency for low doses of immunogen to produce high-avidity antibodies is consistent with current immunologic theory. In order to induce any response, the immunogen first must bind to receptors on the antibody-producing lymphocytes. If the immunogen occurs only at very low concentration (that is, given in a low dose), then the receptor of the lymphocytes must have a high avidity to be able to bind the immunogen molecules (p. 13). The antibodies then produced, as replicates of this primary receptor, will have the same high avidity. This low-concentration immunogen effect is probably also induced by being well mixed with adjuvant, since the retarded absorption of the immunogen over very extended periods from the adjuvant emulsion will eliminate a high initial peak of immunogen in the circulation of the host animal.

For the production of the precipitating second antibody in double-antibody separation assays (for example, in goat against rabbit IgG), we have found that relatively high doses of immunogen (0.5 mg/injection) are necessary and that it may take months before antibodies of sufficient quality and titer appear.

Route of injection

Subcutaneous injection of the antigen has been the standard route of administration. The immunologic response is enhanced by simultaneous injection into many different locations of the animal. In this way, several lymphoid areas are engaged in the production of antibodies. Techniques reported include intraarticular and intrasplenic injections as well as injections into the foot pads of rabbits. The latter method has not proved to give superior results and usually causes serious discomfort to the rabbits. The use of multiple intracutaneous injections over the back of the animal has been associated with good results and has become very popular. If a rabbit is to be injected with 1 to 2 ml of the immunization mixture, it is injected with 20μl to 40μl in each of approximately 50 intradermal wheals distributed over the shaved back of the animal.

Injection schedules

A great variety of injection schedules have been proposed. The advantages of one over another have been difficult to establish, both because of the variation in the response between individual animals and because the response pattern may vary between different immunogens. Most frequently immunization is started with one dose. Sometimes repeated doses are given during the initial period, but it is not evident that this increases the effect. Booster injections are usually given, either relatively early in the schedule, after 1 or 2 months, or later, after several months. Booster injections later in the course of immunization prolong the response and may sometimes induce even higher responses. The immunogen used for boosting may be administered without adjuvant, but the effect is more predictable if given with adjuvant in the same way as the initial injection.

With poor immunogens it sometimes is effective to extend the period of immunization markedly (up to over a year) and to include a rest period of many months before boosting.

Collection and storage of antisera

There is usually no point in collecting any samples earlier than 6 weeks after the first immunization. If a single injection type of immunization is tried, peak titers are usually reached 2 to 3 months after the primary injection (Fig. 2-8). With many immunogens there is a wide variation of responses between animals. Usually animals responding with a high titer initially will continue to do so after prolonged immunization. Those that respond poorly initially seldom improve significantly even after prolonged stimulation. Therefore, to save cost, the animals that show the poorest response during the initial months of immunization can be eliminated.

Rabbits and bigger animals may continue to produce substantial amounts of antisera for long periods. The rabbit may deliver more than 20 ml of blood every other week through the ear veins. If killed, it can be effectively exsanguinated by repeated heart punctures at intervals of a few hours if the first blood loss is replaced with saline.

Smaller animals, such as guinea pigs, must

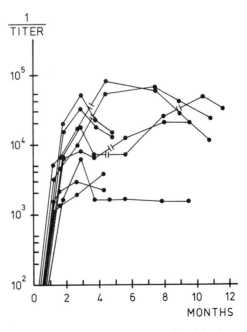

Fig. 2-8. Titer development following injection of 50μg FSH intradermally in multiple sites. Breaks in lines denote booster injections.

be bled by heart puncture, which is associated with a substantial risk of losing the animal. However, in skilled hands mortality is not higher than about 10%. Plain test bleedings in guinea pigs can be done from ear veins to avoid accidental losses that could be catastrophic if antisera from lost animals were found to have unique properties.

Antisera are collected as serum. Large amounts of serum can be retrieved from the sample if, after the first portion of serum is collected, the clot is left in the refrigerator overnight and then centrifuged.

Antisera can be readily stored at $-20°$ C for very long periods (years), although on rare occasions a gradual loss of titer has been found. In the unfrozen state, bacterial growth may rapidly ruin antibody; therefore, preservatives such as thimerosal (Merthiolate) (1:10,000) or 0.2% sodium azide should be included in the sample.

A safer method is to lyophilize the antiserum, after which it is stable at even higher temperatures.

Testing of antisera

Antisera have many different types of qualities (the titer is neither the only nor the most important quality), and there are many different ways to test the properties of antisera. The technique used for testing influences the apparent properties of the antiserum, so an antiserum that is excellent in a gel precipitation or agglutination system may not be as good in an RIA. This dissociation of the different properties of antibodies has two main consequences: the properties have to be tested individually, and the testing has to be performed in an assay that estimates each particular property. Accordingly, there is little value in preliminary testing of antisera for RIA in a gel precipitation system

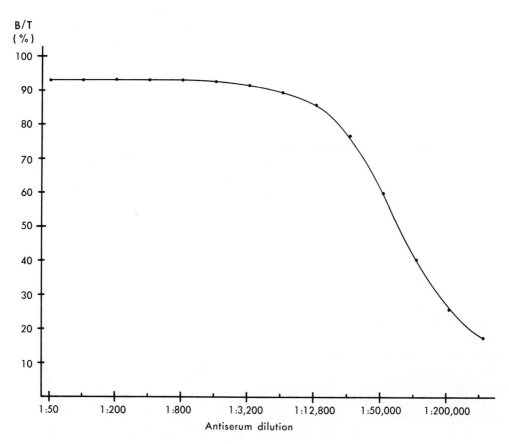

Fig. 2-9. Test of quantity of specific antibody; binding of ^{125}I-labeled insulin to progressive dilutions of the antiserum. The titer (about 1:50,000) is the dilution where 50% of radioligand is bound.

or testing a precipitating second antibody in the same way as the first antibody is tested.

Amount of antibody (titer)

The first step in the characterization of the quality of an antiserum is to get an idea of the amount of specific antibodies. The amount of the binding reagent available does not affect the quality of the assay. Accordingly, the antibody titer (an estimate of the concentration of antibody in a particular antiserum) has no bearing on the specificity or sensitivity of an assay. Although the quantity of antibody is not the most important quality factor, it must be estimated initially to determine whether an antiserum merits further investigation with regard to the more important characteristics of avidity and specificity.

The concentration of a specific antibody is most often expressed as the titer. It is estimated by incubating progressive dilutions of the antiserum with a fixed amount of antigen. Usually it is radioactive, but it may be a mixture of radioactive and cold antigen. At increasing dilutions, the binding capacity of the antibody decreases so that the quantity of antigen present in the tube will begin to saturate the antibody-binding capacity, and part of the antigen will appear as not bound. The titer is then taken as the highest dilution of the antiserum that binds a certain fraction of the antigen. Since the titer is an arbitrary unit for which there are no established standards of calibration, each laboratory must establish its own definition of this unit. It also implies that when one refers to a titer estimation, the method for its determination must be given. Usually the antiserum dilution that binds 50% of the added antigen is taken as the titer. The 50% cutoff point has the advantage that the working range of most immunoassays starts more or less closely to 50% binding of labeled antigen. Thus the titer estimate will give an idea of the dilution of antiserum useful in the assay. A typical antibody dilution experiment is illustrated in Fig. 2-9, and details of the procedure are given in Appendix 8.

The total amount of specific antibody may also be estimated as the total binding capacity. This is measured by addition of increasing amounts of antigen, while the amount of antibody is kept constant. This may be performed with the antiserum undiluted or at a known dilution of the antiserum. The antigen is added either in increasing amounts of radioligand or, more conveniently, in increasing amounts of unlabeled antigen mixed with a constant amount of the radioligand. As with the estimation of the titer, an increasing fraction of unbound radioactivity will appear when the amount of added antigen becomes larger than the binding capacity of the antibodies. If the avidity of the antibodies is not very high, unbound activity will appear before all binding sites are saturated. Therefore, the concentration of antigen has to be further increased to the degree that the binding to the antibodies does not increase further. The binding capacity of the antibody is then calculated as the amount of antigen bound at this saturating concentration of antigen. The determination of the total binding capacity is less suitable for screening of antibody contents in antisera for RIAs. As opposed to the titer estimate done as described previously, it does not give a direct estimate for the working dilution to be used in the RIA. Another drawback for RIA is that low-avidity antibodies are also measured.

Avidity (sensitivity)

As described previously, the avidity of the antibody is usually the important denominator of assay sensitivity. It is not necessary to calculate K_a for every individual antiserum, since for practical purposes it may be sufficient to determine the actual sensitivity (the smallest quantity detectable in the assay). However, K_a is the best term to describe the binding properties of the antiserum, particularly when different antisera are compared, and, as soon as a standard curve is derived, all necessary data for the calculation of K_a are at hand. The avidity or sensitivity is tested by measuring the influence of adding increasing amounts of unlabeled antigen to a constant amount of antibody in the presence of a constant amount of labeled antigen. The inhibition of the binding of radioactive antigen to the antibodies is the parameter recorded. The avidity testing is performed after the titer estimation has established

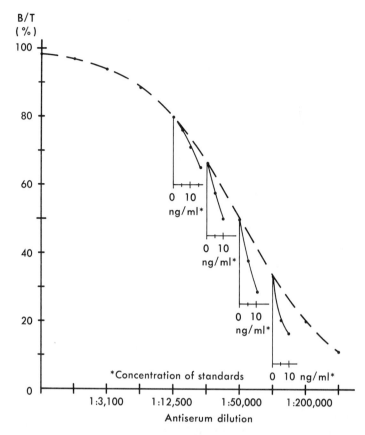

Fig. 2-10. Test for sensitivity of an antiserum to FSH. Short standard curves (continuous lines) are done at some different antisera dilutions (interrupted lines). It is obvious that the best sensitivity is found at a dilution of 1:100,000, when the smallest detectable concentration is approximately 1 ng/ml. However, the working range is restricted to 1 to 20 ng/ml at this antiserum dilution. At lower antisera dilutions the sensitivity decreases, but at the same time the working range increases; thus at 1:30,000 it is approximately 5 to 50 ng/ml.

the approximate working concentration of the antiserum. The sensitivity is then tested at some different antisera dilutions around the titer (dilution). A typical experiment is illustrated in Fig. 2-10. After this initial testing, the full standard curve is prepared to characterize the total working range of the assay. The avidity of the antiserum can then be calculated according to Fig. 2-11.

Specificity

When the titer and avidity determinations have shown that one or several antisera have antibodies in sufficient quantity and with adequate sensitivity, it is important to test their ability to detect only the compound we want to measure, without influence—cross-reactions—from other compounds. The degree of specificity and the presence of cross-reactive material vary from assay to assay. The increasing knowledge about the metabolism of hormones and other biologically active substances has shown that there are very few systems in which no cross-reactions can be anticipated. Thus hormone precursors may be released from the hormone-producing cells together with the active hormone, and the fragments and other metabolites of the hormone may circulate in plasma for a longer time than the active hormone. Such related compounds often have a decreased or absent biologic activity, but since the antibodies may recognize and bind to other parts of the

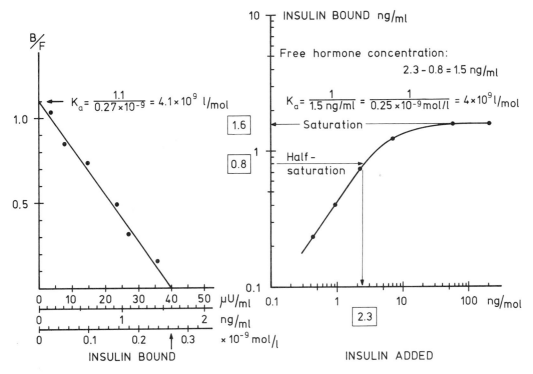

Fig. 2-11. Calculation of K_a by means of a Scatchard plot *(left)* and from the concentration of unbound ligand at half-saturation of antibody *(right)*. In the Scatchard plot K_a is derived from the slope of the line $\left(\dfrac{\text{y-intercept}}{\text{x-intercept}}\right)$. On the abscissa the concentration of bound insulin is plotted. In the actual experiment performed, the concentration of insulin was given in international units. Conversion scales to mass and molar units are noted below. It is mol/liter that is used in the calculation of K_a. In the plot on the right, K_a is calculated as the inverse of the free hormone concentration at half-saturation of the antibody.

Table 2-3. Examples of assays influenced by cross-reactions with material of less or different biologic activity

Assay	Cross-reacting material
Insulin	Proinsulin
Insulin C–peptide	Proinsulin
Parathyroid hormone	Circulating hormone fragments
ACTH	Big ACTH
Glucagon	Glucagonlike activity of the gastrointestinal tract
Growth hormone	Placental lactogen
Thyrotropin	Gonadotropins
Calcitonin	High molecular forms of calcitoninlike activity

hormone than the biologically active site, such precursors or metabolites may be bound by the antiserum with the same affinity as the intact hormone. Therefore, they may be measured to the same extent as the biologically active hormone molecule. Examples of assays where such problems have been particularly prominent are given in Table 2-3.

The greatest problem associated with cross-reactivity between compounds with different biologic activities has occurred in steroid radioassay, where the receptors (antibodies, plasma transporting proteins, and cell receptors have been used) did not have sufficient specificity to recognize the small differences among the different groups of active steroids. Therefore,

Table 2-4. Serum estradiol-17β (pg/ml) found in three plasma samples analyzed with four different RIAs utilizing antisera produced against different estradiol-17β-albumin conjugates*

Sample no.	Sample treatment	Immunogen conjugated at carbon no.			
		3	6	11	17
1	Ext	141	125	73	120
	Ext + Ch	78	70	75	73
2	Ext	94	95	40	67
	Ext + Ch	40	42	45	40
3	Ext	580	372	161	500
	Ext + Ch	210	178	159	183

From England, B. G., and others: J. Clin. Endocrinol. Metab. **38**:42, 1974.
*Comparison between the samples that had been extracted only (Ext) or extracted and chromatographed (Ext + Ch). Only the antisera to the C-11 conjugate had sufficient specificity to permit adequate assay of unchromatographed samples.

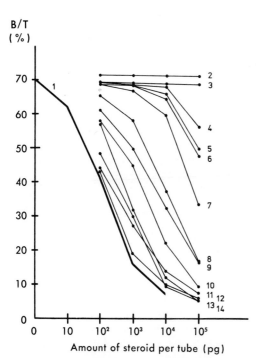

Fig. 2-12. Specificity testing of a progesterone rabbit antiserum. The inhibition of the following steroids was tested: *1*, progesterone; *2*, estradiol-17β; *3*, pregnanediol; *4*, cortisol; *5*, 11-deoxycortisol; *6*, testosterone; *7*, pregnenolone; *8*, corticosterone; *9*, 17α-hydroxyprogesterone; *10*, 11-hydroxyprogesterone; *11*, 11-deoxycorticosterone; *12*, 5β-pregnan-3,20-dione; *13*, 11α-hydroxyprogesterone; *14*, 5α-pregnan-3,20-dione.

these assays included one or more initial purification steps for separation of the various interfering steroids. Recent development has produced antisera of higher specificity, and there are now a number of steroid assays reported in which no initial purification step is needed. Typical results from specificity testing are illustrated in Fig. 2-12. In order to elucidate the cross-reactivity as thoroughly as possible, all chemically related compounds that could occur in the sample to be assayed should be tested. However, cross-reactions may occur not only to structurally related compounds but also to other material possibly contaminating immunogens and ligands (p. 20). For example, a hormone preparation from the pituitary is likely to contain trace (or substantial) amounts of other pituitary hormones. For this reason, cross-reaction testing should not be restricted to structurally related compounds only but should include compounds that otherwise may occur in, or will interfere with, the active reagents of the assay.

Often it is difficult to forsee all possible compounds that may cross-react in an assay. Additional indirect tests for cross-reacting material may be used. One has been used in steroid assays, where it is difficult to test all possible related steroids. In this method, a comparison is made of the results when the biologic samples (plasma) are assayed, directly or after quite extensive purification of the sample. If these two different procedures give the same

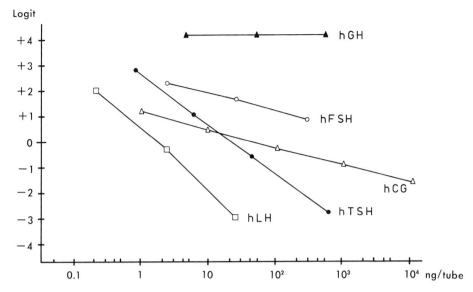

Fig. 2-13. Specificity testing of a rabbit hLH antiserum. Note parallel curves with TSH, which corresponds to a known contamination of TSH standards with LH and the nonparallel curves with the other related but not identical glycoprotein hormones.

results, one has reason to believe that no cross-reacting material of importance occurs in the sample. This approach is illustrated in Table 2-4.

Another indirect test that is influenced by the specificity is the comparison of slopes of inhibition curves, when produced with standards or with dilutions of biologic samples that contain a high concentration of the compound to be assayed. If either of them contains material that binds with different avidity because of structural differences, the inhibition curves may have a different slope. This is a relatively insensitive test but is at times helpful. The procedures and results from such testing are illustrated in Fig. 2-13.

PLASMA TRANSPORTING PROTEINS

Plasma transporting proteins are tested following the same principles as testing of antibody. Particularly when a new method is set up, the same extensive testing must be performed. However, when the period of initial testing is past, new batches of these proteins may not require the same extensive testing, since the properties of different batches of transporting proteins usually show less variation than different batches of antibodies. Thus, testing of a new batch of plasma protein is restricted to finding the appropriate dilution of the reagent.

3 RADIOLIGAND

A detailed review of the basis for radioactive decay, the detection of radioactivity, and radiation protection is beyond the scope of this book. However, a short survey is given here that covers the minimum of background knowledge necessary to perform radioassay work. The reader who wants a more thorough knowledge is referred to the many standard textbooks that cover this subject. This section is restricted to the use of radioactive tracers in radioligand assays and will therefore deal mainly with aspects of radioactive labeling of biologic material.

RADIOACTIVE DECAY

Radioactive decay of an element is principally the result of instability in the configuration of the nucleus. During radioactive decay, a rearrangement of the nucleus occurs, usually toward a more stable nuclear configuration, and energy (radiation) is released.

Isotopes of elements that do not undergo spontaneous radioactive decay are said to be "stable." One consideration in determining the stability of the nucleus is the ratio of protons to neutrons in the nucleus. If the neutron number ("N number") in the nucleus is plotted against the number of protons in the nucleus ("Z number"), the stable isotopes fall along the line seen in Fig. 3-1. For lower Z number stable isotopes, $Z = N$. With increasing Z number, the number of neutrons relative to Z number increases. Radioactive elements above the line of stability have too many neutrons for nucleus stability.

BETA DECAY. Decay of such isotopes involves the spontaneous disintegration of a neutron into its component parts: proton, a beta particle (electron), and a massless neutral particle called a neutrino. The proton does not leave the nucleus, whereas the beta particle and the neutrino are accelerated from the nucleus with an energy characteristic for the decay of

the particular radioactive isotope. The energy given off is partitioned randomly between the neutrino and the beta particle. If all of the energy is given to the beta particle, this is described as E_{max} for the beta particle. A spectrum of beta particle energies is observed with an average beta particle energy (E_{avg}). The energy of beta particle decay for a particular isotope may be described either as an E_{max} or as an E_{avg}. For example, tritium (^3H) has an $E_{max} = 0.018$ meV and $E_{avg} = 0.0055$ meV. It is the energy of the beta particle only, and not the energy of the neutrino, that is detected in a liquid scintillation system. Usually, $E_{avg} = E_{max}/3$ (see Table 3-1).

ELECTRON CAPTURE. If a nucleus contains too many protons relative to neutrons for nuclear stability, radioactive decay will involve reduction in the

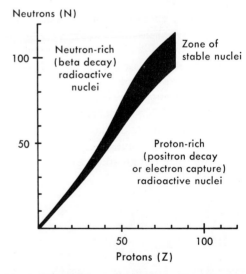

Fig. 3-1. Plot of neutron number (ordinate) and proton number (abscissa) showing the zone of stable nuclei (dark band). Elements that are relatively neutron rich tend to decay by beta decay, whereas those that are relatively proton rich tend to decay by positron decay or electron capture.

neutron/proton ratio. Electron capture is one decay mode in this situation. The nucleus captures an electron from an orbital outside the nucleus; usually either the K shell (K capture) or the L shell (L capture). Electron capture increases the number of neutrons and decreases the number of protons, turning protons into neutrons. Since there is a vacancy in the electron shell of the nuclide undergoing electron capture, characteristic x-radiation or auger electrons may be also given off during this process, as an effect of electrons from outer shells going in to fill the vacant positions.

POSITRON DECAY. Spontaneous transformation of a positron to a neutron may also occur in nuclei that are relatively proton rich. During this process, a positron and a neutrino are ejected. Analogous to beta decay (see above), the energy of decay is partitioned between the neutrino and the positron particle.

GAMMA EMISSION. Radioactive decay of either a proton-rich or neutron-rich nucleus often results in a daughter nucleus that still is in an excited (unstable) state. As this nucleus decays to a less excited state, a gamma ray is released from the nucleus. The change in energy in this case is not accompanied by any change in mass number, proton number, or neutron number. The transition is usually described as *isomeric transition.*

INTERNAL CONVERSION. Isomeric transition usually is accompanied by release of electromagnetic radiation from the nucleus in the form of a gamma ray. Sometimes, however, an electron from one of the inner orbitals (K or L) is released instead, with a kinetic energy that is equal to the energy of the nuclear transition minus the binding energy of the electron in its shell. Accompanying this decay process, characteristic x-rays or anger electrons are given off as the electrons of higher orbitals fill the vacancy left by the internal conversion electron.

X-RAYS. Accompanying electron capture and internal conversion, electromagnetic radiation in the form of x-rays is given off with energies characteristic of the orbital from which the original electron was removed. Gamma radiation is used to describe electromagnetic radiation emitted from the nucleus by nuclear rearrangements; *x-ray* describes radiation emitted from the electron shells. Both types of radiation are physically identical and are emitted with energies that are characteristic of the particular atomic rearrangements that have occurred during the decay process. Both of these radiations will be detected by standard ''gamma'' counters.

Half-life

The probability that a particular nucleus of a radionuclide will undergo spontaneous decay is characteristic of the particular isotope. This is usually described as the half-life and is defined as the time required for one half of the atoms of a radioactive element to undergo spontaneous decay. Another frequently used expression that is related to the half-life ($T_{\frac{1}{2}}$) is the decay constant (λ). This relationship is mathematically expressed as follows:

$$\lambda = \frac{\ell n\ 2}{T_{\frac{1}{2}}} = \frac{0.693}{T_{\frac{1}{2}}}$$

It represents the fractional rate of spontaneous disintegration per unit time, that is, the shorter the half-life, the more disintegrations per unit time. The decay constant may therefore be used to calculate the radioactivity remaining after an isotope has decayed for a certain time, according to the formula

$$A = A_0 e^{-\lambda t}$$

where A is the activity remaining at time t in a preparation that had activity A_0 at time 0; e is the basis for the natural logarithm.

EXAMPLE. ^{125}I activity on July 8, 1977 was $2\mu Ci$. What will the activity be on August 8, 1977?

$$A = A_0 e^{-\lambda t}$$
$$A = 2\mu Ci\ (e^{-0.0115 \times 21})$$
$$A = 2\mu Ci\ (0.7077)$$
$$A = 1.41\mu Ci$$

In practice, it is usually convenient to refer to a table or chart, such as that shown in Fig. 3-2, to determine the activity of a particular radionuclide at the time of use.

Activity

The amount of radioactivity present is expressed as the number of disintegrations per second (dps). The unit of measurement is the curie.

> 1 curie (Ci) = 3.7×10^{10} dps
> 1 millicurie (mCi) = 3.7×10^7 dps
> 1 microcurie (μCi) = 3.7×10^4 dps

The new International System unit is the Becquerel (1 Bq = 1 dps).

> 1 Ci = 37,000 MBq
> 1 mCi = 37 MBq
> 1μCi = 37 kBq

Activity (dps) should be distinguished from the number of counts (cps) obtained in a particular detector instrument since this is determined by the efficiency of the particular instrument. The efficiency is the ability of the instrument to detect the radiation and is expressed as the ratio of the number of counts obtained in the instrument per unit time (for example, cps) divided by the activity (dps) of a par-

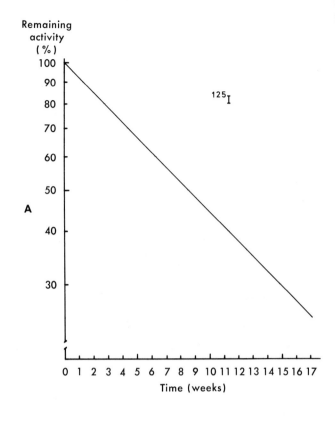

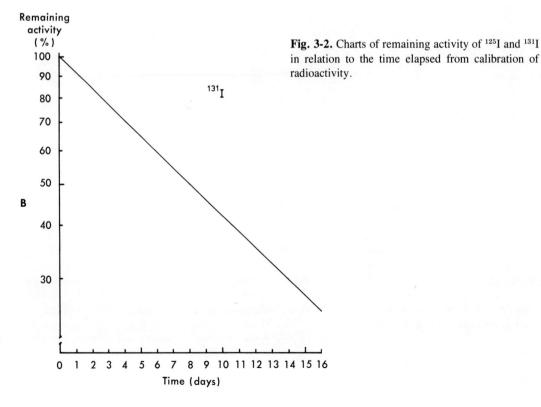

Fig. 3-2. Charts of remaining activity of ^{125}I and ^{131}I in relation to the time elapsed from calibration of radioactivity.

ticular sample. For gamma counters with ^{125}I the efficiency is about 50% to 60%.

RADIOACTIVE ISOTOPES OF NATURAL ELEMENTS

The isotopes carbon 14 and tritium have been used extensively in biologic research. Since they are isotopes of common elements of biologic compounds, one might assume them to be the most useful radioactive tracers for radio-

Table 3-1. Radioactive isotopes of the most common elements in biologic material

| Isotope | Half-life | Main radiation | |
		Type	Energy (keV)
^3H	12.3 years	β^-	18.6
^{10}C	19 s	β^+/γ	1,900/720
^{11}C	20 minutes	β^+	970
^{14}C	5,760 years	β^-	156
^{15}C	2 s	β^-/γ	4,500/5,300
^{13}N	10 minutes	β^+	1,200
^{16}N	7 s	β^-/γ	4,300/6,100
^{17}N	4 s	β^-/γ	4,100/870
^{14}O	71 s	β^+/γ	1,800/2,300
^{15}O	2.1 minutes	β^+	1,700
^{19}O	29 s	β^-/γ	4,600/200
^{20}O	14 s	β^-/γ	2,700/1,100
^{29}P	4 s	β^+	4,000
^{30}P	2.5 minutes	β^+	3,200
^{32}P	14.3 days	β^-	1,700
^{33}P	24.4 days	β^-	250
^{34}P	12 s	β^-/γ	5,100/2,100

ligand assays. However, these radionuclides have disadvantages that make them less suitable for radioassay work, although they are still used in certain assays.

Most radioactive isotopes of the organic elements are pure beta emitters (Table 3-1) and as such must be measured by means of liquid scintillation counting. This is inconvenient and expensive in comparison with the measurement of gamma radiation with crystal scintillation well counters. The low energy of the beta radiation of ^3H also reduces the counting efficiency. The low decay rate of ^3H and ^{14}C with long half-lives gives them low specific activity and correspondingly low count rates (Table 3-2). This reduces their utility for high-sensitivity assays. Unfortunately, as shown in Table 3-1, all other alternatives of isotopes occurring in biologic material also have suboptimal characteristics for use in radioligand assays. Either the half-life is very short, which makes their use impractical, or the type of radiation is less suitable, as in the case of phosphorus 32 with its high beta energy. Certain biologic compounds contain other elements with radioisotopes that are more suitable for in vitro detection; examples are cyanocobalamin labeled with cobalt 57 and the thyroid hormones in which natural iodine 127 is exchanged for ^{125}I or ^{131}I.

RADIOACTIVE ISOTOPES OF IODINE

The lack of suitable radioactive isotopes of the major elements of biologic molecules has

Table 3-2. Radiation characteristics of radioactive nuclides used for labeling of biologic compounds

| Nuclide | $T_{\frac{1}{2}}$ | Chief radiation | | Specific activity* | |
		Decay type	Energy (keV)	mCi/μg	mCi/μmole
^{14}C	5,760 years	β^-	β^-158 No γ	0.0044	0.062
^3H	12.3 years	β^-	β^-18 No γ	9.7	29
^{125}I	60.2 days	EC†	No β γ 28 + 35	17.3	2,200
^{131}I	8.1 days	β^-	β^-608 γ 364	123	16,100

*Carrier-free material.
†Electron capture.

made it necessary to use isotopes of elements other than those present in the native molecules. The occurrence of tyrosyl residues in almost all proteins is the basis for the widespread application of radioactive iodine isotopes for protein labeling. In the same way as occurs naturally in thyroid hormones, the ring structure of tyrosine may incorporate one or two atoms of iodine. The great number of iodine isotopes, no less than 24, offers a variety of decay modes and radiation types, of which a few of practical importance are shown in Table 3-3. The principle for the iodination of the tyrosyl residue is essentially the same as when iodine is incorporated into thyroid hormones (Fig. 3-3). Other amino acid residues, such as histamine and tyramine, may also be iodinated. Recently, many new methods have been devised to iodinate compounds that do not contain tyrosine. This has increased the usefulness of iodine tracers considerably.

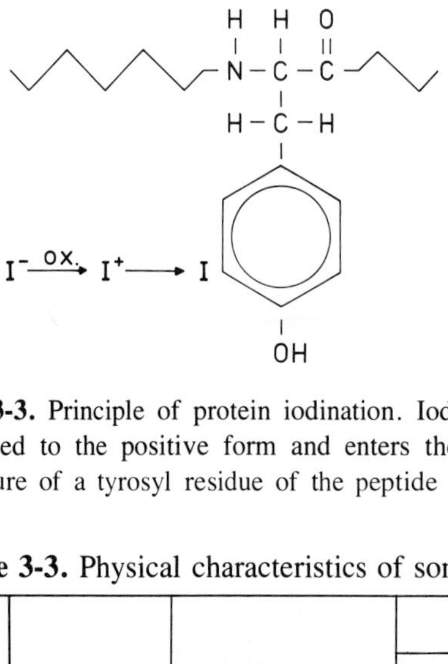

Fig. 3-3. Principle of protein iodination. Iodide is oxidized to the positive form and enters the ring structure of a tyrosyl residue of the peptide chain.

The pioneering work of McFarlane for radioiodination of protein was done considerably before the development of the RIAs. However, these methods did not produce tracers with the high specific activities needed. The main breakthrough that markedly facilitated the development of RIAs was the chloramine-T method for radioiodination of Hunter and Greenwood in 1961. Since then, other methods have been devised for the purpose of minimizing the denaturing effects on proteins during the iodination procedure, such as electrophoretic and enzymatic iodination methods.

Physical properties of iodine isotopes used for labeling

Two iodine isotopes have been widely used for labeling, ^{125}I and ^{131}I. As described in Table 3-3, ^{131}I has 7.5 times higher decay rate than does ^{125}I. However, the ^{131}I preparations available do not give correspondingly higher count rates. This is because the isotopic abundance of ^{131}I is less than 20% of the total iodide content of these preparations; the rest is ^{127}I (stable iodide). Thus the specific activity is reduced correspondingly. The main radiation energy of ^{131}I is the 368 keV peak, which is produced in 82% of the decay events. ^{125}I photon energy is 27 to 35 keV, but as many as 144 photons are produced for 100 decays. With modern equipment, the counting efficiency for both ^{131}I and ^{125}I is high, although a fraction of the ^{125}I is undoubtedly attenuated and therefore lost in test tube walls and detector shields. The net effect of these factors is that freshly prepared ^{125}I will

Table 3-3. Physical characteristics of some iodine isotopes

Iso-tope	Half-life	Mode of decay	Principal photons		Principal β-particle	
			Energy (keV)	Frequency (%)	Energy (keV)	Frequency (%)
^{123}I	13.0 hours	Electron capture	28	87		
			159	84		
^{124}I	4.2 days	Electron capture and β$^+$	28	56	1,550	14
			511	51	2,150	11
			603	62		
^{125}I	60.2 days	Electron capture	28	140		
^{127}I	Stable	—				
^{131}I	8.1 days	β$^-$	364	82	608	87

Data from MIRD/Dose estimate report no. 5: J. Nucl. Med. **16:**857, 1975.

produce more counts per unit of iodide than will ^{131}I. The short half-life of ^{131}I reduces its radiation about 9% every day, so that very soon it becomes a much less active tracer than ^{125}I. In addition to the short shelf life, the high-energy β^- radiation of ^{131}I has a tendency to cause more radiation damage than the pure gamma emitter ^{125}I. Accordingly, ^{125}I is the iodine isotope of choice in most cases. The wide difference between the energies of photon peaks of ^{125}I and ^{131}I makes it possible to measure them simultaneously in a counter with two windows. This has made it possible to develop combined RIAs that simultaneously quantitate two different antigens by having one labeled with ^{125}I and the other with ^{131}I (see Box 8-4). In Appendix 10 a method is given for calculation of radioactivity emitted from the individual isotopes when a mixture of them is counted.

EFFECTS OF RADIOLABELING

The radioactive labeling of any compound will cause a number of secondary changes in the compound that may affect its properties and its behavior in an assay system. Such changes are caused by several different mechanisms. They should be minimized as far as possible to decrease undesirable alterations of the compound as a result of the labeling. The most common untoward effect of labeling is to reduce binding affinity and stability of the labeled compound compared with the unlabeled compound. Some compounds, such as glucagon and prolactin, are particularly sensitive to iodination effects. The shelf life of such material is often significantly shortened in comparison with the native material.

Effects of radiation

If the radionuclide used for tagging is an isotope of an element present in the native unlabeled molecule, and if the labeling involves the simple substitution of a nonradioactive residue with a radioactive isotope of the same chemical species without any alterations in the molecular structure, then the labeled compound might be assumed to have identical chemical and immunologic properties with the unlabeled. However, this ideal situation is seldom realized.

The decay of the radioactive nuclide releases an amount of energy that is much higher than the energy involved in the chemical bonds that maintain the molecular structure. Therefore, decay is likely to break adjacent bonds and cause disintegration of the molecular structure, an event for which the expression "decay catastrophe" has been coined. The decay of the radionuclide also changes its chemical identity (except in isomeric transition decay). The change in the charge of the nucleus (and thereby the place of the element in the periodic system—Z number) will make it a new element (for example, ^{125}I becomes stable tellurium, ^{131}I becomes xenon, ^{14}C will be nitrogen, and ^{3}H becomes helium). Accordingly, the composition and structure of the molecule in which the radioactive isotope is contained will be changed. The effect of this event varies, but not infrequently when a new element is formed, it will alter the structure of the original molecule to the extent that the molecule will disintegrate. Furthermore, the energy released by the decay not only affects the molecule in which it resides but may also interfere with surrounding molecules, inducing changes in their structure and composition.

If the labeled molecule contains only a single radioactive atom, the molecule remaining after the decay will not be the site of any further decay events; thus, no matter what changes occurred as an effect of the decay, the remnants will be nonradioactive and will not contribute to the properties of the radioligand. However, if the labeled molecule contains two or more radioactive atoms, they will not decay simultaneously. After the first one has decayed, the second decay will occur in a molecule that probably has acquired different chemical properties as an effect of the first decay event. This produces labeled material that is nonhomogeneous, with a part of it being dissimilar to the original material. This altered material probably does not have the same immunologic properties as the original material. A jargon term for these influences is "radiation damage." The greater the number of radioactive atoms per molecule, the greater the risk of such damage. The likelihood of multiple decays within one molecule will also increase with decreasing half-life of the radioactive isotope.

The overall effect of the decay events is that essentially no radioactively labeled preparation (radioligand) will remain unaltered over a period of time. However, some of the alterations occur so slowly that they do not cause appreciable changes during the period the radioligand is being used. Because of these radiation effects, as well as the effects discussed in the two following sections, the stability of the labeled preparation is usually reduced in comparison with the unlabeled material. Therefore, one must expect that the useful period of such material is shorter than could be expected from the decay rate or half-life of the radioisotope alone.

Chemical effects

If it is necessary to perform the labeling by introducing a radioactive isotope that is not a normal component of the unlabeled material, not only will radiation change the ligand, but the chemical compositon of the radioligand will be different from that of the unlabeled material.

Iodine isotopes with molecular weights of 121 to 133 have a mass that is larger than the sum of all other constituents of the tyrosyl ring into which it is introduced. If the ring structure of the tyrosine residue projects off the surface of the protein molecule, the introduction of iodine into it will cause a significant alteration of the outer configuration of the protein and thereby influence binding to antibodies or other biologic receptors. The introduction of the iodine also changes the overall charge of the protein. The pK of the tyrosine residue is altered, and the immediate environment of the substituted tyrosine may be changed (for example, by electrostatic forces).

It has been shown that iodination as such (with nonradioactive iodine) influences the potency of biologically active material. Iodinated insulin, for example, retains its biologic effect when less than an average of two atoms of iodine is incorporated per molecule of insulin, but biologic activity is progessively lost at higher degrees of iodination. Studies with many materials have shown that the incorporation of 1 g-atom of radioactive iodine per mole of protein usually does not affect biologic potency or immunologic properties.

The adverse effect of iodination on the binding reactivity of the radioligand to antibodies (immunoreactivity) and other receptors can be lessened to a certain degree. The location of the iodine within the molecules should be as far away as possible from the part of the molecule that takes part in the binding to the receptor (antigenic site). In large molecules, the likelihood is small that the localization of the iodine will coincide with the binding site. However, for small molecules, such as oligopeptides or steroids, the site of iodination must be carefully considered in relation to the binding site.

The location of the iodine substitution can be directed by different means. The unlabeled material can be allowed to react with antibodies coupled to a solid phase (matrix). This complex is then iodinated. Now, iodine will tend to react with tyrosine residues most easily accessible, that is, pointing out from the matrix (and away from the antigenic binding sites). Another mechanism also operates to select labeled antigen molecules with intact binding sites in this procedure. If a tyrosine residue that is an essential part of the binding site happens to be iodinated, the affinity of the iodinated antigen to the antibody will be reduced. This antigen will then be more easily dissociated from its antibody. After iodination, the solid material is washed to remove unreacted iodide as well as iodinated material with decreased affinity that is no longer bound to the antibodies. Accordingly, only labeled antigen maintaining an intact binding site will remain bound to the antibody after labeling. After washing, the bound labeled antigen is dissociated from the antibody by lowering the pH.

Another approach may be used for steroids and other small molecules not containing any tyrosine residue. They may be iodinated after coupling with a tyrosinelike or tyrosine-containing compound that can house the [125]I. Antibodies to these small molecules are usually produced by conjugating them to a carrier protein to make them act as haptens. The antibodies formed against the hapten are essentially directed to the part of the hapten molecule that projects away from the carrier protein. The part of the hapten that faces the carrier protein is therefore not likely to be a part of the binding site. When the molecule is to be iodinated, the tyrosine moiety is coupled to the same part of the molecule as that joined to the carrier protein for the production of antibodies. The iodinated residue will then be located in a part of the molecule that does not participate in the antigen-antibody binding.

A similar technique may be used with antigens that are not used as haptens. A new tyrosine residue is coupled to the molecule, and this is iodinated rather than iodinating a tyrosine present in the native molecule. By such labeling methods the localization of the labeled tyrosine may be selected to occur in a less critical part of the molecule than might have been the case if a native tyrosine were iodinated.

Influences of labeling procedure

The chemical properties of the radioligand may be altered not only by the presence of a radioactive element that is not a constituent of the native molecule but also by the procedures used to introduce the radionuclide into the compound. Most iodination procedures involve an oxidation step and sometimes a reduction step in addition. Unspecific oxidation may cause changes in proteins by interfering with free sulfhydryl (SH) or amino (NH_2) groups. In steroids, unsaturated rings may be changed to saturated rings, and hydroxyl (OH) groups may be changed to keto (O) groups. Unspecific reduction may split disulfide (SS) bridges of proteins.

In addition to these well-understood influences, there are other causes for denaturation of a protein during the labeling procedure. For example, it has been a widespread experience that certain batches of radioiodine may have a denaturing effect on the proteins to be labeled, the reason for which is unclear. The yield of the iodination reaction may be adequate, but the labeled protein has a decreased immunoreactivity and a decreased stability.

TRITIATION

A large variety of biologic compounds tagged with ^3H or ^{14}C are available for radionuclide procedures, but few radioligand assays utilize these tracers today. Therefore, there is little need for the synthesis of ^3H or ^{14}C preparation within the radioligand assay laboratory. Because of the restricted use of these techniques in radioassay work, these techniques will not be discussed here. The reader is referred to the special literature on this subject.

IODINATION

Several iodinated compounds are available from commercial sources. However, the number available does not cover the wide variety of radioiodinated tracers used in radioligand assays. The relative simplicity of iodination procedures may also make attractive the preparation of labeled material within the laboratory instead of reliance on commercial material. Some parts of the following section also apply to the use of ready-labeled material, since it may be necessary both to check its properties and make subsequent purifications.

Iodination procedures involve several main steps. Before the iodination can take place, the quality of the reagents involved, such as the ligand and the radioiodide material, may need to be checked and modified. Following the iodination, the yield of the iodination reaction must be checked. Since the yield almost never reaches 100%, the unreacted iodide must be removed from the labeled material. Furthermore, the iodination procedure may have caused changes in the composition and structure of the labeled material, making it necessary to purify it further. Finally, the quality of the labeled product must be assessed. This may require additional chemical or immunologic analytical procedures.

Chemistry of iodination

Iodine occurs in several different oxidation states (Table 3-4). The positive, +1, form is

Table 3-4. Oxidation states of iodine and their binding with oxygen

Valence	Salt
+7	IO_4 (periodate)
+5	IO_3 (iodate)
+1	I^+
−1	I (iodide)

its reactive form for iodination. Two principal methods are used to produce the +1 ion. One utilizes iodine that is already in the +1 form, whereas the other starts from the negative, −1 ion, iodide, which is oxidized by means of an oxidating method. The +1 species occurs in the compound iodine monochloride, in which form it reacts directly with tyrosine. Oxidation of iodide is the most widely used principle.

Several intermediate steps occur when iodide is oxidized in aqueous solutions, the details of which are not fully known. By enzymatic iodination, the enzyme hydrogen peroxide and iodine form a number of intermediate compounds before the iodine is actually introduced into the protein. The higher oxidation states of iodine are highly reactive with oxygen, which is always present in aqueous solutions. The ions formed as a result of the reaction with oxygen— iodate and periodate—are stable and not easily transferred to the +1 form. Therefore, they are not useful in iodination methods. To prevent

formation of iodate and periodate, reducing agents are often added during the processing of the radioiodide. The iodide material purchased may therefore still contain trace amounts of such reducing substances.

The iodomonochloride method has the advantage of not using any oxidating agent. It is usually primarily based on ^{125}I-NaI and ^{127}I– iodine monochloride, which are treated so as to exchange the stable iodine of the iodine monochloride with the radioactive iodine of ^{125}I-NaI. The drawbacks are the relatively complicated procedures necessary to produce the radioactive reagent and the fact that this reagent is not carrier-free but will contain at least 50% stable ^{127}I–iodine monochloride. This reduces the specific activity of labeled compound in relation to the degree of iodine substitution. These drawbacks have made this method less used in radioligand assays.

One of the major breakthroughs in the development of RIAs was the development of the

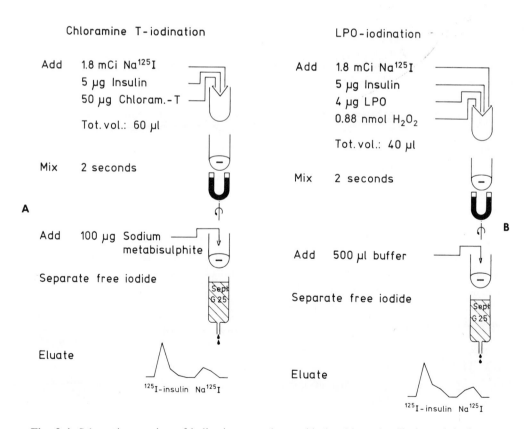

Fig. 3-4. Schematic overview of iodination procedures with the chloramine-T, **A,** and the lactoperoxidase, **B,** methods.

chloramine-T oxidation method by Greenwood and Hunter in 1961 (Fig. 3-4, *A*). This method combines easy handling with the possibility of achieving high specific activities. In the early days of its use frequent failures were encountered with this method, primarily because of variability of the radioiodide preparations available for protein iodination. These products have gradually been improved so that today iodination should be quite reproducible. (See Quality and pretreatment of radioiodide, below.)

The demand for gentler methods of iodination that do not utilize nonspecific oxidating agents has been the basis for the development of electrolytic and enzymatic methods. In the electrolytic method the iodide ion is oxidized in an electrolytic cell. In the enzymatic method, the oxidation (electron transfer) is achieved with the enzyme lactoperoxidase and with hydrogen peroxide (Fig. 3-4, *B*). This reaction is specific in the relation between enzyme and substrate, which implies that nonspecific oxidation reactions that may alter the structure of the protein are less likely to occur.

Practical aspects of iodination procedures

The iodination procedure is perhaps the one single step in a "homemade radioligand assay" that is most likely to cause trouble regardless of whether the assay is in a development stage or established in full production. Since the procedures themselves are quite simple, these difficulties have frequently been blamed on the reagents rather than on the performance of the procedures. The reagents, except for the radioiodide, are easy to standardize, and material from the same batch or bottle may be used for extended periods. However, because the shelf life for ^{125}I is limited, this reagent must be exchanged at intervals. Therefore, unsuccessful iodinations are frequently related to variations in the quality of the radioiodide.

Quality and pretreatment of radioiodide

There are certain differences among the radioiodide preparations presently available. They vary in the concentration of iodide, in the composition of the diluent, and in their contamination with ^{124}I and ^{127}I. It is possible to get very highly concentrated solutions of ^{125}I-NaI, on the order of several hundred millicuries per

milliliter. Since concentrated reactants improve the yield of the iodination reaction (Fig. 3-5), there is an advantage in using a concentrated iodide solution. For most labeling purposes the total amount of radioiodide is on the order of 1 mCi. In the most concentrated ^{125}I preparations, 1 mCi is contained in only a few microliters, which may be difficult to handle with appropriate precision. In our experience a concentration of 100 to 200 mCi/ml is optimal for easy and safe handling. However, it may be preferable to purchase ^{125}I-NaI in the highest possible concentration, so that the appropriate buffers may be added without causing too much dilution.

Most radioiodide preparations are dissolved in NaOH. The concentration of NaOH varies from 0.1 M down to trace amounts, but the pH may be high in nonbuffered solutions (for example, "low pH" iodide solutions may actually have a pH higher than 9 when no buffer is added). Most iodination methods have a rather wide pH optimum, but the reaction rate is clearly reduced at high pH's particularly in the chloramine-T method. Usually the buffer capacity of the iodination mixture is sufficient to maintain the pH of the reaction within the working range (Fig. 3-6). A safe pH control is easily secured by buying a concentrated ^{125}I-NaI solu-

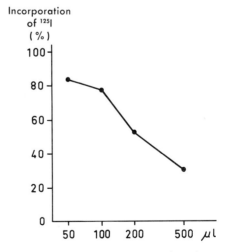

Fig. 3-5. Importance of the concentration of reagents to the iodination procedure illustrated by the effect of diluting the reaction mixture with buffer. The vertical axis shows the yield of the reaction (1 minute reaction time) at increasing total volume of the mixture.

tion, and then adding to it a small amount of a relatively concentrated buffer, such as 0.2 M phosphate buffer (pH 7.5). We like to add this buffer in a 1:1 volume (volume buffer:volume ^{125}I-NaI). When ^{125}I-NaI from the same source is used, there is usually no need for checking the pH before and after addition of the buffer, but this may be necessary when trying a new type of ^{125}I-NaI for the first time or when trouble-shooting difficulties with the labeling procedure. It is easy to check a pH in less than 1 μl of the ^{125}I-NaI solution by placing a tiny drop of the solution on a strip of indicator paper.

Another factor that varies among different preparations of ^{125}I is the degree of contamination with ^{124}I. This does not influence the iodination as such, but the high energy of both the gamma and beta radiation from ^{124}I may cause significant penetration of radioactivity when attempts are made to attenuate the ^{125}I radiation.

As mentioned previously, reducing agents may have been added to the material during the production of the ^{125}I, and significant amounts of these agents may remain in the radioiodide preparation. We have also found that some ^{125}I-NaI contains trace amounts of hydrogen perox-

ide instead of excess reducing capacity. When the chloramine-T method is used in its original form, chloramine-T is added in such excess that small amounts of oxidizing or reducing agents in the radioiodine solution will not influence the results. In the lactoperoxidase method, however, where the substrates for oxidation of the iodide are present in minute concentrations, such variation in the quality of the radioiodide may influence the reaction. For this reason, it may be necessary to test the properties of the particular radioiodine solutions used in this respect.* The presence of trace amounts of reducing substances that may inter-

---

*For example, when we tested the presence of oxidating or reducing capacity of some of the major ^{125}I products in 1973-1974, we found that for ^{125}I from New England Nuclear, an additional amount of sodium peroxide (0.5-2 nmol–1μl-4μl of 1:10,000-dilution 30% hydrogen peroxide) had to be added to compensate for remaining reducing capacity. However, ^{125}I from the Radiochemical Center, Amersham, already contained about 0.2 to 1.0 nmol of hydrogen peroxide. On this occasion we also noted that the Union Carbide ^{125}I sometimes did not work with the lactoperoxidase method. In addition, the properties of the various ^{125}I preparations may change because of alterations in the production methods.

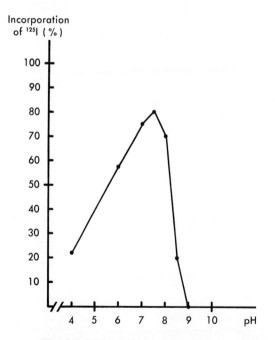

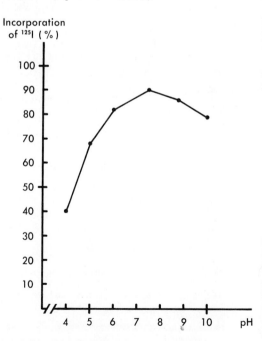

Fig. 3-6. Yield of the iodination at varying pH with the chloramine-T, **A,** and the lactoperoxidase, **B,** methods. (**A,** Data from Hunter, W. M. In Andrews, G. A., Kniseley, R. M., and Wagner, H. N., editors: Radioactive pharmaceuticals, Oak Ridge, Tenn., 1966, AEC Symposium Series no. 6.)

fere in the reaction is easily tested by performing an iodination with an easily iodinated protein, such as serum albumin, starting without addition of any peroxide, and then stepwise adding a couple of microliters of the 1:10,000 diluted hydrogen peroxide and determining the yield of the iodination on a small aliquot of the reaction mixture at each step (see Appendix 11).

In the early days of high–specific activity protein iodination, it was frequently claimed that the radioiodine solution should be very fresh to permit optimal labeling. In our experience, the age of the ^{125}I is not so important, and we do not see any change in the behavior of the preparation during periods up to 1 month after production.

Preparation of material to be labeled

The material to be labeled should be as pure as possible. Contaminating material is likely to be iodinated to the same extent as the material

intended for labeling, and impurities may even be preferentially labeled. It is self-evident that the solution to be labeled cannot contain carrier material such as albumin.

The compound to be labeled should be in a solvent that does not interfere with the labeling. Most generally available buffers are appropriate for this purpose. It may also contain detergents, such as Tween, or agents such as polyethylene glycol, that are used to increase the solubility of the material to be labeled. In enzymatic labeling it is important that the preparation does not contain any enzyme inhibitors. The peroxidases are inhibited by most preservatives used to inhibit bacterial growth, such as merthiolate or sodium azide. Even if these agents were added in several steps before the final preparation of the material to be labeled, trace amounts, particularly of sodium azide, may still remain in the final product and inhibit the iodination reaction. Therefore, it is sometimes necessary

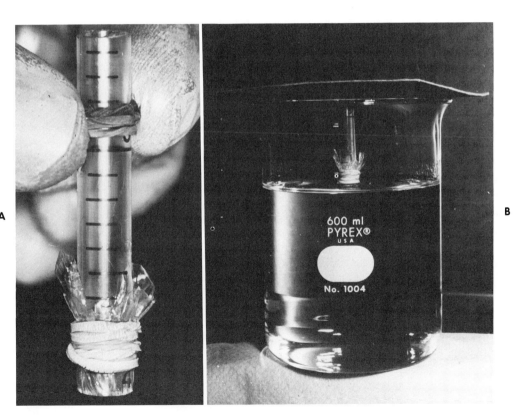

Fig. 3-7. Simple equipment for dialyzing small volumes ($25\mu l$). **A,** The tube is cut from a disposable 5-ml plastic pipette. Its lower end is polished carefully and covered with a film, which is secured to the tube with a rubber band. **B,** Note that the membrane should just barely be immersed into the dialysate. If submerged deeper, the hydrostatic pressure will cause dilution of the dialysate.

to add an extra purification step before labeling. We have found that overnight dialysis against several changes of 500 to 1,000 ml of buffer will remove all such inhibitors. A simple device for dialyzing minute amounts of scarce material is shown in Fig. 3-7.

Iodination procedure

Detailed descriptions of iodination procedures with chloramine-T and lactoperoxidase are given in Appendixes 16 and 17. The pH working range is rather wide (Fig. 3-6), both for the chloramine-T and the lactoperoxidase (LPO) methods, though that of LPO also works at considerably higher pH. However, the optimal pH is also related to the material to be labeled, probably because pH-dependent changes in configuration of the molecule may affect the reactivity of various tyrosines. Therefore, it may be worthwhile to test the pH dependence of the reaction when a new material is tested for labeling. The pH of the reaction also affects the formation of mono- and diiodotyrosines (Fig. 3-8). The yield of the iodination is highly dependent on the concentration of the reagents. Since the amount of radioactive iodide to be used is a limiting factor, in respect to both radiation protection and cost, it is usually necessary to keep the total volume at a minimum if a high specific activity is desired. Not infrequently, the restricted availability of the material to be labeled is another limiting factor. A total reaction volume of $25\mu l$ to $50\mu l$ will give a high yield. This volume is large enough to permit adequate mixing of the reagent and avoid pipetting volumes smaller than $5\mu l$ to $10\mu l$. The amount of radioiodine included in the reaction (1-2 mCi) as described corresponds to about one atom of iodine per mole of protein, calculated on the basis of a protein molecular weight of 20,000 daltons. When new compounds are tried or new assays developed, a lower degree of iodine substitution could be used to assure that the labeled compound is not denatured by overiodination. Even if it is not possible to achieve a lower degree of substitution than one atom per mole, the addition of stoichiometric amounts of radioiodine to the material to be labeled is likely to produce not only monoiodinated tyrosines but also diiodinated tyrosines or multiple-iodinated residues in compounds containing several tyrosine groups. Therefore, an iodine/protein ratio as low as 1/10 is frequently used to increase the probability of monoiodination only. When the behavior of the monoiodinated compound is characterized, further increases in specific activity can be tried.

With the concentrations commonly used, the iodination reaction is almost instantaneous. Thus there is no reason to continue the reaction for a longer period than is necessary for mixing the reagents, although many methods use a 1-minute reaction. Extended periods of incubation may be harmful to the material, exposing it to radiation in highly concentrated volume and prolonging exposure to the oxidating agent or other potential noxious constituent of the radioiodine solution.

The reaction is stopped by addition of a reducing agent or merely by dilution to the point where the reaction rate becomes insignificant. The addition of a reducing agent (sodium metabisulphite) is necessary only with a chloramine-

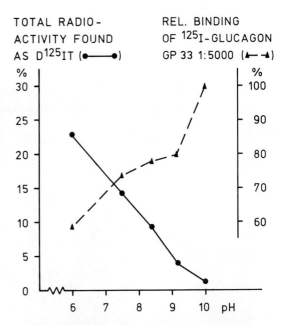

Fig. 3-8. Influences of pH of the iodination reaction on the formation of diiodotyrosine (DIT) as illustrated by iodination of glucagon. At higher pH (abscissa) less DIT is formed (left ordinate), and the binding of the labeled glucagon to antibody is improved (right ordinate). (From Von Schenck, H., Larsson, I., and Thorell, J. I.: Clin. Chim. Acta **69:** 225, 1976.)

T reaction, when a protecting agent such as albumin is added directly to the reaction mixture. If the labeled material is purified from unreacted radioiodide, as in gel chromatography, both the chloramine T and the unreacted iodide will be separated from the protein and therefore will not cause any further iodination. The gel material in the column may be iodinated; however, column iodination is unimportant, since columns are usually used for one iodination only because of the difficulty of washing them free from high activities.

The addition of the enzyme in the LPO method implies that a second protein is present in the reaction mixture. However, the self-iodination of LPO and other peroxidases is minimal. The reason for the resistance of these enzymes to iodination (even with chloramine-T methods) is not clear. However, a small fraction of the LPO, on the order of a few percent, may be labeled as well. In some of the methods used to remove unreacted iodine, such as adsorption chromatography on cellulose or thin-layer chromatography, the peroxidase is also removed. However, even if it remains together with the labeled material, it does not influence the assay. The use of peroxidase coupled to a solid phase, such as polyacrylamide, makes it possible to avoid contamination with LPO. This may be important when one is dealing with material that is difficult to iodinate and where the yield is very low. The insoluble enzyme is then easily removed after the iodination. With chromatographic purification methods this insoluble enzyme preparation will not be able to penetrate the column. The preparation of LPO coupled to polyacrylamide by means of glutaraldehyde and its use in an iodination procedure is illustrated in Appendix 18. The choice of matrix for coupling the LPO is important in high–specific activity labeling of small amounts of protein. Carbohydrate-based matrix material is self-iodinated to a degree, which will reduce the yield of the iodination. Such losses are much lower with noncarbohydrate material, such as the polyacrylamide.

Purification of labeled material

In most cases the labeled material must be purified after the iodination because of the presence of radioactive components with properties other than those desired for the radioligand. Since the iodination rarely causes incorporation of all of the radioiodide added, it is usually necessary to remove unreacted iodide. In addition to removing the unreacted iodide, this step sometimes further purifies the radioligand. Various separation methods have been used for this purpose, such as gel filtration chromatography on Sephadex or Biogel columns (Appendix 19), batch adsorption (Appendix 22), adsorption chromatography on cellulose (Appendix 20), thin-layer chromatography, ion-exchange chromatography (Appendix 23), and dialysis (Appendix 21). This step may also involve an evaluation of the yield of the reaction, a quantitation of the proportion of radioactivity in the labeled material and in the form of iodide. The accurate estimation of the iodination yield may be important, since subsequent quantitations of the amount of radioligand are indirect and based on the measurement of the radioactivity. It is associated with certain problems because of the low concentration of the labeled material.

Of the various methods for estimating the yield of the iodination, dialysis is probably most appropriate, provided that the labeled material is large enough to be excluded by the dialyzing membrane. Carrier ^{127}I-NaI should be added to assure that the radioiodine is not adsorbed to the dialysis bag.

The yield of the reaction may be tested by precipitation of a small aliquot of the reaction mixture with 10% trichloroacetic acid (TCA). To assure the formation of precipitate, a drop of 1% serum albumin may be added before addition of the TCA. This is the most rapid method for checking the yield of the iodination during the iodination procedure and may be performed within 1 or 2 minutes. Most accurate estimation by TCA precipitation makes it necessary to wash the precipitate twice.

Methods that combine the removal of iodide with purification of the labeled material are illustrated by techniques for thin-layer chromatography of labeled progesterone and testosterone (Appendixes 13 and 15). A special form of separation is used in methods where excess amounts of protein are iodinated to assure the formation of monoiodotyrosine only. The specific activity of the labeled material can then

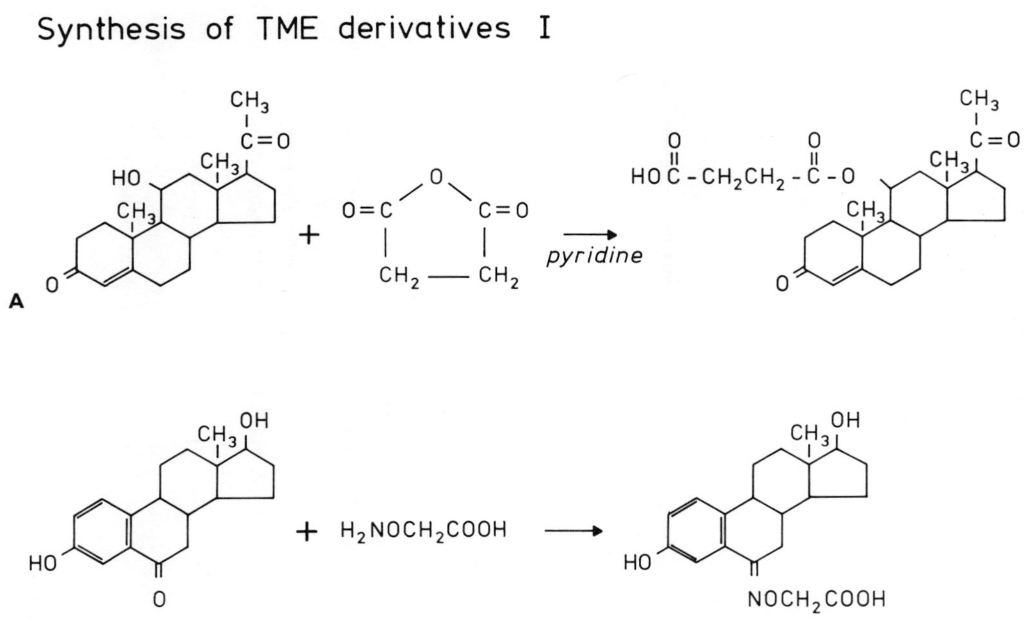

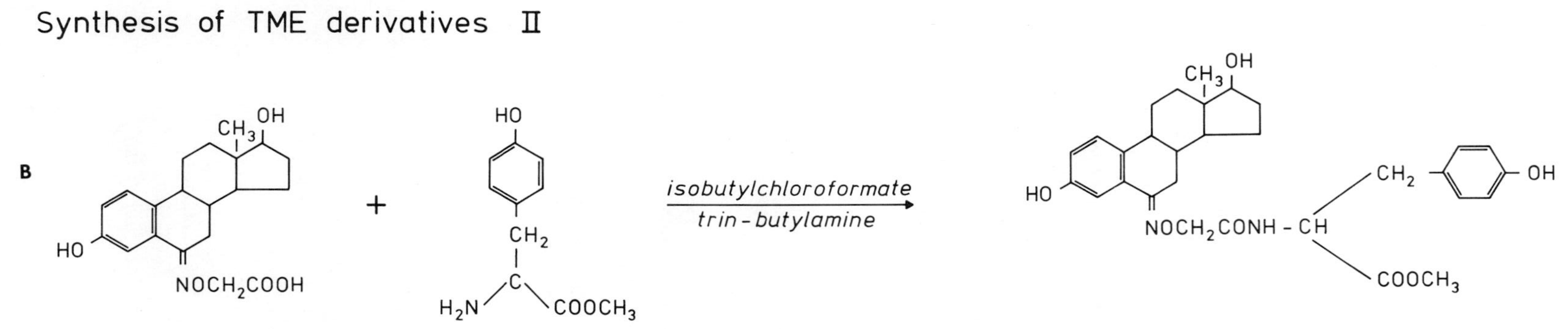

Fig. 3-9. Principle reactions for the synthesis of tyrosine methyl ester (TME) derivatives of steroids. **A,** Production of a hemisuccinate derivative from the C_{11}-hydroxyl group of cortisol (top) and of a carboxymethyloxime derivative from the C_6-keto group of 6 keto-17β-estradiol (bottom). This keto derivative was first produced by oxidation of 17β-estradiol with chromium trioxide. **B,** The final step as illustrated with conjugation of TME to estradiol conjugate. This reaction is identical with either of the derivatives produced in **A.**

be increased considerably by separation of the iodinated compound from the unlabeled material. This can best be performed with relatively small molecules where the introduction of one iodine alters the charge to the extent that they can be separated on this basis. Such methods have been reported for relatively small peptides, such as angiotensin (Appendix 23).

Iodination of compounds not containing tyrosine

Two different methods have been used for iodination of compounds not containing tyrosine: one involves the synthesis of a material containing a tyrosine and the iodination of this material, and the other consists of the conjugation of the material to be labeled with a compound that already contains the radioactive iodine. The latter approach has the advantage of avoiding the direct influence of the iodination procedure on the whole radioligand.

Several different compounds have been utilized for supplying a tyrosine or tyrosinelike residue. These range in size from a whole albumin molecule to a single tyrosine. The residues used for this purpose are tyrosine methyl ester (TME), tyramine, and histamine. The methods used for coupling the tyrosine residue are the same as those described for conjugation of a hapten to a large protein, as discussed on p. 22. If the compound to be conjugated contains a reactive amino or carboxyl group, it is utilized for the coupling. With steroids and similar compounds not containing such groups, hydroxyl or keto groups are utilized by preparing their corresponding hemisuccinate or *O*-carboxy-methyloxime derivative. The essential steps for coupling the residue to a steroid via a hydroxyl or a keto group are illustrated in Fig. 3-9. The tyrosyl residue or the tyrosine conjugate is iodinated by means of chloramine-T or lactoperoxidase (Fig. 3-10).

The most common reagent used for labeling with a preiodinated compound is *N*-hydroxysuccinimide ester of 3-(*p*-hydroxyphenyl)propionic acid. This reagent is commercially available in both labeled and unlabeled forms. The only obvious drawback with this method is the relatively low yield in the conjugation step. However, this does not necessarily prevent achieving relatively high specific activities. The principal steps of this procedure are shown in Fig. 3-11. Detailed descriptions of these methods are given in Appendixes 12 to 15.

When steroids are iodinated, all of these methods will produce a variety of iodinated compounds with varying degrees of immunoreactivity; these will require further purification steps after iodination.

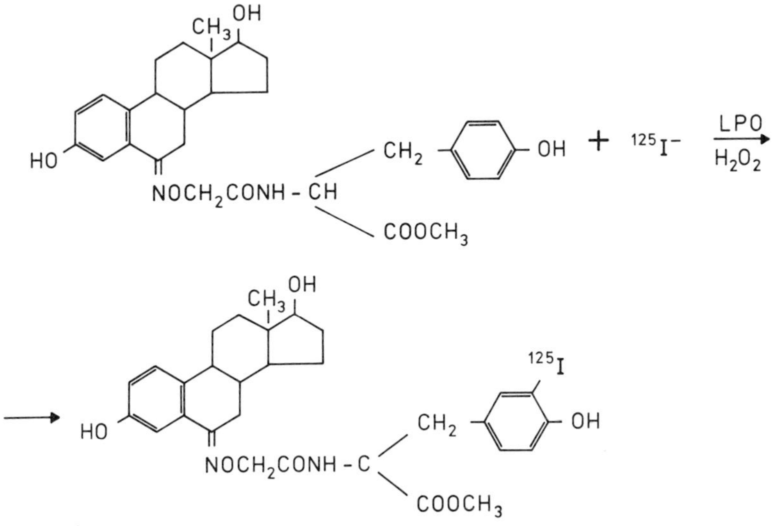

Fig. 3-10. Lactoperoxidase iodination of the estradiol TME derivative.

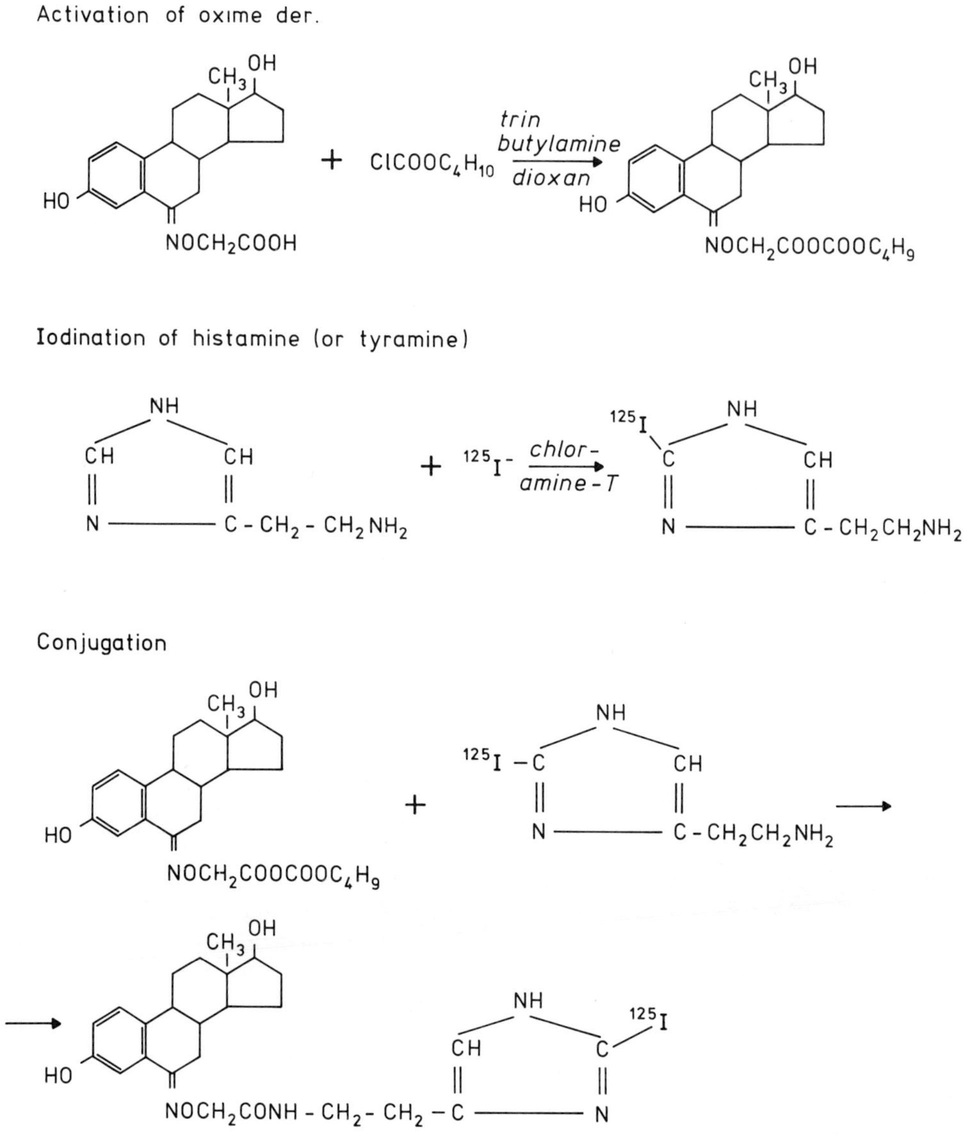

Activation of oxime der.

Iodination of histamine (or tyramine)

Conjugation

Fig. 3-11. Principal reaction of the iodinated histamine conjugation method (Nars-Hunter).

Storage of iodinated material

As soon as possible after iodination, some protecting material, such as 1% serum albumin, should be added. This reduces the adsorption to tube walls and has also been shown to reduce the tendency of the labeled protein to become denatured. It is performed by collecting the column effluent after purification in tubes containing a 2% albumin solution of the same volume as the fraction collected. The concentration of radioligand in the fractions to be used is estimated from its content of radioactivity. The material is then diluted with a serum albumin solution to achieve a concentration and volume convenient for aliquoting the material into multiple small vials, the number of which is about the same as the number of assays it is intended to be used for, so as to prevent repeated thawing and freezing. Most material is adequately stored at $-20°$ C without the addition of any preservative. Lyophilization may increase storability, but the procedure must be appropriately performed so as not to harm the material during freeze-drying. Materials, such as glucagon, that are sensitive to proteolytic enzymes, may be more stable if stored with an enzyme inhibitor, such as Trasylol.

Evaluation of the radioligand

Two properties of the radioligand must be established: the specific activity of the tracer, as discussed previously, and the reactivity of the radioligand toward the assay receptor. Although the radioligand need not be identical to the ligand to be assayed, it must have an affinity to the receptor of the same magnitude as the ligand to achieve the highest possible assay sensitivity. The most appropriate test of the radioligand is in the same test system as it is to be used in. In RIAs the radioligand should be tested for its immunoreactivity, and in other receptor assays it should be tested for its receptor-binding properties. Sometimes a preliminary test by means of other properties may give an indication of the quality of the material. Systems utilized for that purpose have been the adsorption to solid material, such as cellulose, glass, or silica powder. For example, Yalow and Berson found in their first insulin studies that undegraded labeled insulin adsorbed to the Whatman 3 M paper used in their buffer-flow electrophoretic system, whereas the degraded material moved with albumin. The same principle is used as the basis for the adsorption methods sometimes employed to separate labeled material from unreacted iodide and degraded labeled material. This and similar methods are not generally applicable, since many substances do not show this marked adsorption to cellulose or other adsorbents. There is also considerable variation in cellulose quality with regard to its adsorptive power.

Testing of receptor or immunoreactivity can be performed both at receptor excess and with the amount of receptor that is used in the actual assay system. These two tests evaluate two different properties of the radioligand.

The binding of radioligand to a large excess of receptor essentially reflects the amount of contaminated labeled material. This test may not detect minor changes in the radioligand. Fractions with moderately decreased affinity to

the receptor may still be bound to excess receptor. However, radioactive contaminants that do not share the binding properties of the radioligand will effectively prevent the binding from reaching 100%, irrespective of the amount of receptor present. The antibody or receptor excess method of testing has the advantage of being relatively fast; thus it can be used as a preliminary check on the quality of the radiolabeled material immediately after labeling, before it is put into routine use.

The other method estimates the binding of the radioligand to a restricted amount of the receptor. In a more elaborate form it compares the affinity of unlabeled and labeled ligand. The radioligand is tested as a standard by adding increasing amounts of radioligand; the binding should be inhibited to the same extent as if it were not labeled. A rough estimate of this property may be assessed by determining the degree of binding of the 0-standard (B_0).

The quality of the radioligand must be tested not only immediately after labeling but during its whole period of use. Information in this respect can usually be retrieved from the results of the assays by continuously checking the amount bound when no unlabeled ligand is added (B_0), the slope of the curve, and the precision of the assay. In our experience, when an assay is run by an experienced technician, deterioration of the radioligand is most frequently shown by decreased precision in the assay in combination with a tendency for control sera to drift. We have found that when such signs occur, problems are avoided if the batch of radioligand is exchanged for a freshly made preparation. Certain laboratories prefer to repurify the radioligand rather than substitute it with a new batch. We have not found this worthwhile. The iodinated radioligand may be expected to be sufficiently stable for most routine assays for at least 1 month. We have found that routine labeling once a month gives a good margin of safety, since most of the material can be used for up to 2 months. This implies that there are always at least two different batches available, which permits a safe overlap between old and new preparations. This practice reduces problems in routine assays.

4 SEPARATION TECHNIQUES

The methods used to separate free from receptor-bound radioactivity are based on chemical or immunologic differences between the free ligand and the ligand bound to the receptor. Generally, the properties of the bound ligand are determined by the properties of the receptor. The differences utilized for separation of receptor from the free ligand include charge, size, solubility, surface configuration (immunologic determinants), and the adsorption to solid material. Many methods primarily isolate the receptor-bound activity. Adsorption procedures, on the other hand, generally remove the unbound ligand from the solution.

An ideal separation method should not affect the distribution of the radioactivity between bound and free forms. It should give an absolute separation with no overlap of bound and free radioactivity (deficiencies in this respect have been called "misclassification errors"), be rapid and easy to perform, and once done, be stable in time. It should not be influenced by the presence of serum or plasma.

The pioneering radioligand assays of the early 1960s utilized several different separation methods. The chromatoelectrophoretic method used by Yalow and Berson in their first RIA took advantage of differences between free and antibody-bound insulin in two properties: adsorption to cellulose and charge. Electrophoretic separation was used by Ekins in his TBG-based thyroxine assay and by Hunter and Greenwood in their first growth hormone RIA. The double-antibody methods were first developed by Hales and Randle and by Morgan and Lazarow for the insulin assay and by Utiger and associates for the growth hormone assay.

Since then, a great variety of separation methods have been developed. This diverse methodology reflects the fact that RIAs are so universally applicable that no single separation method fits the properties of the multiple combinations of ligand-receptor that can be used as bases for an assay. Furthermore, the performance demanded of a method depends to an extent on the purpose of the procedure. For example, an assay may be optimized for speed and ease of performance or sensitivity and reproducibility. These requirements will determine the methods selected. In addition, the large number of different separation methods reflects technical problems encountered during development of many RIAs. Modification of the separation method has frequently been used as a means of overcoming such difficulties.

PRINCIPLES OF DIFFERENT SEPARATION METHODS
Separation methods based on differences in solubility

These methods are borrowed from protein chemistry, where they were developed for differential precipitation of proteins. In RIA they have mainly been applied to assays of small proteins. Immunoglobulins, with about the lowest solubility of all proteins, are precipitated in solutes such as ethanol, dioxane, and polyethylene glycol, or are salted out by ammonium sulfate or sodium sulfate. IgG is almost completely precipitated in 33% saturated ammonium sulfate, in 70% ethanol, in 15% zirconyl phosphate, and in 15% polyethylene glycol. Most small polypeptides remain in solution in these fluids. These precipitation methods have the advantage of being rapid and usually do not require any special incubation period. They are inexpensive and well suited to automated pipetting systems. Ethanol precipitation has been used in assays for insulin and human chorionic somatomammotropin. Ammonium sulfate has been used for assays of angiotensin, vasopressin, cyclic AMP, steroids, prostaglandins, and so forth. Polyethylene glycol is applied to an increasing number of different types of hormones, such as growth hormone, thyroid hormones, steroids, and so on. Detailed descriptions of these methods are given in Appendixes 24 to 26.

The result of the separation is usually influenced by the presence of plasma or serum, since the volume of the precipitate is greatly increased by precipitating the immunoglobulins of the sample as well. To make standards and samples as comparable as possible, plasma or serum should be added to the standards (and the same volume of diluent to sample tubes to make volumes identical) immediately before the addition of the precipitating agent, if not present from the beginning of the assay procedure.

Separation methods utilizing differences in adsorption to solid material

Many small proteins have a high tendency to adsorb to solid material, which is believed to depend on interaction between cyclic amino acid residues and the rough surface. Polypeptides and proteins containing many such amino acids adsorb more actively. Materials with a high adsorptive power include cellulose, glass powder, silica powder, talc, active charcoal, and fuller's earth.

Of the adsorption methods, the activated charcoal technique, first described by Herbert and associates for the vitamin B_{12} assay, is the one most extensively used. It may be used coated or uncoated. The coating, particularly with dextran, has been assumed to work like a molecular sieve, permitting only the small molecules from coming into contact with the adsorptive area. However, it has been shown that other substances, such as serum albumin, may work equally well to reduce the binding of gamma globulin to the charcoal. Accordingly, the dextran probably works in this system not as a molecular sieve but to reduce the adhesiveness of the adsorbing area of the charcoal surface.

Charcoal adsorption techniques have been extensively used in assays of small molecules, such as steroids and thyroid hormones. One such procedure is described in Appendix 27. Some of the difficulties and inconsistencies experienced with this technique have been blamed on variations in the quality of the activated charcoal. More probably, many of the difficulties relate to the exactness of the technique, since it is not difficult to find preparations of charcoal that work well. Some investigators have found it necessary to perform the centrifugation at cold room temperatures, whereas others have not found this necessary. Undoubtedly, the adsorption process is a dynamic event, and the adsorption increases in proportion to the length of time of incubation of the reagents and adsorber. The adsorption also increases with the amount of adsorber but decreases with heavier coating of the charcoal. Thus the adsorbing material must, to a degree, be regarded as a second receptor system in the reaction that may potentially strip the ligand from its binding to the receptor. Therefore, in order to achieve reproducible results, it is important to rigidly standardize these procedures.

Other adsorption methods have gained less general application, and reference is made to the original description for their performance and evaluation. The chromatoelectrophoretic separation of Berson and Yalow utilized the adsorptive property of cellulose in the Whatman 3MM or 3MC paper strips, which retained the unbound radioligand at the site of application, while the flow of buffer caused by evaporation from the strip, in addition to the electric potential, moved the other reactants away from the origin. This effect can also be achieved without applying any electrical current over the paper strips. Some difficulties with this technique have been caused by uneven properties of different batches of the chromatography paper. A modification of this technique that is more suitable to a large series of tubes is wick chromatography. The utility of this technique, however, is restricted to relatively small sample volumes.

Double-antibody methods

In contrast to many other immunologic systems, no precipitates are formed during the primary reaction between antigen and antibody

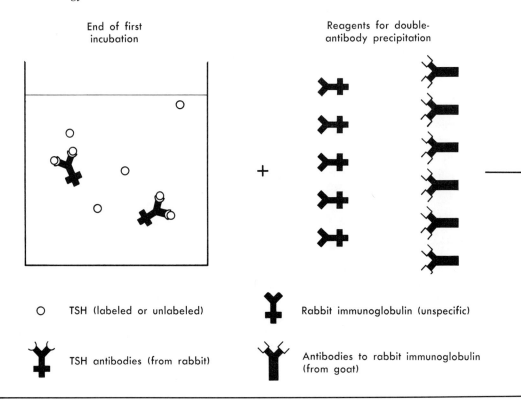

End of first
incubation

Reagents for double-
antibody precipitation

+

○   TSH (labeled or unlabeled)

Rabbit immunoglobulin (unspecific)

TSH antibodies (from rabbit)

Antibodies to rabbit immunoglobulin
(from goat)

in RIAs. The reason for this is that the low concentrations of antibodies and antigens do not permit the lattice formation that is the structure of the immunologic precipitate. It has been shown in gel precipitation systems that below a concentration of 10^{-8} g/liter of antibodies or antigen, no precipitation occurs. This is well above the working concentrations of most RIAs. This problem is circumvented in the double-antibody separation technique in which a second antigen-antibody reaction at a higher concentration of immunoglobulin is included. In this step the antibodies (immunoglobulins) of the primary reaction act as antigen. The second antibody as directed against immunoglobulins of the species in which the primary antibody was produced and therefore from a different species. (This is illustrated in Fig. 4-1 with a thyroid-stimulating hormone [TSH] assay.) Details for production of goat antisera are given in Appendix 29 and for performing the separation in Appendix 28. Since the immunoglobulin making up the primary antibody of the assay may have been diluted extensively, it is usually necessary to add more immuno-

globulin from that same species to achieve optimal precipitation with the second antibody added. In the example in Fig. 4-1, serum from rabbits not immunized against TSH is added for this purpose. Usually, normal serum with its content of immunoglobulins is added. In this way, the concentration of immunoglobulin (antigen in the second system) may be adjusted at will to achieve optimal precipitation with the second antibody. The second antibody will not recognize any differences between the primary specific antibody or the nonspecific immunoglobulins added, so both will be part of the precipitate formed.

The double-antibody separation can either be performed as a postprecipitation method, which is the most frequently used variant, or the precipitation may be done before the primary reaction (preprecipitation). The preprecipitation method works if the antibody-binding sites of the primary reaction are not sterically hindered, after the precipitate has developed, which otherwise will prevent the primary reaction from taking place. This modification can actually be regarded as a solid phase coupled antibody sys-

Precipitation of rabbit
immunoglobulin (including TSH
antibodies)

Removal of supernatant
Precipitate is counted

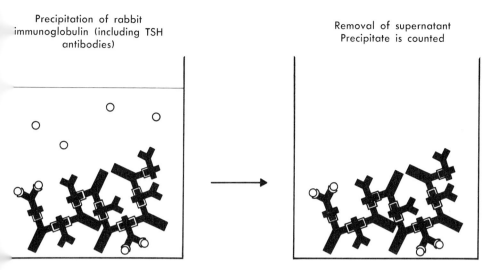

Fig. 4-1. Principles of double-antibody precipitation applied to TSH assay. The addition of the unspecific rabbit immunoglobulin increases the overall concentration of reactants so that a precipitate can develop with the second antibody.

tem where the immunoglobulin precipitate constitutes the solid phase. This method does not work with all double-antibody precipitating antisera and may have a tendency to decrease the sensitivity of the assay.

An alternative in which the double antibody is coupled to a solid phase (DASP) avoids some of the variability of the precipitation reaction.

The major advantage of the double-antibody method is that it can be applied to almost any assay. It achieves a rather complete separation between bound and free ligand, with relatively little overlapping and nonspecific coprecipitation of free ligand. It has very little influence on the distribution of the ligand between the bound and free forms. The main disadvantages are the interferences of plasma in the precipitation, the additional time required for development of the precipitate (a short time with good antisera), and the variation of the properties of various precipitating antisera. Every batch of antisera (which, when it is known that one or several animals consistently produce good antisera, may consist of pooled antisera collected at different occasions) must be carefully characterized before it is employed in an assay.

Frequently, an overnight incubation is used to produce a complete precipitation, but with good antisera the same result may be achieved within an hour. The shorter the incubation period needed, the less the precipitating antiserum can be diluted, so the consumption of the double-antibody antiserum may be considerable. For this reason, it is usually produced in large animals, such as goats or monkeys.

The testing of a double-antibody precipitating antiserum can be performed with ^{125}I-labeled immunoglobulin as a tracer, or usually more conveniently, with the labeled antigen of one of the assays for which the precipitating antiserum is intended to be used. To assure that an incomplete reaction of the first antibody step does not influence the evaluation of the second antibody, the concentration of the first antibody may be increased to the extent that the labeled antigen is completely bound in the first reaction step. This method for testing is best suited for assays with high titer and high-avidity antibodies in the primary step, in which the dilution of the first antiserum is so high that an increase in its concentration will not influence the precipitation. The method is illustrated in Appendix 29. In Fig. 4-2 typical results for testing a rabbit IgG–precipitating antiserum from goat are shown.

Separation based on molecular size

In many assays there is a significant difference in the size of receptor and ligand. Antibodies have a molecular weight of about 160,000 daltons, which is markedly greater than that of protein hormones but smaller than that of many macromolecular proteins. This dif-

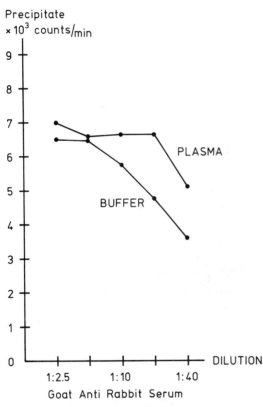

Precipitate
$\times 10^3$ counts/min

PLASMA

BUFFER

DILUTION

1:2.5   1:10   1:40

Goat Anti Rabbit Serum

Fig. 4-2. Results from testing a double antibody. Two series of tubes containing FSH antibody (1:10,-000, a 10× higher concentration than used in the FSH assay) were preincubated with ^{125}I-labeled FSH overnight. The concentration and amounts of the reagents were otherwise the same as in the final assay. One of the series also contained 100μl of plasma, substituted by buffer in the other series (with BSA). Then normal rabbit serum (1:200) and a dilution series of the second antibody were added to the tubes and incubated another night. Note the precipitation-promoting effect of plasma.

ference in size has been used to separate free ligand from the receptor-bound activity by means of gel filtration. This method has the advantage of giving a well-defined separation with little influence on the distribution of bound and free ligand. But to achieve optimal separation it may be necessary to collect several fractions of eluate; even if this can be overcome by standardizing column performance, it is quite tedious to perform on a mass scale. The type of column bed used depends on the size of the ligand. Antigens with molecular weights less than 50,000 daltons are easily separated from antibodies by means of Sephadex G-50 or Bio-gel P-100 gels.

Solid phase receptor systems

In solid phase receptor assays, antibody or cell receptor is coupled to a nonsoluble phase. This coupling is done in advance so that the receptor is insoluble from the beginning of the assay. Antibodies coupled to such a solid phase or matrix are often referred to as immunoadsorbents or immunosorbents. Various kinds of insoluble material have been used as matrix. They may either be in powder form, discs or strips, or coupled to the inside of the test tube. Cell membrane receptors may be regarded as a special type of solid phase system. The "solid phase" consists of disintegrated fragments of the cell membrane, containing specific receptors.

Various methods have been used for the coupling of antibodies to the solid matrix. Covalent binding can be achieved by different methods. Antibodies are usually coupled by peptide bonds by means of reagents, such as glutaraldehyde or carbodiimide, to polyacrylamide (Appendix 30), or with cyanogen bromide to carbohydrate material (such as Sephadex or Sepharose, Appendix 31).

Antibodies may also be made insoluble by physical adsorption to solid materials, such as glass or plastics, such as polystyrene or polypropylene. The adsorption is strong and very little of the adsorbed antibody is eluted from the solid material. Coupling of antibodies may be performed with whole serum or with immunoglobulins isolated by different methods, such as precipitation with ammonium sulfate (Appendix 32) or separation by means of gel filtration or anion exchange chromatography (Appendix 33), or with specific antibody populations isolated by affinity chromatography. The solid phase preparations must be washed extensively after the coupling procedure to remove all noncoupled receptors. In physical adsorption of antibodies to solid material, all adsorptive capacity is usually not occupied by the antibody. To prevent further binding of other proteins when the coating with antibodies has been completed, the remaining adsorption sites of the solid material are saturated by adding either serum albumin or immunoglobulins that do not contain the specific antibody.

The binding of antibodies to a solid phase may change the binding characteristics of the receptor. Therefore, immunosorbent antibody must be tested after coupling of the antibody. Both changes in avidity and significant loss of antibody quantity (titer) have been reported as effects of coupling to solid material.

Insoluble antibodies may also be produced by polymerizing the immunoglobulins with the same type of reagents used for coupling haptens to carrier proteins, such as ethyl chloroformate or glutaraldehyde. Antibodies entrapped in polyacrylamide gels have also been described for use in RIAs.

SELECTION OF SEPARATION METHODS

The factors that primarily govern the choice of separation method are the physical and chemical properties of the ligand and the receptor. Usually, the less chemically similar, the wider the choice of methods. Then, need for rapid separation, for automation, cost, and convenience, as well as the resources and experience of the individual laboratory will determine the selection. Other factors to consider are: how the separation works for denatured labeled material; the degree of overlapping between the phases or of coprecipitation of unbound activity with the receptor; the stability of the separation, and so forth.

For the purpose of developing new assays, it is helpful to have a number of separation methods "in stock" that depend on different principles of separation and in which all reagents and their behaviors are well character-ized. When applying one of these methods to a new assay, one at least knows that the separation method works in a predictable way and that assay difficulties are related to other factors. In our experience, the double-antibody technique, although associated with certain drawbacks, is the most widely applicable method. The availability of a well-standardized and controlled double-antibody method in the laboratory, therefore, facilitates the development of new assays and may be used as a preliminary separation technique for almost all new assays developed. Then, when the assay works with this separation, other separation methods that may better suit the practical conditions are considered.

ERRORS OF SEPARATION
Overlapping (misclassification)

Most separation methods achieve the separation by transferring the bound or the free radioactivity into an insoluble form (if it is in a soluble form from the beginning). The quantitation of unknown ligand is then actually based on the distribution of the radioactivity between the solid (insoluble) and the soluble phase. The solid phase may have different forms, such as a double-antibody precipitate, an ethanol precipitate, a charcoal powder, or the matrix of solid phase conjugated antibody assays. All solid materials have a tendency to adsorb small amounts of polypeptides or of any substance dissolved in the suspension containing the solid material. If the adsorbed substance is labeled with radioactivity, even very small quantities adsorbed will be recognized. Such nonspecific adsorption of soluble radioactive ligand to the insoluble phase will influence the apparent distribution of the radioactivity between the bound and free form. The degree of this nonspecific adsorption or coprecipitation is affected by the type of diluent, the concentration of the radioactive material, the volume of the solid phase material, pH, ionic strength, other reagents present, and so forth. Nonspecific adsorption is influenced (decreased) by the protein concentration of the diluent.

In addition to the nonspecific adsorption to the solid material of the separation method, the inside of the test tube in which the method is performed will also act as a nonspecific adsorber. The effect of this adsorption of radioactivity to the test tube wall will affect the result differently depending on whether the counting of radioactivity is performed in the tube (in which case it will increase) or if counting is performed on an aliquot removed from the tube (it will decrease). Any precipitate or solid material in powder form will include some trapped diluent. If the solid material is voluminous, this trapping effect may be highly significant. For this reason, it usually is better to achieve a small precipitate than a large one. Some of these problems may be reduced by extensive washing of the solid material after separation. However, this usually will not completely remove the adsorbed activity. Repeated washings are tedious and, like any additional step, add to the total variation of the assay.

The highest degree of nonspecific adsorption is utilized to achieve separation of bound and unbound radioactivity; it is active charcoal separation. Such adsorbers have a tendency to adsorb small amounts of almost any macromolecular material present. Thus antibodies are also adsorbed to a degree. Accordingly, the separation of unbound or bound radioligand is not absolute, but it is highly dependent on the conditions of the separation and the quantities of the various reagents. The amount of the separator must be carefully optimized to achieve maximal adsorption of free ligand and minimal adsorption of the receptor. The magnitude of the adsorbing area of the separator is also influenced by other substances present, such as protein or dextran coating of the adsorber.

At present all separation methods involve the physical removal of one of the phases to permit counting of radioactivity associated with the other. Usually it is sufficient to count only one of the phases, since by accurate pipetting the amount of total activity added to the tubes can be assumed to be constant; thus, if necessary, the amount of radioactivity associated with the phase not being counted is easily calculated. In a few separation systems where there is great variability in the quantity of the sample introduced for separation (such as in chromatographic separation), it may be necessary to count both the bound and free fractions, since

the total radioactivity added to the chromatogram varies from sample to sample.

The physical separation of the bound and free phases is often one of the main sources of assay imprecision. When the soluble phase is decanted from the solid phase, a smaller or larger part of the fluid is left in the tube after decanting. If it constitutes a substantial fraction of the soluble phase, variations in its volume can cause considerable assay variation. Accordingly, this type of error is particularly prominent if the total volume of the assay is small. In our experience, decanting of volumes of 0.5 ml or more can be done reproducibly. Another error is that part of the precipitate may pour out of the tube with the supernatant. It is important that the decanting be performed in exactly the same way for all tubes of the assay. Decanting errors may be reduced by increasing the volume of the incubate (for example, by adding 1 ml buffer to the tubes just before centrifugation). Also, if the precipitate is loose and has a tendency to slide out of the tube when decanted, it may be safer to suction off the supernatant. An alternative is to remove an aliquot of the supernatant and perform the counting on this instead of on the precipitate. This involves more work, but it is a relatively precise procedure. Centrifugation in the cold (4° C) may improve precipitate stability and thereby improve the precision of decanting. Another possibility is to perform repeated centrifugation and washing steps and remove only part of the supernatant by suction after each washing.

INFLUENCE OF SEPARATORS ON DISTRIBUTION BETWEEN BOUND AND FREE FRACTIONS

If the separation procedure itself tends to disrupt the receptor-ligand bond, significant change in the distribution of radioactivity between receptor-bound and free fractions may occur. Therefore, the separation procedure should preferably not affect the binding characteristics of the receptor preparation. For this reason, precipitation methods that denature proteins, such as TCA precipitation, cannot be used for separation.

The binding of the ligand to the receptor is a reversible reaction. Thus, if the reaction conditions are changed during the separation step, the equilibrium reached at the end of the primary incubation may change. Some separation methods have a tendency to influence the distribution of the radioligand between the free and bound state, mostly tending to dissociate the bound ligand from the receptor. For example, any significant increase in the total reaction volume during separation will decrease the concentration of the unbound ligand and tend to dissociate the bound material. However, the possible influence of such a dilution is related to the avidity of the binding between receptor and ligand. The higher the avidity of the binding, the less is the tendency toward such effects. If the avidity is sufficiently high and the assay works as a true saturation analysis, the ligand and receptor may still interact at saturation conditions up to a certain degree of dilution. With double-antibody assays, if the second antibody is contained in a small volume, the total volume of the reaction does not appreciably increase; thus this procedure rarely alters the binding conditions. All assays involving repeated washings have the potential risk of dissociating bound ligand from receptor, but generally the dissociation rate is so slow that this effect is negligible. Similarly, in solid phase bound antibody assays, if centrifugation is the only separating step performed, there should be no changes in the primary binding reaction.

In separation methods involving the adsorption of the free ligand, the added adsorber must be regarded as a secondary receptor system with an unlimited binding capacity. Accordingly, by removing all free ligands from the solution, the condition for the binding to the receptor is drastically shifted, tending to dissociate bound ligand from antibody. These types of methods, therefore, have a marked tendency to disrupt binding. The lower the avidity of the receptor (antibody) and the faster the dissociation rate, the greater the tendency toward such problems. In a given assay system, it is difficult to predict the effect of the separation step. Thus the separation system of every individual assay must be checked for time effects and nonstability of the separation in relation to the practical performance and routine of the laboratory.

BEHAVIOR OF DAMAGED RADIOLIGAND

Radioligand that has been altered during radioiodination, prolonged storage, or incubation in the assay procedure usually binds to the receptor with less affinity and remains in the unbound fraction. Damaged radioligand may behave differently from undamaged radioligand in relation to the phases produced by the separation. Also, free iodide may be present and partitioned variably between the fractions. Both free iodide and damaged radioligand may have a tendency to nonspecifically coprecipitate with the receptor in precipitation methods and thereby falsely increase the apparent bound fraction. They may or may not bind to absorbers for free radioligand and thus bias the estimate of binding of intact radioligand to the receptor. The behavior of damaged radioligand or free iodide can be estimated by studying the binding to excess antibody and the nonspecific binding in samples not containing any specific antibody. Such controls should be included in all assays (p. 68).

INFLUENCE OF COMPETING SPECIFIC RECEPTORS

The presence of receptors in a sample other than the primary receptor (antibody) of the assay, such as plasma transporting proteins or endogenous antibodies, will influence the binding of the ligand to primary receptor of the assay as well as the distribution of radioactivity between apparent bound and free forms after the separation. For example, in an assay of a sample from an insulin-treated patient, where plasma contains insulin-binding antibodies, part of the radioligand will bind to these endogenous antibodies. If the presence of these antibodies is not recognized by the assayist, the result of the assay may be highly misleading. In this instance the apparent outcome of the assay depends on the type of separation method used. In a double-antibody system, only the antibodies added in the assay (such as insulin antibodies from guinea pig) are precipitated by the double-antibody antiserum (to guinea pig immunoglobulin from goat). The radioligand (^{125}I-labeled insulin) bound by the endogenous human antibodies will not precipitate and therefore is misinterpreted as free ligand; thus the amount of insulin is overestimated. In an assay with ethanol precipitation of the antibodies, both the added exogenous guinea pig antibodies and the endogenous human antibodies will be precipitated, increasing the apparent bound fraction and thereby falsely reducing the quantity of insulin recorded.

INFLUENCE OF PROTEIN CONCENTRATION

It is a rule rather than an exception that the protein concentration of the reaction mixture influences the results of the separation. For assays to be used with plasma or serum, the influence of plasma and serum on assay results must be investigated. These effects are often more complex than what could be expected from the protein concentration of the sample alone. For that reason, there may be marked differences in the results of the separation in tubes containing plasma samples and those containing standards in a buffer diluent that often are not appropriately compensated for just by the addition of HSA to standards. Several different methods have been proposed to supply the standards with a diluent that is sufficiently similar to that of the unknown sample so as not to cause any systematic errors in the results. These problems not only apply to the separation methodology but also to other stages of the assay.

Chemical protein precipitation methods are also affected by relative protein concentration, since in the presence of serum or plasma the precipitate is heavier because of the coprecipitation of other serum proteins.

Some precipitating antisera of double-antibody assays are markedly sensitive to the presence of serum or plasma. This can cause precipitates to increase or decrease. A number of possible reasons for these effects have been suggested, such as the influence of complement or cross-reaction with human immunoglobulins. The presence of anticoagulants, such as EDTA or heparin, that interfere with the complement activity has also been shown to influence some double-antibody systems.

Adsorption systems are highly influenced by the protein concentration, which must be well matched in standards and samples. At low protein concentrations, even the antibodies may be adsorbed by activated charcoal.

If only the separation is affected by the presence of plasma or serum and not the previous steps of the assay, plasma or serum effects can often be compensated for by the addition of plasma or serum to the standards (and a corresponding volume of buffer to the samples to compensate for the increase in volume) just before the separation. In an assay with a relatively long incubation time and a low dissociation rate, such as most assays performed with overnight incubation for the first reaction, the presence of small amounts of homologous antigen in this late added plasma will not appreciably alter the equilibrium between antigen and antibody.

5 ASSAY PERFORMANCE

The optimal approach for performance of a particular assay depends on many factors, such as available resources (equipment and personnel), the assay sensitivity and/or specificity required, whether or not there is a need for rapid results, whether the number of samples is small or large, and so forth. Of great importance also are the properties of the reagents, such as avidity of antibodies and stability of the ligand and whether it is liable to degradation or affected by serum constituents.

In the previous sections of the methodology, the individual constituents and steps of the assay have been discussed. The aim of this section is to consider how these individual building blocks should be put together to achieve an assay with optimal properties.

Radioligand assays may be performed according to one of the following different principles:

A. Competitive systems
   1. Equilibrium type
   2. Nonequilibrium type
      a. Parallel
      b. Sequential
B. Noncompetitive systems

The properties of an assay will vary according to the principle chosen. Each has its advantages and drawbacks for a particular application. It is therefore impossible to select one that is the best for all purposes; the selection must be made in relation to a particular situation and its needs.

The results of any assay are influenced by many factors, including concentration of reagents, temperature and length of incubation, serum effects, damage of reagents, blank problems, and the separation method used. Consid-

ering the influence of each of these factors individually facilitates the choice of the optimal principle as well as the best working conditions for a particular assay. Each of these aspects of assay performance is discussed in this chapter.

Finally, it should be remembered that there is no method, based on kit material or homemade reagents, that will produce good results if the laboratory work is not performed with meticulous care. It is particularly important that day-to-day assay procedures strictly adhere to the established methodology. Any deviations from established procedures or shortcuts in relation to variations in work load tend to cause instability of the methods. Tendencies toward unplanned individual initiatives and "improvements" in running methods by the technician performing the assays should usually be discouraged if not a part of the systematic development programs. As elaborated at length on pp. 283-284, it is necessary that the procedures be described in detail in a laboratory manual that is always kept in the laboratory and that is continuously updated as changes in the procedures occur.

REAGENTS
Amount of radioligand

Two considerations influence the choice of the amount of radioligand. One is related to problems associated with counting radioactivity and the other to effects of the concentration of ligand in the binding reaction with the receptor.

The higher the radioactivity of the sample to be counted, the more exact the measurement of the radioactivity. With ^{125}I-tagged radioligands as used in most of today's RIAs, high count rates are usually achieved. In counting only a few minutes, so many counts are registered that statistical variation becomes almost negligible (Table 5-1). Other sources of variation usually contribute much more to the overall assay variation. For example, even in a good assay the intraassay variation is rarely below 5%, of which the counting error is only a small part. Therefore, the time used for counting each tube should be considered in relation to other errors of the method. There is no reason to aim at very high precision in counting if other parts of the assay are associated with much higher imprecision. Since the counting capacity of the laboratory is often a major capacity-limiting factor, there is good reason to restrict the counting time. The count rate of most assays permits a sufficient number of decays to be registered within a couple of minutes. A counting time of 2 minutes permits the measurement of about 25 samples per hour. This implies that rather large assays may then be counted during a workday or overnight with a counter with an automatic sample changer. However, considerably improved utilization of available counter capacity can be achieved if the counting time is adapted to the demand for precision in the counting step. There are more or less sophisticated methods available for this purpose. The use of a combined preset count and preset time in the scaler (such as 4,000 counts and 2 minutes, respectively) may be timesaving. Counting time longer than 10 minutes is usually impractical.

It is obvious that it is not the total radioactivity of the assay tube but the amount in the phase to be counted, either bound or free radioactivity, that is the important determinant of how many counts should be collected. However, the radioactivity of these fractions is not constant but varies with the concentration of the unlabeled ligand. For example, in Fig. 1-1, *C*, when no cold ligand is present, the bound activity is 4,000 counts, whereas at a high ligand concentration, it is as low as 1,000 counts. This gives a counting error of 1.6% at low ligand levels and 3.2% at the high levels. In comparison with the other errors of the assay, a 1.6% counting error is probably quite acceptable, but the 3.2% counting error may make up a significant part of the total error (for example, at high concentrations of unlabeled ligand when the bound fraction is small and the standard curve often relatively flat). In noncompetitive assays (see Fig. 1-2), however, the bound activity is smallest at the low-concentration end of the scale. With less than 1,000 counts, the counting errors become larger than 3% and increase rapidly with decreasing counts. This implies that the confidence limits (95%) of within-assay variation may be relatively high (see Table 5-1).

Usually both the bound and free radioactivity will increase if a larger total activity is added to the system (even if the bound activity, expressed as a fraction of the total activity, decreases). For this reason, improved counting statistics may be achieved by increasing the total activity. However, there are certain limitations to this approach, mainly because of "misclassification errors" in the separation step, such as nonspecific binding of radioactivity to antibody precipitate or nonadsorption of free radioligand to the absorber in a charcoal separation method. Such misclassified activity is pro-

Table 5-1. Influence of counting statistics at different count rates*

Count rate from radioactive source (cpm)	Coefficient of variation at a counting time of (min)					
	0.2	0.5	1	2	10	20
100	31.6	20.0	14.1	10.0	4.5	3.1
500	10.9	6.9	4.9	3.5	1.5	1.1
1,000	7.4	4.6	3.3	2.3	1.0	0.7
2,000	5.1	3.2	2.3	1.6	0.7	0.5
4,000	3.6	2.2	1.6	1.1	0.5	0.4
8,000	2.5	1.6	1.1	0.8	0.4	0.2

*Background is assumed to be 100 cpm. The variation is calculated as the square root of the total number of counts collected and is expressed in percent of total counts from the radioactive source. Note that at low count rates the variation in background counts will influence the total variation significantly.

portional to the total radioactivity of the sample. In an assay with a high bound fraction this effect is not too important. For example, if the bound activity of an assay has a working range of 50% to 10%, a nonspecific binding of less than 4% will influence the result only at the highest concentration of unlabeled ligand (at the lower end of the standard curve). However, with a proportionally higher total activity, where the working assay range of bound activity covers only 15% to 5% of the total activity, the results may be influenced by a nonspecific binding (or blank) of 4%. Such misclassification errors limit the amount of radioactivity that can be added to the system. Otherwise, very high activities could be added as a means of amplifying the sensitivity of the system. In certain assays, particularly with solid phase coupled receptors, the optimal working range utilizes relatively small fractions of the total activity. It is then important that nonspecific binding be low and have a small variation.

The other effect of the amount of radioligand is related to the amount of ligand that it adds to the system. This effect is closely interrelated with the amount of receptor present and influences the sensitivity of the assay. In competitive assays the receptors should already be close to saturation when only the radioligand (no unlabeled ligand) is present. Otherwise, if unoccupied receptor sites remain, any unlabeled ligand added will bind to the empty sites without inhibiting the binding between radioligand and receptor. If the avidity of the receptor (association constant) is very high, the best sensitivity and counting conditions are achieved when the binding sites are just saturated (see Fig. 1-1), that is, when the amount of radioligand corresponds to the binding capacity of the receptor. Any further increase in the amount of radioactivity in this system would only contribute to increased nonspecific binding without adding to the sensitivity. However, most antisera have a lower avidity than in this ideal case. Then, it has been found both empirically and with computer models that the highest sensitivity is achieved when the amount of radioligand markedly exceeds the binding capacity of the receptor at the actual concentration of ligand. Usually, the highest sensitivity occurs when there are binding sites available for no more

than 50% of the radioligand, that is, when less than 50% of the added radioactivity is bound when no unlabeled ligand is added. (Compare discussion on binding kinetics, p. 14.) In some assays the highest sensitivity has been found by such an excess of radioligand that the working range of the assay only covers a bound activity of 15% to 5% of the total activity. Because of nonspecific bound radioactivity or other types of misclassification errors, it is usually not possible to decrease the bound fraction below 15% of the total radioactivity. Since the potential sensitivity of an assay is influenced not only by the plain kinetics of the ligand-receptor binding but also by the many "errors" of the individual assay, it is impossible to have any precise rule regarding the concentration of radioligand that is valid in all assays. However, as a general rule, the amount of radioligand should be as large as possible.

Amount of receptor (antiserum concentration)

As discussed above, optimal conditions for competitive assays usually are found when the receptor sites are almost saturated by the radioligand. This implies that the amount of receptor should be as small as possible and that antisera should be correspondingly diluted. Especially when receptor avidity is very high, antibodies may be diluted, so that the radioligand just saturates all binding sites, that is, almost all added radioactivity is bound when no cold ligand is added. Examples of assays that work in this way are vitamin B_{12}, thyroxine, and cortisol assays. In most instances, however, the receptor avidity does not permit the assay to work at perfect saturation, because the binding capacity cannot be saturated at the low concentrations in which the ligand occurs. As discussed in the previous section, the receptors have to be diluted to less than 50% binding to achieve the highest possible sensitivity. As a general rule (with certain limitations), higher dilutions of receptor (antibody) give higher sensitivity; lower dilutions give a wider working range with some loss of sensitivity. Another advantage of high dilutions is that when antisera are highly diluted, low-avidity antibodies are "diluted out," and their influence in the assay is decreased.

From the above it is evident that the concentrations of the receiver and ligand are very closely interrelated and that the concentration of one must be judged in relation to the concentration of the other. It must also be understood that it is usually the avidity of the receptor that is the primary limiting factor of assay sensitivity.

Another factor that is also influenced by the concentrations of receptor and ligand is the speed of the reaction. The higher the concentration of the reactants, the more rapidly the reaction approaches equilibrium. Since highest sensitivity usually is reached at low receptor concentrations, short incubation times tend to restrict assay sensitivity. Therefore, speed and sensitivity must be balanced against each other.

Theoretical models for estimating optimal concentrations of the active reactants of the assay have been reported. However, in most instances, it is as easy and effective to establish assay conditions experimentally as long as the principles are understood.

Noncompetitive systems

The effects of the concentrations of the reagents are different in assays based on noncompetitive principles. In a sandwich-type radiometric assay (see Fig. 1-2) all reagents could be added in excess, since the rate-limiting step of the binding should be only the amount of *un*labeled ligand to be assayed. Thus, from a theoretical standpoint, the quantities of the reagents should be much less critical in optimizing the properties of noncompetitive systems, because of the reagent excess conditions. In the two-site assay, the first antibody, coupled to the matrix (immunoadsorbent), can be used in any amount as long as its binding sites are well in excess of the number of antigens added. The second (labeled) set of antibodies added should also be in excess of the amount of antigen remaining bound to the immunosorbent, since the unbound ^{125}I-labeled antibody will be washed off and will not influence counting. Particularly in assays for very large proteins, such as viruses, where there are many antigenic combining sites on each antigen molecule, a large excess of ^{125}I-labeled antibody would increase the sensitivity of the assay. However, as in the competitive types of assays, the nonspecific ad-

sorption of radioactivity to the solid matrix will affect the blank level count and therefore will restrict the use of unlimited amounts of radioligand. Since the blank count is proportional to the total amount of radioactivity, added limitations on the amount of ^{125}I-labeled antibody are imposed. Such blank levels can be reduced to an extent by washing the immunosorbent after completing the reactions, but this will not remove all nonspecifically bound radioactivity and may cause a dissociation of bound antigen or ^{125}I-labeled antibody. For this reason the potential sensitivity of this assay depends not only on the overall avidity of the antibodies but, as in nonequilibrium types of competitive assays, to a great extent on the dissociation rate.

In regard to the amounts of reagents used in the so-called immunoradiometric type of noncompetitive system, the same theoretical conditions occur, in that the only rate-limiting factor is the amount of antigen present, and unbound labeled antibody is removed before counting. However, the amount of the specific antibody that can be added depends on the efficiency of the immunoabsorbent in removing unreacted labeled antibody after completing the binding reactions. The complex between antigen and labeled antibody remaining in the supernatant cannot be effectively washed in the same way as in the two-site assay. The amount of labeled antibody may influence the occurrence of ^{125}I-labeled antibodies with only one combining site occupied by the antigen and the other remaining unoccupied. This antibody may still be able to bind to the immunoadsorbent and therefore cause a misclassification error that will reduce the sensitivity of the assay. Also, the probability of obtaining half-saturated antibodies will increase with increasing amounts of ^{125}I-labeled antibody. However, this phenomenon does not appear to be of any practical consequence, since it occurs only to a slight extent. It has been suggested that such negative influences be avoided by utilizing univalent antibody in the form of ^{125}I-labeled Fab IgG fragments.

Solvents and diluents

The rates of antigen-antibody reactions have a rather broad pH maximum around pH 7.0. The primary reaction is little affected by the ions used in most common buffer systems. Generally, assays can be performed with any standard buffer, such as phosphate, borate, barbital (Veronal), glycine, or bicarbonate. The addition of 0.15 M (0.9%) NaCl to make them "physiologic" in osmolarity does not seem necessary in most systems.

It is important to include an agent that prevents the adsorption of reagents to the walls of tubes, pipettes, and so forth, in all diluents and solvents. Most solid materials have the ability to absorb constituents of solution to their surfaces. The extent of this adsorption varies with different materials. At the extremely low concentrations of active reagents used for radioligand assays, even low-absorbing surfaces tend to remove significant fractions of the reagents from the solution. Certain compounds are excessively "sticky" in this sense. For example, drawing a diluted solution of ACTH that does not contain any adsorption-preventing material in and out of a micropipette may cause a major loss of the ACTH, some of which remains on the inside walls of the pipette. The addition of proteins to the solution in concentrations that are much higher than those of the active reagents will reduce the adsorption markedly, probably by covering the surface with a nonadhesive film. Human or bovine serum albumin in a concentration of 0.1% to 0.5% is most commonly used for this purpose. Albumin binds some active molecules and may serve as a transporting protein in plasma. For this reason albumin should be avoided in some assays. In steroid assays, for example, porcine gelatin is a suitable replacement. The addition of proteins to the diluents also serves to decrease the radiolytic denaturation of the radioactive proteins.

The choice of solvent for standards presents a particularly important problem. The accuracy of radioligand assays relies on comparisons of the unknown sample with the standards, which contain a predetermined amount of the material to be measured. The validity for such comparisons presumes that samples and standards are identical except in regard to the variation in concentration of the ligand. This implies that standards should be contained in a fluid that either is identical to that of the unknown sample or does not influence the binding reaction dif-

ferently. As a rule that binding reaction is influenced by the reaction milieu, although the influence varies from assay to assay. The influence not only affects the binding reaction as such, but also other assay steps, such as the separation of bound and free ligand. For this reason, each individual assay must be investigated to determine the extent to which dissimilarities between standard and sample solvents will influence the results. It is difficult to establish any general rules, since solvent effects can vary not only between different assays but also between individual antisera against the same antigen. In our experience, the primary binding reaction in assays for protein hormones, such as growth hormone and gonadotropins, is influenced relatively little by the solvent. In assays for small peptides, such as thyroid hormones and steroids, the binding is greatly influenced by the presence of plasma or serum in the reaction mixture. This influence is only partly related to the existence of specific binding proteins for these substances.

When the results are affected by the type of solvent used, it is necessary that the standards be dissolved in something that is as similar to serum as possible. For this purpose, it is sometimes possible to find human serum that, for biologic reasons, does not contain the substance to be assayed and therefore can be used as solvent for standards. An example of such material is serum from nonpregnant humans in assays for hormones produced exclusively in the human placenta. Similarly, accurate serum solvents may be collected from patients who, for some reason, are known not to produce a particular hormone, for example, from hypophysectomized patients for assays of pituitary hormones and, for determination of thyroid hormones, serum from patients who have undergone complete thyroidectomies. Another approach, where the degree of identity between sample and standard solvent is lower, involves the use of serum from different species as standard solvents. This may be particularly useful for protein hormones with high species specificity. However, the differences in other constituents of serum from a different species are frequently so great that they will influence the binding reaction (for example, differences in various complement components). A solvent that is even more unlike plasma but sometimes quite adequate is serum albumin. Addition of 7 g/100 ml of HSA gives a diluent that essentially compensates for the difference in protein concentration.

In cases where it is necessary to have standards in serum milieu, a common method is to produce a "hormone free" serum. Since most free ligands absorb quite well to activated charcoal, it has been common to absorb plasma with an excess of active charcoal as described in Appendix 36. The disadvantage of this approach is that charcoal treatment will also remove many other substances, which, although not measured in the assay, may affect the binding reaction and the results of the assay. Despite this objection, the hormone-free serum so produced is an appropriate standard solvent in most assays. The most valid solvent for standards, as indicated above, is that which is devoid of the substance to be assayed but in all other respects similar to the sample. It is possible to come relatively close to this goal by treating plasma with an immunosorbent, that is, an antibody to the substance in question, coupled to a solid phase. When it is added in excess to the plasma, it will remove all the ligand but essentially no other material. However, it is important that the immunosorbent be stable, so that no antibody is released during this procedure.

Not infrequently, there are significant differences between samples from different individuals in terms of their influence on the primary binding reaction (but for that caused by differences in ligand concentration), the degree of nonspecific binding, or the degree of denaturation during incubation. Such effects may in particular influence the results when one is working close to the limit of sensitivity of an assay.

Because of these potential differences between samples and standards, the absolute levels of any substance cannot be accurately measured with confidence until the nonspecific influence of the sample is evaluated. Testing recovery and parallel slopes give certain information but will not completely reveal the degree of such influences. The only adequate way to attack this problem is to find an appropriate "ligand free" serum that is similar to the sample to the degree required for the specific situation. In addition, the possible interference of binders of other types should also be considered (for example, transporting proteins, enzyme inhibitors, and endogenous antibodies).

For some biologic fluid samples, variation in factors such as pH and salt concentration may significantly affect the assay. Plasma samples vary little in this regard, but urine shows such variation in pH, salt concentration, and so forth, that it usually is necessary either to control these factors or to extract the material to be assayed from the urine samples. Such nonspecific influences can also be minimized if the material to be assayed is in such high concentration that urine can be highly diluted with buffer (and carrier protein).

Variation in solvent composition poses a special problem in assays with a tritium-labeled radioligand, since liquid scintillation counting efficiency may be influenced by variations in quenching effects.

INCUBATION CONDITIONS
Incubation temperature

Increased temperature will generally increase the rate of the reaction between antigen and antibody. These binding reactions are reversible; there are two events, association and dissociation, that are affected. The dissociation rate is often more temperature dependent than is the association rate. Since the avidity of the binding depends on the ratio between association and dissociation rates, this ratio is often increased at low temperatures, and thus the overall avidity increases. It has also been shown experimentally that the energy of the antigen-antibody binding increases at low temperatures. Accordingly, the highest avidity and therefore the highest potential sensitivity are achieved by incubation at low temperatures. When sensitivity is less important, it may be more convenient to use incubation at room temperature. It is also a frequent finding that not only the sensitivity but the reproducibility and precision of an assay are improved by extended incubation in the cold.

Other reactions that may affect the assay are

also influenced by temperature. Proteolysis and other adverse reactions occur at much faster rates at higher temperatures. Therefore, it is sometimes necessary to perform the assay at low temperatures to minimize these influences. Protein radioligands in particular are liable to degradation in the presence of serum ("incubation damage") at higher temperatures.

An overnight incubation at 4° C will usually bring the reaction relatively close to equilibrium. A further increase in binding may occur up to several days, but this is usually needed only for high-sensitivity methods. Shorter incubation times, down to less than an hour, have been obtained by incubation at room temperature or at 37° C, in particular with assays for small ligands of nonprotein type that are less liable to degradation. A technique used to increase speed without too much loss in sensitivity involves an initial incubation at high temperature, followed by a period at low temperature. The low temperature reduces the dissociation rate of the already bound ligand and thereby increases its affinity and the sensitivity of the assay.

In practical terms, the slow rate reactions at low temperature (4° C) have the advantage that timing is less critical in the various procedures. This is particularly important for long assay series. For short incubation times when the reaction does not come close to equilibrium, timing and identical handling of all tubes are much more critical.

Incubation time

The initial rate of the antigen-antibody reaction is rapid. Despite the high association rate, most RIAs approach equilibrium relatively slowly and may sometimes require quite extended incubation periods to achieve equilibrium. The reason for this slow reaction is not fully understood. The extended incubation slowly increases total binding over time, but more prominently there is a gradual shift of the binding from one with a relatively rapid dissociation rate to one with a very slow dissociation rate. This phenomenon has the effect of increasing the avidity of binding, which results in the increased sensitivity registered in some assays by such long incubation times. It is believed that this change depends on a transfer of

antigen from a rapidly equilibrated and dissociated order of binding sites to a second order of binding sites with a low dissociation rate. However, secondary changes in the binding may also occur, such as the formation of aggregates between several antigen-antibody complexes, that also alter the kinetics of the binding reaction.

For assays of analytes in relatively high concentration, such as human placental lactogen (hPL), thyroxine, cortisol, or digoxin, equilibrium is achieved relatively rapidly; thus incubation times on the order of a few hours will bring the binding to a plateau with little further change with time.

An increasing number of assays are performed as nonequilibrium assays. The shorter the incubation time, the more critical is the exactness of the timing of the various steps of the assay. Usually, this can be managed without much problem. However, one step that sometimes causes difficulties is centrifugation, used for separation of bound and free activity. For example, if the time lag between pipetting the antibodies (that start the reaction) into the first and the last tube of an assay series is 15 minutes and the tubes are incubated for 60 minutes after pipetting into the last tube, the incubation time will be 75 minutes for the first tube. To keep the time of incubation constant, the next step in the assay should maintain the same time lag as the pipetting. This may not be readily achieved with certain procedures such as centrifugation, but a workable compromise may be to start the centrifugation of the first, middle, and last third of the tubes at 5-minute intervals. Otherwise, the characteristics of most nonequilibrium assays do not differ from those of the equilibrium type, provided that the timing of the reactions is appropriately controlled.

In most competitive systems the reagents are added at the same time, to permit the labeled and unlabeled material to react with the binder on equal terms. However, it may be advantageous in certain situations to permit the binder to react with the unlabeled ligand in a preincubation step, followed by addition of the radioligand. This type of assay condition is called "sequential" incubation. If the dissociation rate is not too fast, most of the ligand that has

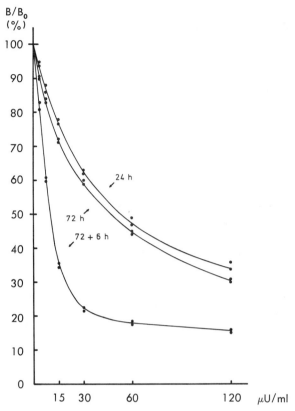

Fig. 5-1. Comparisons of standard curve of (close to) equilibrium and nonequilibrium types of assays, here exemplified by a TSH assay. The increase of incubation time from 24 to 72 hours in the equilibrium system causes a minimal increase in sensitivity (two upper curves). In the nonequilibrium assay, standard TSH and TSH antisera are preincubated for 72 hours before addition of ^{125}I-labeled TSH, after which incubation is continued for 6 hours. This gives a marked improvement in sensitivity.

bound in the first step will remain bound even after addition of the radioligand and will not completely equilibrate with the radioligand in the second step of incubation. In this way, such a procedure may increase the sensitivity considerably (Fig. 5-1). The obvious reason for this is that when the radioligand is added, binding sites are already occupied in proportion to the amount of ligand initially present. In tubes containing little or no ligand, more sites for binding the radioligand will be available than in tubes containing larger amounts of ligand from the beginning.

A sequential type of incubation may also be used to reduce the time during which the radioligand is incubated together with plasma. This may be particularly valuable for assays where the radioligand is sensitive to degradation effects from serum or plasma constituents.

Noncompetitive assays are affected by temperature and incubation time in a manner similar to competitive assays. However, the kinetics of the antigen-antibody reactions may be markedly influenced by the drastic change in the reaction conditions that occurs when the free ligand is washed off (as in the two-site, sandwich-type assays). This effect is less marked if the reaction between antigen and antibody is near completion, since at that time there is often a very slow dissociation rate. Accordingly, prolonged incubation time increases sensitivity in noncompetitive assays also. When sensitivity is not the most essential assay feature, assays may be performed with a shorter incubation. Not only sensitivity but specificity may be improved by extended incubation, probably because the binding shifts to antibodies of higher avidity and specificity.

The incubation times of assays used in clinical practice are often influenced more by the need for urgent results than for optimal sensitivity or precision. The assays used for decision making in acute medicine, such as digoxin, estriol, or drug assays, must be performed within a few hours if the results are to be clinically useful. The incubation time is then frequently restricted to 1 or 2 hours. In some instances, incubation times of even less than an hour may suffice. In nonacute clinical settings it is often practical to perform the assay with overnight incubation. With the exception of small sample number assay series, it may be difficult to complete all procedures, ranging from collecting the patient's sample to delivery of the final results, within the 8-hour workday, even if the incubation time spans only a few hours. We have found it more convenient in such assays to have sufficient time available on day 1 for collecting samples and transporting them to the laboratory during the morning hours; the afternoon is used for making up the assay series. The separation step is performed the following morning after an overnight incubation. Counting is done during the late morning hours; calculation and delivery of results are made during the afternoon of day 2. If the counting facilities are in demand, we delay counting of nonurgent assays to the night after day 2 and thereby distribute the work load of the counters more evenly during the day and night.

COMMONLY ENCOUNTERED ASSAY PROBLEMS
Degradation of ligand

The active reagents used in radioligand assays vary in stability. In certain assays the ligand may be actively degraded by enzymes in the sample. Examples of such ligands are angiotensin II, bradykinin, and glucagon. In these cases enzyme inhibitors must be added at the time the blood sample is taken from the patient in order to prevent rapid degradation of the ligand. Trasylol, benzamidin, and ethanol are used as such inhibitors.

Degradation of radioligand

Degradation of the radioligand is recorded as a reduced immunoreactivity. The apparent effects of such degradation depend on the method used for separation of bound and free activity and how the degraded material behaves in the system. If the separation technique isolates and counts the bound fraction, there will be an apparent increase in the free fraction when radioligand degradation has occurred. If this degradation is of the same magnitude in all assay tubes and is not excessive, the actual calculated results may not be significantly affected. Frequently, however, if part of the radioligand has lost its immunoreactivity completely, it is likely that the remaining radioligand has been somewhat altered also. This will decrease the affinity of the radioligand for the binder and cause a decreased assay sensitivity.

When the degradation of the radioligand is marked, particularly if it occurs during the incubation period, the degree of damage to the radioligand is likely to vary between different tubes and in particular between tubes containing samples from different patients. The effect of this will be that in samples containing the same amount of analyte, the degraded fraction will vary and thus cause variation in the apparent free fraction. This in turn will be falsely interpreted as a variation in the amount of cold ligand.

In assays using a separation method that adsorbs free radioligand, such as coated charcoal, the effect of radioligand degradation on the results depends on whether the degradation is also associated with decreased adsorption. If this is the case, an apparent (false) increase in the bound fraction will be observed. Not infrequently, some of the degraded material may partially retain its adsorption, whereas the rest of it will lose it. In such cases the effect will be unpredictable.

For this reason, assays should include some check to ascertain that the radioligand retains the properties expected. The most obvious effects of radioligand degradation are usually a decreased slope of the standard curve and decreased precision of the assay. This latter effect shows also that the degree of degradation varies between sample tubes, with decreased reliability of the results, as discussed above.

The degradation of reagents is usually more rapid with higher concentrations of serum. Therefore, most assays work with a serum concentration less than 10% to 20%. Degradation is also highly temperature dependent. Stability may increase considerably if the incubation is performed at 4° C instead of at room temperature. At 37° C degradation may be quite pronounced even with material that is relatively stable at room temperature. Sequential incubation, as mentioned in the previous section, is one way to reduce the time that the radioligand is in contact with serum. The sandwich type of noncompetitive assay has a significant advantage in this sense, since, following the first incubation of serum with the first set of receptors, all serum components except those bound to the antibodies are washed away; thus the radioligand will not be in contact with the serum.

Nonspecific binding

At the low concentrations of reagents used in radioligand assays, there is a tendency for reagents to adsorb to any kind of solid material. The degree of adsorption varies between different adsorbers as well as between different reagents. Antibodies, for example, have a relatively small tendency to adsorb, which is utilized in methods such as coated charcoal for separation of bound and free activity. The term nonspecific binding usually denotes the occurrence of adsorption of free radioligand to antibody precipitate or solid phase antibody. This has been called misclassification error in the separation of bound and free activity. This effect occurs irrespective of whether the solid phase is produced before the assay as solid phase coupled antibodies or precipitated in the assay (for example, by double antibodies or other precipitation methods). Similarly, there may be some adsorption of antibody-bound activity in separation methods such as coated charcoal adsorption. The nonspecific adsorption also varies with protein coating or other types of coats used in the assay, whether caused by intentional coating of charcoal or simply by the presence of serum albumin or gelatin in the diluents. Accordingly, the cutoff point between bound and free activity is influenced by many factors. Usually, the larger the amount of insoluble material in the assay, the larger the degree of nonspecific adsorption.

The nonspecific adsorption is the main reason for the blank levels, that is, the binding registered either when there is no specific receptor added to the assay or when all binding sites are occupied by the addition of a large excess of cold ligand. The nonspecific binding should be checked by some means in all assays. In some systems (see example in Appendixes 38 and 39), this is easy to perform by not adding any antiserum to the tube. In other assays, particularly those with solid phase coupled antibodies, this technique does not give any true blank values, since omission of antibody also implies omission of the solid phase. In such systems the best estimation of the blank values occurs after the addition of a large excess of cold ligand. The nonspecific adsorption is often quite small, a few percent of the total radioactivity added in systems such as double antibody or solid phase antibody types. When the precipitant becomes heavy, as in ethanol or ammonium sulfate precipitation techniques, the nonspecific activity may increase considerably and reach more than 10% of the total radioactivity. At this point any variation in the blank

adsorption will cause a considerable difference in the assay.

A slightly different type of nonspecific binding occurs by adsorption to the walls of the test tubes. This is usually a relatively small problem that is avoided by adding materials such as serum albumin to the diluents. However, steroids show a high degree of adsorption to plastic material, greater than to glass. In this case the adsorption may be so high that the tube walls work as a competing binder. For this reason it may be necessary to perform these assays in glass tubes instead of less expensive and more practical plastic tubes. Glass tubes have the additional disadvantage of not infrequently showing considerable variation in thickness of the glass. The low energy of ^{125}I adsorbs to a significant degree in glass, and for this reason glass tubes may contribute to the counting error in the assay. Therefore, in steroid assays counting may be more appropriate if it is done on an aliquot of the supernatant pipetted into a plastic tube, rather than on the charcoal remaining in the glass tubes.

In certain assays the blank values caused by nonspecific adsorption may be so high that they induce considerable variation in the results. If there is a significant variation between individual serum samples in nonspecific adsorption it may be compensated for by correcting every individual serum sample for its nonspecific adsorption. As a general rule, it is better if such corrections can be avoided, since it is difficult to properly make such corrections. This is because the nonspecific adsorption in a blank tube without added antibody is probably not completely representative of the nonspecific adsorption in the plasma sample with antibodies included, since the binding to the antibody changes (usually reduces) the nonspecific binding. Usually it is better to try to make standards and patient samples as similar to each other as possible. This means that the nonspecific binding is the same in standards and samples, which reduces the need for any correction.

Competing binders

Radioligand assays work on the assumption that the added receptor is the only binder present in the assay. Many biologically active materials circulate in plasma bound to transporting proteins that bind both specifically and with high avidity. These proteins may also be present in such high concentrations that their binding capacity greatly exceeds that of the antibodies in an immunoassay. Obviously, a binder in addition to the antibodies in an RIA will completely alter the kinetics of binding. In addition to these specific binders, there is a group of less specific binders among the plasma proteins that have very large binding capacities. Albumin binds many hormones and other biologic substances. The enzyme inhibitors α_2-macroglobulin and α_1-antitrypsin may bind enzymes and coagulation factors.

There are several different ways to avoid the problem of binding proteins. They can be denatured, either by means of proteolytic enzymes or by heating at low pH if the substance to be assayed can resist such treatment. The binding capacity of the protein may be saturated with some analog to the substance to be assayed that is different enough not to cross-react with the antibodies. It is possible to interfere with the binding in a more nonspecific way, and, finally, it is possible to separate the binder from the material to be assayed by extraction from serum. Examples of ways to neutralize the effect of endogenous transporting proteins in plasma are given in Boxes 8-2 and 8-3.

Another group of highly specific binders that will compete in the system are endogenous antibodies produced in response to therapy with exogenous proteins, such as insulin, growth hormone (GH), or TSH. Endogenous antibodies will make it impossible to perform a direct assay in the way in which insulin, GH, or TSH is usually assayed. There are methods for the extraction of insulin from the insulin-binding antibodies that occur in most insulin-treated diabetic patients. The results of the assays of these hormones after extraction from the antibodies are difficult to interpret, since we know too little about the biologic activity of hormones bound to endogenous antibodies and the kinetics of their binding in vivo to be able to draw any accurate conclusions on the biologic importance of a certain concentration of hormone measured in the presence of antibodies. Therefore, it is necessary to ascertain whether or not

samples assayed for insulin contain endogenous insulin antibodies. The effect of endogenous antibodies on the assay results depends mainly on which type of separation step is used. In an insulin assay with ethanol precipitation of antibodies, both the reagent antibodies and endogenous antibodies will be precipitated. Accordingly, the bound fraction will increase, causing the estimated insulin values to be falsely low. If the separation is performed instead with a double-antibody assay, for example, with guinea pig insulin antibodies as the first antibody and goat antisera to guinea pig immunoglobulins as the second antibody, the goat antiserum will recognize and precipitate only the guinea pig immunoglobulins and not the human immunoglobulins. Accordingly, radioactive insulin bound to the endogenous (human) antibodies will be classified as not bound to antibodies. Such an increase in apparent free insulin would falsely be interpreted as an increased concentration of insulin in the sample. This false value could be very high and even be misinterpreted as being caused by an insulin-producing tumor rather than merely as an effect of insulin antibodies developed during prior insulin therapy.

The presence of insulin antibodies may not be suspected if the insulin treatment occurred several years earlier, for example, as part of treatment for a psychiatric disorder. Since insulin antibodies are the most common type of endogenous antibodies that interfere in RIAs, we regularly include blanks without added antibodies, in which the antibodies are precipitated by means of ethanol. The occurrence of endogenous antibodies then immediately appears as an increased blank level.

Separation method artifacts

The choice of separation method may also affect the binding reaction between receptor, ligand, and radioligand, or at least how this reaction is recorded after the performance of the separation. Certain separation techniques directly affect the primary reaction between ligand and receptor.

Certain separation methods tend to rip the ligand from its binding to the receptor. Since the binding reactions are reversible, any method that removes the free ligand from the solution will tend to cause dissociation of bound material. This is the case with coated charcoal and similar adsorption methods. When all free ligand has been removed from solution, the binding reaction will tend to be reversed, with an increased dissociation, since there is no longer any free ligand available for reassociation. This is one reason that such separation methods usually are not stable with time. The longer the incubate is left in contact with the charcoal, the greater the tendency of the antigen-antibody complex to dissociate and the greater the increase in the free fraction.

Precipitation of antibodies with ethanol has a marked tendency to dissociate the binding if the free ligand is readily soluble in ethanol, such as in insulin assays.

Conventional double-antibody separation is regarded as a method with relatively little effect on the binding reaction. This method does not change the concentration of free ligand in the solution, and the receptor sites are still largely available for the primary reaction even after precipitation with the primary reaction. This property of double-antibody precipitation makes it a valuable basic separation technique for developing new assays.

Solid phase coupled antibodies are maintained in an insoluble form from the beginning of the assay, and the concentration of the free ligand is not influenced by the separation if the solid phase is not washed. Extensive washing may dissociate the binding; however, solid phase coupled antibodies have been described as having markedly reduced dissociation rates. Still, knowledge of the behavior of insoluble antibodies is relatively limited, but it is obvious that coupling of antibodies to solid matrices may alter the binding characteristics. Binding capacity may also be lost during coupling, and it is characteristic that many solid phase assays work with relatively small fractions of bound activity.

Preprecipitated antibodies with a second antibody system have been successfully applied to some assays, but in our experience it has been difficult to reproduce such results with antigen other than insulin. The reason may be that the binding sites of the antibodies are partly covered or, for other steric reasons, less available in the antigen-antibody complexes of the precipitate.

PRACTICAL ASPECTS OF PERFORMANCE

Many of the practical details necessary for the successful performance of assays (minor essentials) are usually not covered in the scientific literature. This is probably not because scientists regard them as trivial but rather as unscientific, since these problems are usually approached from a practical rather than a scientific viewpoint. Many of these details are never worked out in a manner that warrants publication, so despite the ever-increasing flow of scientific papers on RIA, practical details of performance are usually spread only by word of mouth.

Preparation for assay

In previous sections, the production and testing of reagents have been covered. The results of any assay, particularly in the routine laboratory, are also highly dependent on the appropriate performance of the immediate preparatory work for the assay. It may not be obvious in all situations that this part of the work must be done with the same care as the assay itself. Accordingly, the preparatory procedures should be performed in a reproducible way day after day. Appropriate time should be allotted for this purpose; the manuals should include this part of the work as well and should be followed as religiously as for the assay itself.

Reagents and samples should be stored well marked, in standardized concentrations and volumes to avoid mistakes such as erroneous dilution or a mix-up of vials. This is facilitated if they are kept in easily accessible places, since it is difficult to maintain reproducible and safe handling if the reagents cannot be found without searching through the entire freeze-storing facility of the laboratory. Reagents are preferably stored in the concentration in which they are to be used in the assay, or in a way such that they require only minimal treatment before being used.

Both for the sake of practical handling and of maintaining high reproducibility, the less treatment necessary at this stage, the better. If the reagent is stored at a higher concentration than used in the assay, we will permit the final dilution after thawing to be at most 100-fold and possible to perform in only one pipetting step. For example, in one assay we regularly use about 20 ml of a 1:100,000 dilution of the antiserum. This is stored in 1.1-ml portions at 1:5,000 dilution. The working solution is then prepared by diluting 1 ml of the 1:5,000 antiserum with 20 ml of the diluent solution. This gives 21 ml of 1:105,000 diluted antiserum. In this way, repeated thawing of the stock solution is avoided, and the degree of dilution required before assay is not excessive. In our experience, it is better to avoid dilution procedures that involve pipetting of volumes less than $100\mu l$ or one-step dilutions of more than 1:100 to 1:1,000.

Deep-frozen reagents are thawed carefully. Rapid thawing in warm water may cause undue elevation of the temperature of the reagents. The reagents are taken out of the freezer a couple of hours before the assay work starts. If thawing in the refrigerator is too slow, the reagents are kept at room temperature; direct sunlight and other heat sources in the area are avoided. The reagent is shaken gently now and then. When only a small lump of ice remains, the vial is transferred to the refrigerator.

It is important that both reagents and samples be equilibrated to the appropriate assay temperature before being combined. This also applies to the empty test tubes. In assays performed at $+4°$ C it may be necessary to keep tubes as well as reagents in an ice bath if the assay is very temperature dependent or the reagents are highly temperature sensitive. Often it is appropriate to keep only the reagents in an ice bath and not leave the rack with the tubes at room temperature for long periods. When temperature control is less critical, it may be sufficient to keep the reagents in the refrigerator until just before pipetting, provided the total reagent volume is large enough to maintain its temperature during each series of pipetting. For assays performed at higher temperatures, temperature equilibration is also important. Reagents normally stored in the refrigerator should be placed in the appropriate ambient temperature for a couple of hours before assay work is begun.

Before the actual analytical work is begun, a report of the procedure is written. This includes identification of the reagents used, the volumes, and the order of pipetting. Identification codes for patient samples, as well as notes on how tubes are numbered, are also included. The preparatory work also includes marking of tubes. The marking of individual tubes may seem tedious and a waste of time but is a worthwhile safety measure that decreases the risk of mix-up errors considerably. Only when the operation is highly organized or automated, for example, by maintaining the tubes in one set of racks through all procedures, should one omit marking individual tubes. In this case, the first tube of the assay series should be labeled so that it also permits identification of the assay.

An example of a procedural report currently used in this laboratory is shown in Appendix 38. Its format is the same as the computer printout of the assay results, so the printout is taped onto the report formula.

Organization of assays

An assay can be set up in several different ways, of which no single one is ideal in all respects. However, some models have certain advantages. The larger the assay and the heavier the work load, the more thought should be devoted to these aspects. Routine assays are built up from the following main components:

1. Standards
2. Controls
3. Samples

It may be convenient to have the standards and controls at the beginning of the assay. This permits an early check of assay qualities and also permits starting some calculations before all tubes have come out of the counter. However, if only one set of standards is used, these will be more representative of the whole assay if they are placed in the middle of the assay series.

The assay should not be so large that systematic errors or drifts occur within the series but small enough so that the time for pipetting throughout the series is no more than a small fraction of the total incubation time and procedures such as centrifugation can be performed simultaneously with all the tubes. Therefore, centrifuge capacity often becomes the size-limiting factor of the assay. The particular features and problems involved in nonequilibrium assays with short incubation periods are discussed on p. 65.

To ascertain the assay stability, the sample controls (pools) can be run twice in each assay, once at the beginning and again at the end of the assay.

The number of standards needed depends on the linearity of the standard curve. If completely linear within the working range (irrespective of whether the plot is linear in lin-log, log-log, logit-log, or any other type of linearization), it can be completely defined by only two points. However, most curves are not strictly linear, but in most assays, the standard curve can be sufficiently well defined by five to seven different concentrations of the standards. Even with linear curves it is a good quality control to make certain of the linearity by additional points on the standard curve. In assays based on commercial kit reagents, the cost of the reagents may impose certain limitations on the number of "nonproductive," tubes, such as standards and controls. When bulk reagents are used, whether homemade or purchased, the reagent cost often contributes relatively little to the total cost.

Practical handling of the assay

The wet part of the assay performance essentially involves only three different types of procedures: addition of reagents (pipetting), mixing of reagents, and separation of bound and free activity.

The addition of the reagents should, like all other phases of the work, be carefully organized, since this will improve precision and reduce the risk of error. If this step is not fully automated, the assay is facilitated by having racks for the test tubes in which the replicates for each standard or sample are placed behind each other. If there is an extra row of places in the rack, in front of the other tubes, the tubes containing the samples can be conveniently located in front of the line of replicate test tubes into which the sample aliquots are to be pipetted, which decreases the risk of pipetting into the wrong tube.

The main type of pipetting error is skipping tubes or adding reagents twice into the same tube. This can be prevented by moving a cap along the tubes as an indicator of the last tube into which the reagent was added. We have found it even easier to tilt the tubes over from right-tilted to left-tilted position with the pipette as it goes down into the tube. This is possible provided the holes of the rack are slightly wider than the tubes, permitting them to lean to either side. Tubes into which a certain reagent should not be added are capped before the addition of this reagent is begun. For example, in blank controls where no antiserum is added, these tubes are covered when antiserum is pipetted.

It is also important that the pipetting be performed in quiet surroundings that permit adequate concentration. Technicians should be allowed to perform each series of pipetting without interruption, since interruptions are liable to cause errors despite the above-mentioned precautions.

Following the addition of the reagents, the contents of the reaction mixture are mixed carefully. This is usually performed with a vortex-type mixer, which rapidly swings the bottom part of the tube while the upper part of the tube is held fast by the technician. Each tube is mixed for a few seconds. This type of mixing may be performed without capping the tube if the content of the tube is relatively small in relation to total tube volume. If the tubes are capped, mixing may also be performed by inverting the tube a few times. This procedure can also be performed with many tubes simultaneously if they are placed in a rack to which they are secured with a cover. One alternative is to shake the whole rack horizontally for a somewhat longer period. We have adhered to vortex-type mixing of individual tubes as a very reliable procedure.

In systems with all reagents in soluble form there seems to be no need for further mixing during the incubation, since diffusion of the reagents will maintain a sufficient mix of the reagents within the incubate. With insoluble phase assays, the insoluble reagent is usually distributed in a small part of the incubates, and diffusion alone will not produce a sufficient contact between the soluble and insoluble reagents. Therefore, it may be necessary to mix the reagents physically, either continuously or at intervals during the incubation.

One of the practical details that involves significant work in a large-scale operation is the question of whether the tubes should be individually capped during the incubations. In small series, it certainly is wise to cap the tubes. Otherwise, the evaporation from the tubes may vary (for example, in tubes at the end or in the center of a rack). To avoid such effects when individual capping is impractical, it is possible to cover a whole rack with a lid that will close the tubes efficiently if the tubes are kept in a precise upright position in the rack. We have found it sufficient to put the rack into a plastic bag that fits the rack well.

The incubation is usually performed at room temperature or in the cold. It should be realized that the temperature is not stable in a refrigerator that is opened many times during a day. Therefore, it may be important to have separate refrigerators for storage of reagents and for incubation. All tubes belonging to one assay should be incubated in the same spot within the refrigerator, so that they are influenced by any fluctuations in temperature in an identical way.

One of the most critical parts of most assays is the physical separation of the bound and free phases. The separation procedure may contribute significantly to the imprecision of the assay if not appropriately done.

Solid phase methods with the antibodies bound to macro-size material, such as discs, strips, or the inside of the test tube, are characterized by their easy handling. Separation requires rinsing in water or buffer with relatively limited need for precise handling. Solid phase systems with small particles require more careful handling. This is true for solid phase coupled antibodies with powder-type matrixes, such as Sephadex or cellulose, antibodies precipitated by a double antibody or by other immunoglobulin-precipitating reagents, or any other type of powder separator, such as charcoal or talc. If the counting is performed on an aliquot of the supernatant, this must be very precisely pipetted from the reaction tube. However, this technique is slow and has the drawback that if the supernatant is not to be contaminated with any part of the precipitate, the

fraction removed can be only about two thirds to three fourths of the total supernatant. This causes loss of count and impaired counting statistics.

Decanting the supernatant and counting the precipitate is a much simpler procedure but involves the potential error of either pouring part of the precipitate out of the tube or leaving a varying amount of the supernatant in the tube. The smaller the volume of the supernatant, the larger the risk. The possibility of error can be reduced by diluting the supernatant just before centrifugation of the sample. As shown in the example given on the TSH method, we add 1 ml of buffer to each tube just before spinning. This reduction of the concentration of radioactivity in the supernatant also reduces the background count in the samples. This can be reduced further if the precipitate is washed repeatedly (addition of buffer after first decanting, recentrifugation, and removal of the supernatant). Instead of decanting the supernatant, it may be removed by means of a suction pump, such as an ordinary water tap vacuum pump. Devices are available for removing the supernatant from multiple tubes simultaneously, but in this case the total supernatant cannot be removed, because of the risk of also removing part of the precipitate; thus only a fraction of the supernatant is removed. Then more diluent is added, and one or more centrifugations and washings are done to remove another fraction of the remaining radioactivity in the supernatant. In our experience, repeated washing is not necessary with most precipitates, since they remain conveniently at the bottom of the tube. Decanting can be performed reproducibly enough that the increased background caused by the small amount of supernatant remaining is so similar in all test tubes that its complete removal does not improve either sensitivity or precision. However, in assays working with low bound fractions, as in some of the solid phase assays, it is necessary to remove the supernatant as completely as possible, since even small variation in baseline count may influence the results significantly.

Certain racks that hold the tubes firmly permit the removal of the supernatant from the whole rack in one operation. In this case, one must be very careful to avoid contamination of the rack. Furthermore, this technique is difficult to perform on precipitates that are "loose" and have a tendency to slide out of the tube.

INITIAL CONSIDERATIONS WHEN STARTING RADIOLIGAND ASSAY WORK OR A NEW RADIOIMMUNOASSAY

Radioligand assays are simple in principle. However, from the standpoint of actually developing an assay, every individual step of the assay may be associated with problems, both in regard to the reagents used in the assay and to the performance of the assay. We have seen many cases where a laboratory without previous experience in this field, about to begin working with such assays, could have saved much effort and cost by working in association with a laboratory already experienced in running the assay in question. Reagent problems may largely be avoided by using reagents produced by another laboratory (commercial or noncommercial) that has reliable, high-quality reagents. The explosive development of the RIA kit market has shown that this is the route chosen by many laboratories. However, there is no absolute guarantee that everything will work as suggested by the manufacturer's brochure.

Any new immunoassay being developed involves so many steps that can fail that it is wise to reduce the number of unknown factors insofar as possible initially. The problems may be insurmountable when one starts with poorly standardized antigen, an antiserum with unknown qualities, a labeled antigen of unknown antigenic activity after labeling; or a system for separating antibody-bound activity from unbound activity that may or may not work with this particular antigen. It is best to start a new assay by using as many steps as possible from a system with known qualities where behavior can be predicted. In this way "homemade" reagents or modifications may be tested step by step. Some schematic rules for the selection of assay conditions as discussed in this chapter follow.

SCHEMATIC SUGGESTIONS FOR SELECTING CONDITIONS FOR A NEW ASSAY (COMPETITIVE TYPE)
Amount of radioligand

Roughly, the amount of radioligand should be as large as possible. There are certain limiting factors. The amount must be related to the smallest amount of ligand to be assayed; with a good antiserum and an otherwise good assay, radioligand concentration can be up to about 10 times the smallest amount of ligand to be measured (but preferably somewhat less) and about equal to the amount of ligand measured in the middle part of the assay working range.

The amount must also be related to statistical requirements for counting; if the "rule" above gives more counts than needed for good statistics and convenient counting time, the radioligand concentration may be reduced, since this may permit reduction of antibody concentration and thereby give an increased sensitivity.

Amount of antibody

Roughly, antiserum concentration should be as low as possible. It is diluted so that the binding capacity is exceeded by the actual amount of radioligand used. In most instances approximately 50% of the radioligand is bound when no unlabeled ligand is added. When a wide working range is more important than high sensitivity, it may be useful to increase the bound fraction. If the sensitivity is of major importance and the avidity of the antiserum is critical, a lower bound fraction may help.

Time and temperature

Begin with overnight incubation at $+4°$ C with simultaneous addition of all reagents. Demand for higher sensitivity may be met with longer incubation or delayed addition of radioligand. Improved precision may also follow extended incubation. Then modify these conditions to meet other demands, such as turnover time, and so forth.

Separation method

Begin with a double-antibody system or other standard in-house system well characterized in other assays. A double-antibody step working well in other circumstances can be expected to behave well here, too. Then change to the separation method suited to actual assay requirements. A charcoal adsorption method may also serve well for initial trials if this method is in good control in the laboratory.

6 DATA PRESENTATION AND QUALITY CONTROL

The usual method for presenting the data from a radioligand assay is as a *dose-response curve,* in which a response variable, such as change in count rate, is plotted (on the y-axis) against the total ligand (x-axis) present in a series of standard tubes (see Fig. 1-1, *C*). In the practice of radioligand assay, a variety of methods of plotting the data have been developed, with different ways of expressing both the response variable (y-axis) and the dose variable (x-axis). Some examples of common response variables are ratio of bound activity to free radioactivity (B/F), ratio of free activity to bound activity (F/B or $R_{f/b}$), ratio of bound activity to total activity (B/T), ratio of bound activity to bound activity in the zero standard curve (B/B_0), logit y, and so forth. The dose variable, however, is usually plotted as the concentration of dose or the log concentration of dose, where "dose" is taken to mean the amount of the substance used as standard in the assay.

In this chapter we give examples and discuss the common methods of graphic presentation of dose-response curves. These variants have developed in part because of different mathematical formulations of the dose-response relationship, which we have included as background for those readers interested in the kinetics of the interaction.

MATHEMATICAL BASIS FOR DOSE-RESPONSE RELATIONSHIP

The mathematical basis of radioligand assay has been developed by several authors. Although each has taken a somewhat different approach and has arrived at slightly different conclusions, the differences are of detail. The fundamental assumptions are similar for all of these systems. Each author is concerned with the concepts of sensitivity and precision in RIAs; in particular, the following questions are asked: what is the best mathematical description of the most sensitive and precise RIA system, and what is the best description of the smallest detectable quantity for RIA and similar methods.

Basic assumptions

The basic underlying assumptions as expressed by Rodbard are as follows:
1. The ligand is present in homogeneous form and consists of only one chemical species.
2. The receptor (antibody or binding protein) is present in only one homogeneous chemical form.
3. Both ligand and receptor are univalent; that is, one molecule of ligand can react with one molecule of receptor, but no other combinations can occur.
4. No allosteric or cooperative effects are present, and the ligand and receptor react in a simple bimolecular interaction.
5. Ligand and radioligand behave identically with respect to binding to receptor.
6. Ligand and receptor react until equilibrium is reached.
7. Bound and free forms of radioligand can be completely separated without disrupting the equilibrium.

Formulation of Berson and Yalow
Mathematical formulation

The mathematical considerations for the first-order mass action law are applied to RIA as follows.

$$[Ag] + [Ab] \underset{k_{-1}}{\overset{k_1}{\rightleftharpoons}} [AgAb] \tag{1}$$

$$\quad\quad F \quad\quad\quad\quad B$$

K = association constant at equilibrium

$$\frac{k_1}{k_{-1}} = K$$

and is defined as

$$K = \frac{k_1}{k_{-1}} = \frac{[AgAb]}{[Ag][Ab]}$$

where

[Ag] = concentration of antigen
[Ab] = concentration of antibody
[AgAb] = amount of complex formed
[Ab⁰] = molar concentration of total antibody combining sites
[Ab⁰] = [Ab] + [AgAb]

It can be shown that

$$B/F = K([Ab^0] - B) \qquad (2)$$

where

B = amount of bound antigen
F = amount of free antigen

This description of the interaction of Ab and Ag follows the Scatchard solution of the formula and is linear. From this relationship it should be a simple matter to empirically determine K, the equilibrium constant.

Sensitivity

The ability to detect a hormone concentration depends on the relationship between K and [H], where [H] is the concentration of hormone.

$$B/F = b/(1 - b) = K([Ab^0] - b[H]) \qquad (2a)$$

where b = bound fraction of hormone

From this relationship, the concentration of receptor binding sites should be of the same order of magnitude as the concentration of hormone that we wish to measure if a significant change in B/F is to occur, with a change in the bound fraction of hormone.

This consideration determines one assay condition, namely, that the concentration of antibody should correspond to the concentration of hormone. This usually means a very dilute concentration of antibody.

A B/F ratio of about 1.0 is readily used for assay when no stable ligand is present in the assay system. At low concentration of hormone, [H] → 0, so now (2a) becomes $1 \leq K[Ab^0]$, when [Ab] ≈ [H]; then $K \geq 1/[H]$. By resubstitution in (2a), it can be shown that if K ≈ 1/[H] when we wish to measure a hormone concentration of [H], then B/F will decrease by 39%; if K is tenfold lower, then the B/F will decrease 5%. The greater the change in B/F for a given change in [H], the more sensitive the assay.

This determines another assay condition—that the sensitivity is limited by the K value, which characterizes the binding of antibody and ligand.

If one considers sensitivity as the slope of the dose-response curve, it is evident from (2a) that

$$db/d[H] = -\frac{Kb(1 - b)^2}{1 + K([H](1 - b)^2)} \qquad (3)$$

db/d[H] is the slope of the standard curve when b, the fraction of hormone bound, is plotted against [H]. This expression is at a maximum when [H] → 0. Thus, to find the conditions of maximal sensitivity, [H] → 0, and the derivative of the right-hand side of the equation is set to zero.

$$\frac{d}{db}[(-Kb)(1 - b^2)] = 0$$

$$-K(1 - b)^2 + 2Kb(1 - b) = 0$$

b = 1/3, b = 1, the solution to the binomial equation

Thus sensitivity is at a maximum at (the bound fraction) b = 1/3 and when b = 1, sensitivity is at a minimum. Sensitivity is maximal when

$$b = 1/3, [H] \to 0, \text{ and } db/d[H] = \frac{-4K}{27}$$

Precision

Optimal precision may be defined in relative terms, as related to a standard expression of variance about any particular assay value. An example cited by Berson and Yalow is as follows. A stock solution of hormone (1 mg/ml) is assayed with reference to a standard containing $1,000\mu U/mg$ of activity. The stock solution is measured at three different dilutions, for example, $1:10$, $1:10^3$, and $1:10^5$. The results are $100 \pm 0.5\mu U/mg$, $1 \pm 0.1\mu U/mg$, and $0.01 \pm 0.005\mu U/mg$ (mean ± standard error of the mean for several replicates). The relative uncertainties of these assays are 0.5%, 10%, and 50%. The relative uncertainty is least for the highest dilution of stock solution.

Thus the "precision" is greatest when the relative uncertainty is least.

This definition of uncertainty can be expressed in mathematical terms as follows. For a hormone concentration [H], the uncertainty is Δ[H], and the relative uncertainty is Δ[H]/[H].

The goal of optimizing precision in an assay is to make Δ[H]/[H] a minimum at a given change in response, Δb. As a condition that is "essentially" the same the authors look for conditions at which Δb, a change in the bound fraction, will be maximal for any value of Δ[H]/[H]. Mathematically, the authors express precision as db/(d[H]/[H]). Multiplying equation (3) by [H] gives

$$d\frac{db}{[H]/[H]} = \frac{-bK[H](1 - b)^2}{K[H](1 - b)^2 + 1} = \qquad (4)$$

$$-\frac{b}{1 + \cfrac{1}{K[H](1 - b)^2}}$$

For any given value of b, equation (4) increases with increasing [H] and is a maximum when $K[H](1 - b)^2 >> 1$.

Then,

$$1 + \frac{1}{K[H](1 - b)^2} \to 1$$

and equation (4) becomes

$$\frac{db}{d[H]/[H]} = -b$$

This situation of maximal precision is thus independent of K and in theory is the same for all antibodies. The main requirement is that the expression $K[H](1 - b)^2 >> 1$.

Thus, maximal precision is attained when both the concentrations of antibody and hormone are high.

However, it is only at maximal precision that [H] is independent of the K value. Under other conditions, for any desired degree of precision, the concentration [H] can be calculated in relation to K, as follows, from equation (4). If a precision of 99% of the optimal is desired, then $1/K[H](1 - b)^2 \le 0.01$ and the following equations hold.

$$[H] \ge 100/K(1 - b)^2 \text{ or } [H](1 - b)^2 \ge 100/K$$

This shows that the higher the K-value, the lower the concentration of hormone required to reach a given level of precision.

EXPERIMENTAL ERRORS. Throughout these derivations, it has been assumed that experimental error is random and not a function of the experimental condition. Thus, at any given level of statistical confidence, it is the slope of the dose-response curve and the experimental errors that determine sensitivity. This is illustrated by an example in which b, the bound fraction, can be determined to within 0.02 units over the range of b = 0.05 to b = 1.0. Over a particular range of hormone concentration, 10^{-10} M > 0, a linear relationship is observed ($b = 1 - 0.8 \times 10^{10}[H]$); over this range $\Delta b = 0.8 \times 10^{10} \Delta[H]$, so that when $\Delta[H] = 2.5 \times 10^{-12}$ mol/liter, $\Delta b = 0.02$. This could be considered the detection limit but only under these particular experimental conditions. *Thus the detection limit is in part dependent on the experimental errors of the procedure.*

LIMITATIONS TO THEORETICAL CONSIDERATIONS. Experimental data in general do not fit a linear relationship as expressed in equation (2a). This is the result of a population of antibodies that is heterogeneous with respect to K. This heterogeneity makes it difficult in practice to determine an absolute K. However, as discussed in Chapter 2 (p. 18), the upper portion of the Scatchard plot can be used to determine K to a first approximation. This heterogeneity also actually decreases the precision at some concentrations of hormone. Thus, in practice conditions, optimal precision must be empirically determined. For optimal sensitivity, these theoretical considerations serve as useful but not perfect guidelines for selection of assay conditions.

Summary

1. The relationship between the response variable B/F and the antibody binding sites concentration is linear.

$$B/F = K([Ab^0] - B)$$

where

B = amount of bound hormone, ligand, or antigen

F = amount of free hormone, ligand, or antigen

K = association constant for antibody, antigen interaction

$[Ab^0]$ = molar concentration of Ab binding sites

A graph of B/F against B is a straight line with a slope of $-K$ that intersects the ordinate at $K[Ab^0]$ (see Chapter 2, p. 29; Fig. 2-11).

2. The assay sensitivity is defined as the smallest measurable change in the slope of the dose-response curve, db/dH. This condition is met when b, the bound fraction of hormone, is 1/3, or the B/F ratio is 0.5.

3. The assay sensitivity is limited by the K-value, which characterizes the interaction of antibody and antigen and ideally is maximal when $db/d[H] = -4K/27$.

4. For sensitive assays $[Ab^0]$ (the concentration of antibody-binding sites) must be low, and $[Ab^0] \approx [H]$, the concentration of hormone.

5. Conditions for optimal precision occur when $[Ab^0]$ and [H] are high.

Approach of Ekins

Mathematical formulation

Throughout the analysis, Ekins has preferred to use F/B, rather than B/F, versus dose concentration, since the former method of plotting is more likely to give a straight line.

$$[P] + [Q] \rightleftarrows [PQ]$$

$$K = \frac{[PQ]}{[P] \times [Q]} \qquad (1)$$

where

[P] = concentration of univalent hormone

[Q] = concentration of univalent antibody

[PQ] = concentration of complex

$$R_{f/b} = \frac{[P]}{[PQ]} \qquad (2)$$

$$[P] = p - [PQ] \qquad (3)$$

$$[Q] = q - [PQ] \qquad (4)$$

where p and q are the initial concentrations of hormone and antibody.

$$R_{f/b} = \frac{p - [PQ]}{[PQ]} \qquad (5)$$

$$[PQ] = \frac{p}{R_{f/b} + 1} \qquad (6)$$

When combined and rearranged, this becomes

$$R^2_{f/b} + R_{f/b}\left(1 - \frac{p}{q} - \frac{1}{Kq}\right) - \frac{1}{Kq} = 0 \qquad (7)$$

When plotted, the curve F/B ($R_{f/b}$) versus concentration gives a hyperbola that asymptotically approaches a line whose slope is $1/q$, the reciprocal of the receptor concentration (Fig. 6-1). This line intercepts the $R_{f/b}$ axis at $[(1/Kq) - 1]$. If $R_{b/f}$ is plotted

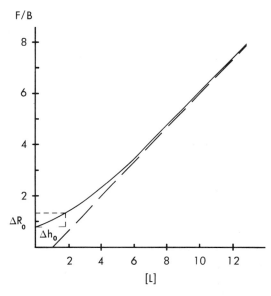

F/B

[L]

Fig. 6-1. Plot of the ratio of free to bound activity versus concentration of ligand. The plot of the standard curve tends to become a straight line at high concentrations of ligand. Δh_0 is the standard deviation of the determination of this ratio at zero added hormone concentration. Δh_0 is the smallest amount of added hormone that will change the measured $R_{0\,f/b}$ by $> \Delta R_0$, the least detectable change in the F/B ratio.

against q, a hyperbola is also observed; it has as its asymptote a line whose slope is $-K$. This line intercepts the ratio axis at $R_{b/f} = Kq - 1$. Thus, for a plot of $R_{f/b}$ versus p, the lower the concentration of q, the steeper will be the slope of the curve (given by a reciprocal $1/q$). On the $R_{b/f}$ curve, a change in K can be seen to cause an increase in the slope and height of the intercept on the y-axis.

Ekins has also considered the situation in which there is more than one receptor binding site, with a K given by K_i and concentration q_i. The details are not presented here, but the basic conclusions from the mathematics are:

If a number of receptors of differing affinities and concentrations of binding sites are present in the reaction mixture, the slope of the curve in Fig. 6-1 will be proportional to the weighted mean of the binding K-values. The weighting will be given by K_iq_i.

For low hormone concentrations, the slope of the binding curve will predominantly reflect the K-value of the most avid receptor.

In other circumstances, the slope of the binding curve may be weighted primarily to the low-avidity binding site. This circumstance would hold if the product K_iq_i is much greater for this site than for all others.

This also implies that isolation of receptors to improve the concentration of high-affinity sites in comparison with low-affinity sites may significantly improve assay sensitivity.

Ekins has also considered the situation in which the standard hormone (s), the unknown hormone (u), and the tracer hormone (P*) react with the same binding site but with K-values that are different (K_s, K^*, K_j, respectively). This situation occurs relatively frequently in RIA. It can be shown that:

At low values of $R_{f/b}$ (lower end of the standard curve), the shape of the response curve is not affected very much by the K-values, so the standard curves are superimposed. However, at high values of $R_{f/b}$, the two curves cannot be exactly superimposed.

Thus, for substances with different K-values, the standard curves cannot be made to coincide over the entire range of hormone concentration.

This fact implies several general points:

1. In the strictest sense, cross-reaction between hormones that are not identical (such as two different species) cannot be used in an assay system, except in the special circumstance that the two have identical immunologic reactivity.

2. In regard to specificity, if a cross-reacting compound (u) differs with regard to K-values of binding from the primary hormones (s), it will be relatively underestimated by a factor that is approximately equal to K_u/K_s.

One of the limitations of this theoretical approach is that only one binding site is assumed. In fact there are several orders of binding sites in the antibody mixture, with varying degrees of cross-reactivity (p. 17).

The interference of plasma, salt concentration, and so forth, may also cause what in effect is a lack of specificity between standard hormone and endogenous hormones. Various extraction techniques may also influence the apparent specificity between unknowns and standards.

For further details, see Ekins and others in the bibliography for Part 1.

Sensitivity

The treatment of Ekins differs fundamentally from that of Berson and Yalow by according a different definition to the concept of sensitivity. Instead of considering sensitivity as the smallest measurable change in the response variable with a small change in hormone concentration (that is, the smallest measurable change in slope $\Delta(B/F)/\Delta p$), Ekins has defined sensitivity as the quantity of unlabeled hormone ($\Delta'p$) that will change the distribution of radioactivity by an amount $\Delta'R$ that is just equal to the standard deviation (ΔR_0) of the experimental determination of R_0, where R_0 is the ratio of free to bound activity at zero concentration of hormone.

If the only error that is included in the estimate of $R_{0\,f/b}$ is that of counting, it can be shown that if

S = specific activity of labeled hormone (counts/minute/unit weight)

V = the volume of the reaction mixture that is fractionated and counted

$R_{0\,f/b}$ = distribution ratio, free to bound activity at the zero point on the standard curve

P^* = concentration of labeled hormone

b_0 = activity in the bound fraction

f_0 = activity in the free fraction

and

$$\frac{(\Delta R_{0\,f/b})}{(R_{0\,f/b})} = \text{the standard error of the determination of } R_{0\,f/b}$$

then

$$\Delta'p \sqrt{SVT} = \left(1 + \sqrt{R_{0\,f/b}}\right) \tag{8}$$
$$\left(qR_{0\,f/b} + \frac{1}{KR_{0\,f/b}}\right)\sqrt{\frac{K}{[(KqR_{0\,f/b})-1]}}$$

The minimal detectable quantity of hormone ($\Delta'p$) for any value of antibody concentration (q) or radioligand concentration (p^*) is given by this equation.

This quantity is at a minimum when

q $= 3/K$

$p^* = 4/K$

and

$R_{0\,f/b} = 1$

Then,

$$\Delta'p = \frac{4\sqrt{2}}{KSVT}$$

This equation gives the conditions of maximal sensitivity. The optimal concentrations of radioligand and antibody are independent of the specific activity of the tracer hormone, and the minimum detectable hormone concentration is thus inversely proportional to the square root of the tracer's specific activity, the binding constant of the reaction (K), and the volume of the incubation mixture, and the time of counting.

Thus maximum sensitivity occurs at $R_{0\,f/b} = 1$.

If errors other than counting are considered, the situation is as follows:

$$\Delta'p = \left(qR_{0\,f/b} + \frac{1}{R_{0\,f/b}K}\right) \tag{9}$$
$$\sqrt{\frac{R_{0\,f/b}+1}{R_{0\,f/b}p^*\,SVT}\left(1 + \sqrt{R_{0\,f/b}}\right)^2 + \epsilon^2}$$

where ϵ is the minimum experimental error (relative error) in the determination of $R_{0\,f/b}$

If this expression is differentiated to determine a minimum for $\Delta'p$, the minimum detectable hormonal concentration, at $R_{0\,f/b} = 1$,

$$\epsilon^2\,SVT\left(q - \frac{1}{K}\right)^2 + 2\left(q - \frac{1}{K}\right) - \frac{4}{K} = 0 \tag{10}$$

This equation shows the relationship between the optimal concentration of receptor binding sites, K, and the parameter $\epsilon\sqrt{SVT/K}$.

Fig. 6-2 is a graphic representation of the relationship of the parameter $\epsilon\sqrt{SVT/K}$ versus optimal concentrations of receptor and radioligand. In this equation, as ϵ (the relative error of measurement of $R_{0\,f/b}$) approaches zero, the quantity $K \times q$ tends toward 3, and the quantity p^*K approaches 4; thus where ϵ is zero, the optimal concentrations of radioligand and receptor are $4/K$ and $3/K$, respectively. If ϵ is not zero, however, the optimal concentrations of radioligand and receptor sites may be significantly different from this, depending on the values that ϵ, S, T, V, and K actually take if these are known. Then, from Fig. 6-2, a prediction of the minimum quantity detectable can be made by substitution of the values of q and p^* into equation (9). According to Ekins, the

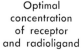

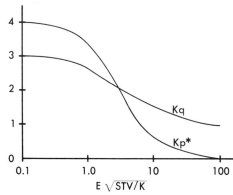

Optimal concentration of receptor and radioligand

$E \sqrt{STV/K}$

Fig. 6-2. Graphical relationship between the parameter $\epsilon\sqrt{STV/K}$ and the optimal concentration of receptor (as expressed by the parameter Kq) and radioligand (as expressed by the parameter Kp*) for maximal sensitivity of radioligand assay. See text for details.

value of the quantity $\epsilon\sqrt{SVT/K}$ is roughly about 1 to 10 under most assay circumstances that are practicable. For this reason, this value is quite small when compared with K in determining the minimal detectable concentration of hormones; thus, for reasonable experimental errors, a value for K of 10^{11} liters per mole (L/M) is a minimum for detecting the usual plasma concentration of insulin, for example. These relationships also imply that beyond a certain limit increasing the specific activity gives a correspondingly smaller improvement in the minimum hormone concentration detectable.

Optimizing assay conditions

From the foregoing analysis, Ekins has concluded that optimization of assay conditions (such as concentration of radioligand, receptor, optimal ratio of free to bound activity) may be very important in the laboratory or clinical situation, in which radioligand and ligand interact significantly differently from each other with respect to the receptor site and the errors of measurement are not zero. (For further details see Ekins and others.) In practice it is usually possible to achieve a reasonable approximation of these optimal conditions by empirically seeking conditions that allow reasonable assay precision, as determined by the ability to measure a known concentration of hormone in serum.

Summary

1. A general formulation for the relationship (dose-response curve) between a change in amount of bound radioligand and changing total concentration of ligand is

$$R^2_{f/b} + R_{f/b}\left(1 - \frac{p}{q} - \frac{1}{Kq}\right)$$

$$-\frac{1}{Kq} = 0$$

where

$R_{f/b}$ = ratio of free to bound ligand
   K = association constant between receptor and ligand
   p = initial concentration of ligand present
   q = initial concentration of receptor present

2. Sensitivity of an assay should be defined as the smallest detectable hormone concentration and not as a slope of the dose-response curve—that is, the smallest change in hormone concentration above zero ($\Delta'p$) that results in a change in the response variable ($\Delta'R_{0\ f/b}$) equal to the standard error of measurement of $R_{f/b}$ at zero hormone concentration.

3. Assay conditions can be specified to achieve optimal sensitivity and precision. In general (neglecting experimental errors), the concentration of radioligand is equal to 4/K; that of receptor binding sites is equal to 3/K, where K is the equilibrium constant and $R_{f/b}$ = 1. In this situation the minimum detectable hormone concentration becomes $\dfrac{4\sqrt{2}}{\sqrt{KSVT}}$ where K = the reaction constant for interaction between ligand and receptor, S = the specific activity to tracer, V = the volume of the reaction mixture, and T = time available for counting.

4. In addition to determining K from a Scatchard plot, K may be determined from the basic form of the equation relating the response variable ($R_{f/b}$) and hormone concentration by determining the slope of the asymptote to the curve, which is 1/q; this intercepts the ratio axis at $R_{f/b} = [1/Kq - 1]$, where q is the concentration of receptor binding sites.

5. In practice, receptor preparations are characterized by a number of different binding sites, each with a different and unique K. In this case, the slope of the asymptote will be proportional to the weighted mean of all the K-values. The weighting factor is related to the amount of a given species that is present (K_iq_i), where q_i is the concentration of the ith species of receptor and K_i is the association constant that characterizes the antibody-binding site.

6. At low concentrations of receptor, the highest-affinity K will predominate. For higher concentra-

tions of receptor, the lower-avidity receptors may predominate.

7. In terms of specificity, if a cross-reacting compound (u) differs with regard to K-value from the standard (s), the concentrations of the unknown will be underestimated by the proportionality factor Ks/Ku.

8. Consideration of experimental errors at the point where $R_{f/b} = 1$ permits a prediction of the optimal assay conditions in terms of concentration of receptor and radioligand where the error (ϵ), the specific activity S (counts/minute/unit weight), T (minutes), V (volume of sample), and K (association constant at equilibrium) are known (see Fig. 6-2).

9. Under optimal assay conditions and known ϵ, S, V, T, and K, the smallest detectable concentration of hormone may be calculated.

COMMON METHODS OF GRAPHIC PRESENTATION OF THE DOSE-RESPONSE CURVE (BOUND/ TOTAL VERSUS DOSE)

The most commonly used method of graphic presentation is the B/T versus dose (Fig. 6-3), since counting the bound fraction is the technique most frequently used to estimate the distribution of radioactivity between bound and free fractions. This technique of plotting shows the same relationship as simply plotting raw counts versus dose (Fig. 6-3). One popular method to illustrate this is to normalize the estimate of the bound fraction in relation to the bound activity in the zero standard tube (B_0) by dividing the fraction bound at each concentration of the standard series (B) by B_0 (Fig. 6-4). Since this method of data presentation hides some of the important characteristics of the assay, the total amounts of radioactivity added to the tube should also always be indicated. In addition, the inclusion of a value for a blank N when no receptor has been added is an important indicator that determines the quality of the assay. Another term for this parameter is "nonspecific binding" (NSB). The B/B_0 response parameter, corrected for NSB, may be calculated as follows:

$$\left(\frac{B - N}{B_0 - N}\right)$$

The dose of cold ligand can be expressed in various ways: for example, as final concentration in the test tube, as the total amount of li-

gand in the test tube, or as the concentration of ligand in the standard solution. The latter mode is frequently used, since it then serves as a direct indicator of the concentration in the unknown sample, provided that the same volume of the standard and sample are added to the tubes.

The plot of B/F versus dose is also used (Fig. 6-5). This makes the y-axis highly nonlinear and expands the y-axis scale. Therefore, it is a method of plotting that does not increase the informational content. B/F is primarily useful when the primary standard curve serves as a basis for calculating the Scatchard plot (see Chapter 2, p. 15).

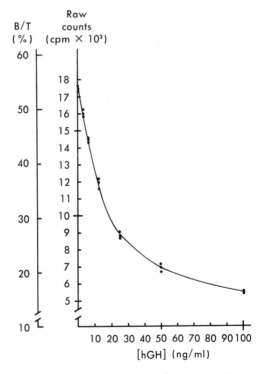

Fig. 6-3. B/T (bound counts/total counts × 100) and raw counts (counts uncorrected for nonspecific binding and background) versus concentration of human growth hormone (hGH). The concentration of ligand in this and the following figures is given as the concentration of the standard solution (of which $100\mu l$ is added to each tube; the volume of each sample is also $100\mu l$). This curve gives a direct reading of the concentration in the sample. B/T and raw counts give essentially the same standard curve information.

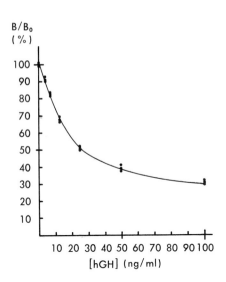

Fig. 6-4. Percent B/B_0 versus concentration of hGH. B_0 is the amount of bound activity in the absence of added ligand.

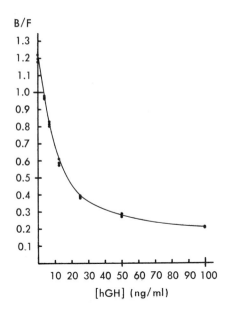

Fig. 6-5. Bound to free ratio (B/F) versus concentration of hGH. Note the relatively steep standard curve at the lower concentrations of ligand in the standard tubes.

A number of methods have been proposed for linearizing the curve, since normal interpolation of the concentration of ligand is performed more readily in regions where the dose-response curve is linear. This is because it is easier to manually draw the appropriate straight line connecting the standard points and to detect incorrect results in the standard tube series. Furthermore, slopes of curves may be more readily compared, and automated calculations are simplified greatly when a linear relationship exists between the response and dose variables.

However, none of the methods proposed for this purpose is completely successful, and, as a rule, the linear part of the curve is restricted to only a portion of the curve.

Those mathematical relationships that have been useful in estimating linear response in biologic systems have also been useful in RIA. Bound/total versus log dose is widely used (Fig. 6-6). This relationship tends to prolong the linear section in the midportion of the curve. Another way to linearize the curve is to plot F/B versus dose (see Fig. 6-1). In the lower end of the curve, at low concentrations of dose, the curve is quite nonlinear. With increasing con-

centration of dose, the curve will approach an asymptote, which is a straight line.

A widely used method for linearization of the standard curve is the "logit plot" (Fig. 6-7).

Rodbard and his associates have developed an empirical linear relationship between a response variable and the dose, as follows:

$$\text{logit } (B/B_0) = \log_e \left[\frac{(B/B_0)}{(1 - B/B_0)} \right]$$

or

$$\text{logit } (Y) = \log_e \left(\frac{1}{1 - Y} \right)$$

where

$$Y = \frac{B - N}{B_0 - N}$$

where N represents the nonspecific counts bound in the absence of receptor (the "standard" or "plasma blank," p. 67), B_0 = counts bound in the absence of labeled hormones, and B = counts bound in the sample determinations.

When logit Y is plotted against the log dose, a linear curve is usually obtained.

This relationship is theoretically exact under conditions of saturation of the antibody. An as-

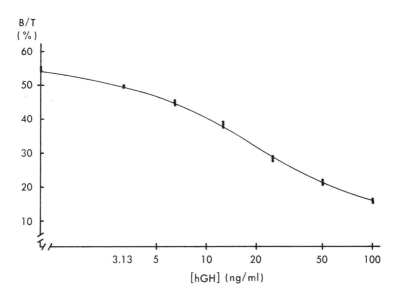

Fig. 6-6. Percent B/T versus log (dose). This method of plotting the data results in a relatively linear response.

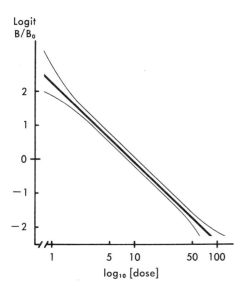

Fig. 6-7. Logit B/B_0 versus log (dose). This method has the advantage of linearizing most RIA standard curves over their entire range. The 95% confidence interval (thin lines) is shown. The errors are greatest at the upper ranges and minimal at the midrange.

sumption of this system is that most assays will be operating near saturation and that in any event the logit transformation will result in a useful approximation in most systems.

A problem with the logit Y transformation is that the variance is not uniform along the entire curve, being least in the midrange and greatest at the ends (Fig. 6-7). For this reason, simple linear regression techniques are not applicable, and a weighted regression must be applied.

The weighting factors must be derived from a consideration of variance of logit Y.

$$\text{Variance of logit (Y)} = \frac{\text{Var Y}}{Y^2 (1 - Y)^2} \qquad (1)$$

The variance of Y defined as

$$\text{Var (Y)} = \frac{\text{Var (B)}}{(B_0 - N)^2} \qquad (2)$$

must be calculated.

In order to do this properly, the total error variance of the determination of B in the sample measurements is determined from a consideration of the following sources of error:

1. Pipetting of the radioligand
2. Pipetting of the antibody
3. Pipetting of standard and unknown
4. Misclassification of tracer as being in the bound or free state due to errors of separation

5. Counting errors (see Rodbard and Rodbard and Cooper)

A detailed consideration is outside the scope of this review (see the work by Rodbard).

In practice, it is usually simpler to empirically determine the variance of Y by calculating the variance of Y among several replicates at various ligand concentration steps from several assay runs (for example, 10 assays).

The regression line (logit Y versus log X) may be plotted and the 95% confidence determined by calculating the value of logit Y for $Y \pm 2 \sqrt{\text{Var} (Y)}$ at various values of log X. This allows one to plot the "envelope" of variance about the logit curve as shown in Fig. 6-7.

The reciprocals of the variance of logit Y are used as weights in the calculation of a weighted least-squares regression line. (In practice, a weighted and unweighted line will be very similar.) The 95% confidence envelope is minimal between 0.25 and 0.50 for logit Y.

For routine assay performance one method is usually as good as another. There may be some advantages in a relatively linear standard curve if this suits the assay conditions and if computer interpretation of the data is to be employed. More sophisticated automated techniques are being employed. These methods have the advantage of ease and convenience in high-volume operations.

QUALITY CONTROL

Quality control is a term used to describe the way in which a laboratory assures that its operation continuously produces highly reliable assay results on clinical samples. This process is usually thought of in terms of the assay system itself as the final point of reference. How "good" is the testing system in terms of producing an assay result that truly reflects the concentration of the analyte? To describe the "goodness" of the assay system, four terms are used.

1. *Precision.* An estimate of assay reproducibility. An assay is "precise" if a series of repeated measurements on the same sample gives the same result.

2. *Sensitivity.* The minimum quantity of a substance that is detectable. An assay is "sensitive" if it is able to detect very tiny amounts of a particular analyte in a biologic sample.

3. *Specificity.* The ability to measure one particular compound or group of compounds without interference from other related material.

4. *Accuracy.* Closeness to the real or true value. A test result is "accurate" if the measured value is very close to the "true" concentration in the biologic fluid.

Thus, quality control is concerned with both establishing and maintaining the highest possible quality in these respects.

As we have defined quality control, it is something that mainly concerns internal laboratory operation and procedures. There are other legitimate concerns regarding the particular assay result that fall outside the usual quality control considerations. One of these is the efficiency of a particular test result. A result may be precise, accurate, and have no relevance to a particular clinical problem. A result may be precise and accurate but, in fact, misleading if proper consideration is not given to patient preparation before sampling or if the referring physician draws unwarranted conclusions from a particular test result. To describe the efficiency or "value" of a particular test the terms *diagnostic sensitivity* (frequency that a test is positive when a particular disease is present) and *diagnostic specificity* (frequency that a test is negative in the absence of a particular disease) are used. For most diagnostic tests, the diagnostic sensitivity and specificity are interrelated variables; thus, when the diagnostic sensitivity is increased, the diagnostic specificity is decreased and vice versa. The predicted value of a positive result is the percentage of all positive results that are true positives. The *predictive value* of a particular test can be shown to be a function of the diagnostic sensitivity and specificity of the testing system and the *prevalence* of the disease in a particular population.

Even "very good" diagnostic tests (such as those with high diagnostic sensitivity and diagnostic specificity) will have little or no predictive value if the prevalence of disease is very low in the population being studied by this testing system. For this reason the value of a particular laboratory test can usually be increased by selecting the population that will be studied through appropriate history, physical diagnosis, pedigree, and so forth. As a general rule, "screening" examination, even with "very good" diagnostic tests performed with high quality control, have a low predictive value, simply because the disease being tested for has a very low prevalence in the population.

In practice, quality control is a program for providing systematic review of the entire laboratory operation. Such operation may be considered to have the following components:
1. Equipment
2. Reagents
3. Sample collection and handling
4. Assay performance
5. Personnel
6. Administrative practices

Equipment

The equipment that is essential for the operation of an RIA laboratory is described in Chapter 7. Proper operation of all of these items is important. Two types of equipment have a particularly profound effect on the assay results: pipettes and counting instruments. Proper upkeep and maintenance of these devices are all too frequently neglected.

PIPETTES. Special attention should be directed toward the proper cleaning of conventional pipettes; their decontamination should be checked with a counter to avoid contamination with trace amounts of radioactivity that might be inadvertently transferred into a critical assay reagent. A rule that may save much trouble is that different sets of pipettes are used for high- and low-activity work.

In the performance of RIA, manual set-volume pipettes (Eppendorf type) are frequently utilized. These pipettes are calibrated to deliver a fixed volume of between $10\mu l$ and 1 ml. The ability of these instruments to repeatedly deliver a fixed volume is essential to the precision of RIA results. For this reason, these pipettes should be checked for accuracy and precision at the time of purchase and, more important, they should be serviced periodically thereafter.

The precision of the manual set-volume pipettes is evaluated by repeated pipetting of a radioactive solution; 20, preferably up to 100, tubes are pipetted and counted in a gamma

counter. At least 50,000 counts should be contained in the pipetted solution to make counting errors negligible. The precision is expressed as the coefficient of variation (standard deviation/mean) $\times$ 100%. The coefficient of variation should be less than 2%. Automated pipettes, dispensers, and diluters are also used in RIA. These devices are serviced regularly, either at the intervals recommended by the manufacturer of, if not specified, monthly. These devices are checked for accuracy at the time of purchase. Testing for precision is performed as described above after these instruments are serviced and reassembled.

COUNTERS. Gamma counting provides the basis for the quantitation in most radioassay systems. The reliability of gamma counting is affected by fluctuations in the *background counting, calibration* of the instrument to the energy settings optimal for counting a particular radionuclide, and the *stability* of the electronics of the machine. The extensive use of ^{125}I in RIAs has resulted in the need for a long-lived radionuclide with a spectrum similar to the shorter-lived ^{125}I. ^{129}I ($T_{\frac{1}{2}} = 1.6 \times 10^7$ years) and single 38-keV gamma photons are used for the purpose of providing a convenient "instrument standard." A background count is included at the beginning and end of each run, and a record is kept of the background count to ensure that no major changes have occurred. The calibration of the gamma counters is checked daily with the instrument standard. Every 3 months the calibration is checked with a higher energy source, such as cesium 137. Every year *efficiency* and *energy resolution* of the instrument are checked by standard methods.

The mechanical components of automated counters are the parts most liable to cause trouble. Whereas their malfunction most often stops function completely, problems such as inappropriate positioning of the sample in the well detector may result instead, which are as serious but may be more difficult to detect.

Reagents

The degree of quality control that is required varies to an extent with the source of the reagents to be used in the assay procedure. However, some in-laboratory checks are mandatory even for kit assays.

NONKIT ASSAY. With an assay that has been developed totally in house, new reagents must be thoroughly characterized as discussed in detail in previous chapters. Once this is done, the controls can be restricted to those used for monitoring assay performance, in addition to regular checks that the properties of the reagents have not deteriorated. This applies in particular to the radioligand, which in some assays has a tendency to deteriorate more rapidly; for this reason it may need testing quite frequently, often as a part of every assay run.

KIT ASSAYS. Assays based on kit material might appear to require less quality control than nonkit assays, since one purchases a certain quality control from the manufacturer. However, as long as kit producers do not provide complete test protocols of the individual reagent batches, such material may require more extensive testing than that actually necessary for "homemade" reagents.

One must be aware of the fact that it is the laboratory that performs the test that is responsible for the relevance of the results reported. Therefore, the laboratory supervisor must have the competence to critically evaluate the information given by the manufacturer (as well as to realize any shortcomings of these reports).

Another important aspect of quality control in the use of kits is the need to ensure that the reagents supplied have not been damaged during transportation. Each newly delivered kit should be tested before use on clinical samples. This is most easily done by the "kit overlapping" procedure, in which individual reagents from the new kit are tested against the reagents in the currently run kit. The receptor and radioligand from the new kit are substituted in the assay procedure for the reagents in the currently run kit. Also, individual standard concentrations (usually at the midpoint of the standard curve) are assayed with the new kit materials. The "normal pool" (see Chapter 5) is also run with new kit reagent. In this way a new kit will be appropriately evaluated with respect to standards, receptor preparations, and radioligand before its incorporation into the clinical routine.

Quality of ligand
Standards

All radioligand assays depend on comparisons between the unknown samples and standards for quantitation of the assay data. Therefore, it is necessary to have a preparation of the ligand that can serve as an appropriate standard for this purpose.

Well-defined compounds that are generally available in "pro analysis" quality with established high purity and stability will serve as adequate standards. For many biologically active substances, however, the substance to be assayed is poorly chemically characterized and available only in crude form. This is exemplified by the hepatitis B antigen assay. An intermediate position in this respect is occupied by the pituitary hormones, although developments in recent years have produced reagents of steadily improving quality that consequently have served to improve assay quality. For such substances, special reference preparations have been established to improve accuracy. Three types of such reference preparations are used.

INTERNATIONAL STANDARDS. Materials for these standards are collected, tested, and aliquoted by responsibility of the World Health Organization International Laboratory for Biological Standards. They have been extensively tested in regard to potency and stability. A unit for activity has been assigned to these preparations after extensive collaborative effort by several different laboratories. Accordingly, these reference preparations are to be regarded as the most reliable standards. They are associated with the drawback of the time lag involved in the acquisition of all the necessary data. They are available in limited quantity free of charge for calibration of national or laboratory standards or reference preparations. They are not available in sufficient quantity for routine use as standards. A list of the international standards available and extensive discussion of their application to immunoassays have been presented in the Technical Report Series No. 565 from the WHO Expert Committee on Biological Standardization, Geneva, 1975.

REFERENCE MATERIALS. These have not been as extensively tested as the established international standards but have certain potency and purity data, primarily provided by the producer. They are distributed by such institutions as the Division of Biological Standards, National Institute of Medical Research, London, and the National Institute of Arthritis, Metabolic and Digestive Diseases, Bethesda, Maryland. These preparations are widely used; thus substantial data on their quality accumulate and are reported in many publications. Accordingly, they constitute a valuable tool for calibration of the assays.

IN-HOUSE OR ''WORKING'' REFERENCE PREPARATIONS. These are preparations that may have been produced by the laboratory performing the assays or acquired without any reliable potency estimates. In this case the individual investigator is responsible for the potency of a particular working standard. Frequently these materials are ''calibrated'' by reference to an international standard.

Standards in quality control

The working standard is in many respects the most important form of standard, because it constitutes the basis for the accuracy of the routine assay. Therefore it must have certain characteristics. However, in contrast to the case of international standards, the laboratory itself must take responsibility for maintaining its appropriate quality; there is no official agency that guarantees its performance. For this reason, it is important to acquire as high-quality standards as possible in regard to purity, homogeneity, and stability. It is also important that the standard be as similar to the material to be assayed as possible. For example, standards for assay of human pituitary hormones should be extracted from human pituitaries, since it has been shown that corresponding material extracted from human urine has different immunologic properties.

When a new standard is first used, it may either have been calibrated by some external laboratory or agency or within the laboratory against some material with an established potency and purity. However, it is important to remember that immunologic potency sometimes is markedly influenced by the properties of the antiserum or receptor used in the assay. For this reason, immunologic potency calibra-

tions must be performed with the same assay as that in which the standard is to be used. Such calibration should be performed over a range of different concentrations of the standard, and the test should be repeated to ascertain consistency of the results. This will also permit a check on the parallelism of the dose-inhibition effect (see Chapter 2).

After the initial testing, one should not forget the possibility of deterioration of such materials. First, they should be stored under optimal conditions. They should be aliquoted to avoid repeated thawing. Dissolved material is kept at $-20°$ C or preferably at $-70°$ C. Second, signs of gradual deterioration should be noted. Maintenance of continuous records of standard curve slopes, pool values, and average results on patient samples collected in certain situations (or, better, on samples from the normal population) permits the detection of changes in the quality of the standard. Gradual degradation of standards will result in a corresponding increase in the values determined on samples.

Cross-checks of the working standards against established standards should, if possible, be performed once a year. Standard calibration should also be checked when new antisera are introduced in an assay, since small differences in antisera specificity may alter the apparent potency of the working standard.

The accuracy of the calibration of an assay may also be ensured by the use of control sera. They may be sold by the commercial reagent producers and have usually been assayed by several unrelated laboratories that have supplied their analysis data, or they are distributed to assaying laboratories as part of a quality control program (for example, within the framework of the College of American Pathologists or the National Immunoassay Service in Britain).

The diluent used for the standard is also important. It should contain an appropriate amount of carrier material to prevent its adsorption to glassware and so forth. The carrier material may also help to prevent degradation of the standard.

Another important quality of the diluent for the standard is that it should be as similar as possible to the solute in which the sample is contained, most frequently plasma or serum. This problem is discussed at some length in Chapter 5.

Samples

It is not only the reagents which contain impurities that may affect the assays adversely. The complex composition of most biologic materials that constitute the sample to be assayed may sometimes influence the method significantly; thus differences in the composition of samples and standards must be taken into account. Occasionally, the sample must be purified before it is introduced into the assay. Purification steps such as extraction or chromatography have been particularly necessary in steroid assays.

Although certain impurities or variations in the properties of various components of the assay have marked influences on the assay, it is obvious that most of the complex constituents of biologic samples have little influence. Radioligand assay is an analytical technique that in many respects is exceptionally insensitive to nonspecific influences as long as appropriate precautions are taken to neutralize those that may occur.

SAMPLE HANDLING. In general, for both serum and plasma sampling, the serum or plasma should be rapidly separated from the cellular blood elements. If the storage stability of the particular analyte is not known, the substance should be considered labile. Some substances, such as adrenocorticotropic hormone (ACTH) and folic acid, are rapidly degraded at room temperature in serum. It may be necessary to freeze these samples very quickly after collection. Repeated thawing of samples before assay should be avoided. If there is any doubt as to the stability of the substance to be measured under the collection conditions, the stability is tested by storing at various temperatures for various periods of time. Also, effects of anticoagulant and the influence of hemolysis are checked. All assays performed should be evaluated for effect of severe hemolysis, varying sample size, and stability of the analyte in serum or plasma. The effect of varying sample size on assay performance can be determined by running a range of samples, usually diluted with

the 0-standard. The stability of the analyte in serum is checked by repeated testing of a sample that has been allowed to stand at room temperature in comparison with a frozen sample.

Assay performance control

The details of the procedures employed are written up for each assay performed in the laboratory, including the kit assays. It is important to emphasize that the manuals should be kept up to date and the directions followed exactly to minimize the variation when more than one technician is performing a particular assay.

MONITORING OF ASSAYS. For the purpose of determining variation in the quality of assay performed, several "control" tubes are included in the assay run. These include the *standard blanks* and the *sample blanks* that include blanks for the pools run with the assay. The blank tubes contain none of the specific binding receptor preparation and are a convenient way to assay nonspecific binding in samples. It may be necessary to include individual sample blanks if there is a significant variation in the assay from sample to sample.

In many assays the interindividual variation in blank value is relatively small; thus only a few representative sample blanks are included.

Pooled plasma, preferably several pools in different concentration ranges (a "normal" pool, a "high" pool, and a "low" pool), is included. These pools are used to permit a ready review of the performance of the assay system at various levels of analyte concentration. A 100% tube (total activity, T) is also included, to permit calculation of the percentage of activity bound in the 0-standard. The assay behavior at various levels of displacement of radioligand can also be monitored to get an idea of the sensitivity of the assay. A convenient way to do this is to set the amount of counts in the 0-standard, $B_0 = 100\%$, and then to determine the concentration of ligand that will displace, for example, 10%, 50%, and 80% of the labeled ligand. The mean of the sample values may also be calculated as a further control of assay level. If outlying values are excluded, this mean is quite consistent for relatively large runs.

The results obtained can be expressed in a

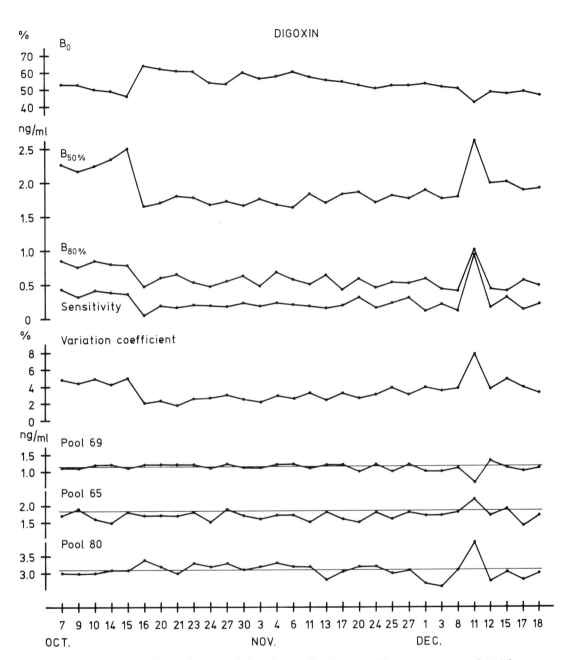

Fig. 6-8. Example of a quality control chart from a digoxin assay. The parameters are plotted for each individual assay run. B_0, binding (percent of total activity) when no cold digoxin is added; $B_{50\%}$, amount of digoxin causing 50% inhibition of the binding ($B_0/2$); $B_{80\%}$, amount of digoxin causing 80% inhibition of the binding ($B_0/5$). Sensitivity = SD of a sample containing no cold digoxin. These three parameters should be as low as possible. The higher the values, the less slope of the curve. A newly made tracer was introduced on October 16, with marked improvement. The assay of December 11 was unacceptable for unknown reason but was adequate when repeated the following day.

variety of ways. One method is to prepare control charts that show the values for a series of different measurements on the pools plotted to a series of individual assay runs. An average value for the pool is determined, and cutoff lines for the control data are established. If the parameters approach these values, it is an indication to the technicians to alert their supervisor. In this way a problem with a particular run can be determined promptly. Examples of various quality control parameters used to monitor assays are shown in Fig. 6-8.

Administrative matters—importance of written procedures

As far as possible, the laboratory operation should be reduced to a written format with a detailed description in cookbook style. In addition to being good laboratory practice, written procedures are requirements of certain accrediting bodies in the United States, including the Joint Commission on Hospital Accreditation. Although details of the requirements vary from agency to agency, the following seem to be general requirements. A laboratory manual should be prepared and kept in the laboratory. The following information should be included.

PERSONNEL. A detailed description of the personnel with appropriate titles should be available in writing in the laboratory files. A description of his or her academic qualifications and formal training courses should be included and maintained up to date. In addition, documentation of satisfactory completion of in-service education should be included. Before personnel are permitted to run an RIA, they must demonstrate that they have a basic understanding of the theoretical aspects of the test protocol and the manual dexterity required to adequately carry it out. Knowledge of the theory of RIA can be evaluated by a written questionnaire. Manual dexterity can be evaluated by an exercise in repeated pipetting. On two different occasions, 100 tubes with $500\mu l$ and 100 tubes with $50\mu l$ of a radioactive solution are pipetted. Enough radioactivity is present to make counting errors negligible. The precision is determined by calculating the coefficient of variation for each run. The coefficient of variation must be less than 2%.

EQUIPMENT. A list of the equipment in the laboratory should also be maintained, along with written procedures for critical operation (such as calibration to counting of ^{125}I sources). A description of the quality control programs employed for the equipment, with documentation of the results obtained,

should be included. In addition, service records should be kept, with a listing of maintenance checks that includes dates and results. Dates of equipment malfunction and repair should also be kept.

PERFORMANCE. Written procedures should be kept in the laboratory manual for all of the individual aspects of assay performance. In general these will cover the following aspects.

1. *Sample collection.* A detailed protocol for the collection of each individual sample should be included in the written protocols of assay performance. Remarks regarding general precautions of sample collection and controls for ensuring that the proper procedures are being followed should also be included. One important aspect of sample collection is the use of an appropriately designed radioassay request slip, which may contain information on sampling conditions (for example, on the back of the form).

2. *Written protocols of the assay procedure* (see Chapter 5). These should be available for each assay and include an overview of the technique; a description of the reagents, including standard, used; a protocol for running the assay; and calculation and interpretation of the results.

3. *A written report for each individual assay.* This should include the reagents used and the samples analyzed as well as how the quality control procedures are performed for each assay. It should also include the results of the assay.

ADMINISTRATION. A detailed organizational chart should be available that describes the administration of the laboratory. This requirement is imposed by a number of agencies in the United States and is apparently related to proper assignment of responsibility for the work performed in the laboratory and quality control for efficient laboratory management. In addition, some reviewers may require that job descriptions be available. Although these job descriptions are not usually a part of the laboratory manual itself, it may be good practice to keep written job descriptions in an easily accessible place within the laboratory.

The use of radioisotopes imposes certain safety requirements. A copy of the laboratory license and film badge reports, including exposure records of the personnel, must be available for review. In addition, a radiation monitoring program of radiation control areas and personnel is mandatory. The laboratory manual will not include this information but should state where these items are kept.

7 EQUIPMENT

GENERAL LABORATORY REQUIREMENTS

Because several relatively recent publications have dealt with the problems of space, record keeping, radiation safety regulations, and personnel associated with running a radioassay laboratory, these topics are not discussed at length here. Suffice it to say that in most countries licensing by the appropriate public agency is necessary to purchase and handle radioactive material. In the United States licensing is necessary if the amount of any single radionuclide exceeds the following activities: ^{125}I, 1μCi; ^{131}I, 1μCi; ^{3}H, 1μCi; ^{14}C, 100μCi. An investigator using more than one of these isotopes must also be licensed by the National Regulatory Commission or appropriate state authority. In regard to space planning, the most important aspect is that it should allow the adequate separation of high-activity (labeling) and low-activity (assay performance and sample counting) procedures.

GENERAL LABORATORY EQUIPMENT

A suggested inventory for a radioassay laboratory of moderate size is shown in the outline below. In addition to the assorted laboratory glassware expected in any working laboratory, several specialized items are noted. For solid phase radioassay techniques, rotators and mixers are required. Items of particular importance include pipettes. Major pieces of equipment are centrifuges and radioactivity counters.

EQUIPMENT FOR RADIOIMMUNOASSAY

A. Glassware
   1. Beaker
   2. Erlenmeyer flasks
   3. Graduated cylinders
   4. Volumetric flasks
   5. Tubes (plastic for most assays, size 11-12 mm × 55-75 mm; glass for some steroid assays)
B. Assorted test tube racks
C. Balances
   1. General purpose laboratory precision-type scale
   2. Analytical scale
D. pH meter
E. Water bath
F. Shakers
G. Mixers
   1. Vortex type
   2. Magnetic type
H. Chromatography equipment
   1. Pumps
   2. Fraction collector
   3. Assorted columns
   4. Connectors and tubing
I. Water deionizer
J. Drying oven
K. Centrifuges
   1. General purpose bench top centrifuge
   2. Refrigerated high-capacity centrifuge (to 4,000g)
L. Pipettes
   1. General purpose
   2. Volumetric, or transfer
M. Micropipettes
   1. Constriction type
   2. Hamilton syringe
   3. Capillary pipettes
   4. Manual set-volume pipettes (often called Eppendorf type)
   5. Cornwall type
   6. Automated (with or without automated tube transport)
N. Dispenser
O. Combined sampler/dispenser/diluter
P. Radiation detectors
   1. Portable radiation detector ("cutie pie")

type with low-energy measurement capability for ^{125}I detection
2. Manual single well type
3. Gamma detector (with either rate meter or scaler)
4. Automated radioactivity detectors
5. Gamma counter
6. Beta counter
Q. Computational devices: calculator, portable (with or without programming capability)

Pipettes

Performance of RIA procedures requires rapid and precise measurement of reagent volumes. For most applications, the exact calibration of the pipetting instruments is less important than the precision and reproducibility of the measurement.

Preparation of standards requires the use of volumetric, or transfer, pipettes of various sizes. There are two main types: "to contain" pipettes are calibrated to contain a given volume. "To deliver" pipettes, calibrated to deliver a certain volume, are marked with one or two frosted rings at the top of the pipette. The frosted ring pipettes must have the last drop blown out of the end for complete accuracy. Some "to deliver" pipettes do not have a frosted ring; these pipettes do not need to have the last drop blown out.

For smaller volumes of measurement either constriction pipettes or microsyringes of the Hamilton

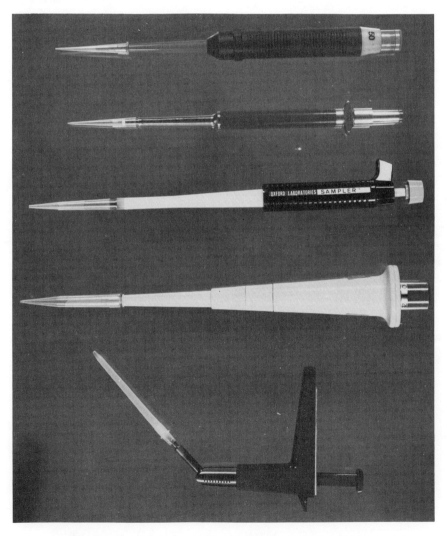

Fig. 7-1. Examples of preset (or fixed) volume manual pipettes.

type may be used. Constriction pipettes are used with a rubber tube, usually with a safety bulb and mouthpiece. The constriction pipettes are filled by suction to just above the constriction point. The tip of the pipette is touched to the side of the container from which the solution was originally taken. The fluid in the pipette is then blown out gently to assure delivery of the proper volume of solution. Radioactive solutions should not be pipetted by mouth.

It is important to clean pipettes properly. This can be accomplished with several standard laboratory detergents. Rinsing of pipettes should be with distilled or deionized water, and the pipettes may be conveniently dried in a drying oven. It is particularly important to clean constriction pipettes properly with a laboratory detergent, rinse them with distilled water, and then dry them only in a drying oven.

For delivery of small volumes, the Hamilton-type syringe is preferred. Accuracy of $\pm 1\%$ can be achieved with even the 1μ to $5\mu l$ sizes of this type of pipetting device. The Hamilton syringe for smaller volumes has an inner platinum wire that serves to push all of the contained fluid out of the tip of the needle of the syringe.

A pipetting device that is important to assay performance is the semiautomated hand pipette (often called Eppendorf type even though there are many different brands and models; Fig. 7-1). Semiautomated hand pipettes are designed for rapid, precise dispensing of volumes from $20\mu l$ to $1,000\mu l$. These instruments are widely used in RIAs. Precision of repetitive measurements are approximately 1%.

Several varieties of Eppendorf-type pipettes are available, which vary slightly in design. All of these have in common the use of disposable plastic tips, a plunger assembly for filling and dispensing a liquid sample. In general, the use of these devices is similar in that the plastic tip should be firmly fixed to the end of the pipette and the plunger should be completely depressed before the end of the plastic is placed below the surface of the sample. This is important in order to avoid trapping an air bubble in the plastic tip, which will interfere with the accuracy of dispensing.

There are two modes in which the dispensing operation can be performed. One type of pipette requires an additional depression of the plunger to fully expel all of the liquid from the plastic tip. The other type has only a single stage in the depression of the plunger at the dispensing step. Thus taking up and dispensing the solution require the same manual operations and degree of depression of the plunger. Most of our technicians prefer the latter type of semiautomated pipettes, although this seems to be a mat-

ter of individual preference rather than a basic superiority of one instrument over another. Some of these units are also able to eject the plastic tip automatically, which may be valuable when radioactive materials are being used.

Automated pipetting systems

Pipetting systems of varying complexity have been developed for automatically dispensing volumes of reagents and samples. The simplest of these devices repeatedly dispenses a fixed volume of solution. Instruments for delivering macrovolumes or microvolumes are available. The next order of complexity is a variable diluter, which dilutes a fixed volume of sample with an appropriate buffer by initially aspirating the sample volume against a column of buffer in the sample tip. The sample in the tip is then flushed out with the desired reagent volume. The volumetric accuracy of the sample volume is $\pm 1\%$ and the reagent dispensing 1%. Some of these sample diluters are also capable of delivering adjustable volumes from $2\mu l$ to 10 ml of two separate liquids, through either a common delivery tip or dual delivery tips into a vessel.

Automated pipetting systems have also been developed that can repetitively dispense or dilute volumes with high precision into test tubes that are automatically advanced across a working surface. Several hundred operations can be performed per hour with these automated units. The types of operations include sample dilutions, in which a sample is aspirated from one tube and then the sample and an appropriate volume of diluent are transferred to another tube. Then, the other reagents needed are added to this tube, through either the same tip or through multiple outlets.

Counting devices

Gamma counting

Gamma counters in current use are primarily based on sodium iodide (thallium-activated) radioactivity detection systems. NaI (Tl) is a crystal that gives off light when x-rays or gamma rays strike the crystal structure. The amount of light produced is directly proportional to the amount of energy from the x-ray or gamma ray that is deposited within the crystal.

A block diagram of the common types of NaI (Tl) gamma scintillation detectors is shown in Fig. 7-2. The NaI (Tl) crystal is encased in an aluminum can to exclude light and air. It must be airtight in order to prevent the hydrophilic

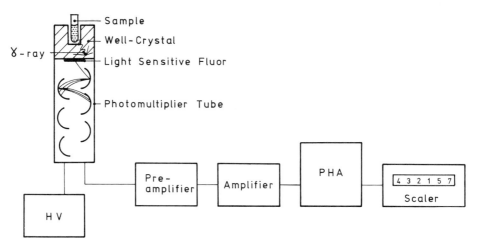

Fig. 7-2. Block diagram of the principal components of a well-type crystal (NaI) scintillation counter for gamma detection. The photomultiplier tube is served with a high voltage *(HV)* from an HV power supply. The pulse leaving the photomultiplier tube is amplified, after which the appropriate pulses are screened in the pulse height analyzer *(PHA)* (sometimes called spectrometer). The pulses then remaining are counted in the scaler, which also contains a very precise timer to set the time interval for the counting.

NaI (Tl) crystals from absorbing water. The crystal usually has a hole punched in it in the shape of a well. The sample sits within the well. A gamma ray or an x-ray penetrates the aluminum, enters the cover and crystal, and gives up some or all of its energy within the crystal substance, which causes the crystal to give off light. Twenty to thirty photons of light are given off per each electron volt of energy absorbed. Since the crystal is transparent, the light produced passes through the crystal to strike against a light-sensitive surface of the photomultiplier (PM) tube; the surface is usually coated with an alloy of cesium. The light photons cause electrons to be released from the surface of the photocathode. The electrons so released are further multiplied within the PM tube by acceleration under a high-voltage electric field. The electrons strike a dynode, a positively charged electrode a short distance from the photocathode. About 3 to 4 electrons are released from the dynode for each electron that strikes it. After passing through 6 to 10 such discrete steps, the current pulse that reaches the anode of the PM tube is large enough to be further amplified and/or detected. The PM tube achieves an amplification of about 10^8, so that

for each electron leaving the photocathode, 10^8 arrive at the anode of the PM tube.

In order to reduce the distortion of the electrical signal produced by the NaI (Tl) PM tube detector system, a following preamplifier is usually employed before the signal from the PM tube is further amplified for energy resolution and counting. The preamplifier produces an electrical signal that is matched to the impedance of the amplifier that follows it. The amplifier then multiplies the incoming pulse from 1 to 50,000 times, depending on the particular detector and counting device employed. Amplifiers may be *linear,* in which case the output pulse is directly linearly proportional to the input pulse, or *logarithmic,* in which case the output pulse is a log function of the input pulse. Logarithmic gain is valuable when simultaneous counting of variable energies is to be employed, as in gamma counting of the 35 keV photon of ^{125}I and the 364 keV photon of ^{131}I or in liquid scintillation counting with simultaneous counting of ^3H and ^{14}C with their energies of 18 and 159 keV, respectively.

The actual output of the amplifier is in the form of a voltage pulse, which has a particular pulse height (Fig. 7-3). For both liquid scintilla-

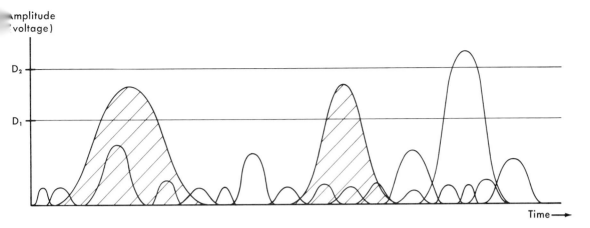

Amplitude (voltage)

D₂

D₁

Time ⟶

Fig. 7-3. Schematic representation of the effect of the pulse height analyzer (PHA). The vertical axis is the energy (pulse height) of the pulses that enter the PHA from the amplifier during the time recorded (horizontal axis). The discriminating levels are set at D_1 and D_2. Only pulses with energies falling in this interval (hatched areas) are permitted to pass through the PHA.

tion detectors and NaI (Tl) detector systems, the height of the voltage pulse provided from the amplifier is proportional to the energy deposited within the detector. Many isotopes produce radiation of several energies and, accordingly, pulses with different amplitudes. A pulse height analyzer sorts out these pulses according to their amplitude (voltage) and allows only those that fall within a restricted range of pulse heights to pass to the counter.

Since the pulse height is proportional to the energy of interaction of a particular photon or particle within the detector system, in principle for monoenergetic gamma-emitting isotopes one would expect a single pulse height to be continuously produced. In practice, however, some of the gamma rays' energy escapes from the detector system without being fully absorbed. Thus a spectrum of energies (pulse height) is recorded by the detector system, even when a unique gamma photon energy is produced by the radioactive decay process. If the count rate detected is plotted as a function of energy (number of pulses of particular voltages), a differential spectrum is obtained (Fig. 7-4). This differential spectrum is characteristic of a given radionuclide and detector system. It consists of the different types of pulses that are recorded since, in reality, except for the pulses coming unaltered from the decaying atoms,

these are recorded pulses from radiation that has been altered on its way to the detector by interference with the material it has passed (Compton scatter) as well as from background radiation and pulses that emerge from the electronics of equipment (electronic noise). The levels D_1 and D_2 described in Fig. 7-3 usually correspond to two settings on the spectrometer (the instrument that distinguishes pulses with different energies: the "lower discriminator," D_1, and the "upper discriminator," D_2). The interval between D_1 and D_2 is frequently called the "window width." D_1 and D_2 are usually calibrated in terms of energy and are set so that D_1 and D_2 include the lower region and the upper region of the photopeak.

Several factors reflect the reliability of counting samples. First there is a certain *background level* of counting, which varies with energy settings of the machine. Under normal circumstances the background level is less than 100 cpm for counters at the photopeak. For ^{125}I the photopeak energy is relatively low, being only 27 to 35 keV (Fig. 7-4). This low-energy radiation is readily absorbed within large samples and even within the walls of thick test tubes (sample self-absorption). Some gamma counters, particularly older models, also have thick enough casings around the NaI crystal that the photons from the ^{125}I do not readily penetrate to

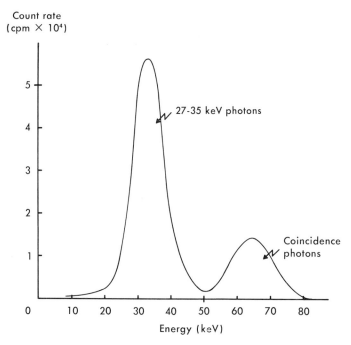

Fig. 7-4. Spectrum of ^{125}I, showing the dominant peak of the x-ray photons (27-35 keV) and the apparent energy recorded in the detector when two photons happen to cause a scintillation simultaneously (coincidence photons).

interact with the crystal. Also, the *volume* through which a sample is distributed will affect the counting rate. This effect is particularly important as the sample size becomes large in relationship to the volume of the detector crystal. For this reason sample volumes should be kept as constant as possible. Samples and standards should always be counted in the same relative volumes. Finally, counting of ^{125}I in glass tubes may cause an undue variation in the count rate, since glass is relatively dense and has a high absorption capacity for the ^{125}I gamma rays. In addition, glass test tubes often show considerable variation in thickness. Plastic tubes are more constant in configuration and absorb less radiation.

All of these factors together determine the counting efficiency of a particular gamma counter. The counting efficiency is the ratio of the number of counts recorded to the number of photons produced in the radioactive material during a certain time. The number of photons produced is not necessarily identical to the number of decays, since the number of photons

usually is higher or lower than the number of decays. (All decays do not produce identical radiation. For example, for 100 disintegrations of ^{125}I, 144 photons are produced.) One should be aware of these distinctions when evaluating the salesman's declarations of counter qualities. The settings of the machine for counting will, to a certain extent, be important in determining the counting rate obtained. Maintaining optimal counts depends on maintaining constant calibration settings for gamma counting. A standard protocol for calibration is shown in Appendix 37.

SAMPLE COUNTING. The window of the discriminator may be set relatively wide so that it includes not only the photopeak but also some scattered radiation, or it may be set so that it covers the photopeak only. Often window width is set rather arbitrarily at approximate levels that will include the photopeak. At low sample count rates, the quantity S^2/B (where S = net sample count rate and B = background activity) should be optimized. This can be done by centering the window at the photopeak and varying the window width. When the quantity S^2/B is greatest, the fractional standard deviation of the net count rate is minimized.

Almost all counting devices in current use are in some way automated. A variety of systems, including conveyer-type systems and mechanical arms, have been employed for changing of samples. In some cases the samples remain stationary, and the crystal assembly moves to the sample. Regardless of the design of the counting instrument, some considerations are common to all such devices.

1. The instrument should be stable; that is, it should not vary greatly in its efficiency for counting of a particular radioisotope. This can be checked by repeated counting of a standard over a period of several days. Stability deficiencies are often effects of disturbances from the surroundings, such as fluctuations in power supply from the main lines. It is sometimes necessary to install stabilizing or screening devices to prevent such effects. The machine itself should be on an isolated power line so that power surges are minimized. Power surges can cause significantly accelerated wear for electronic parts and can also result in shifts of the energy settings of the counter.

2. The background level should be acceptably low and remain constant over a prolonged period of observation.

3. The shielding of NaI detector systems should be sufficient to minimize interference from radioactive background sources, which may occasionally be encountered in the laboratory.

Liquid scintillation counting

On occasion, it is convenient to utilize for radioassay techniques a radioactive element that emits beta particles as part of its decay process. Beta particle decay is usually detected in high-capacity beta counters, which utilize liquid scintillators.

In this type of system the particle interacts with a molecule (fluor) to excite it above its ground state energy. The fluor, or scintillator, has the property of fluorescing with visible light when it returns to ground state energy. The penetration of the beta particle is so short (half-thickness, 0.008 mm) that the scintillator must be mixed within the sample to be reached by any beta radiation. Therefore, the sample is dissolved in a solution, usually in an organic solvent, that contains the fluor. The light from the interaction of the fluor and emitted particle emerges out of the sample and is collected into a PM tube, and amplification takes place in the same manner as for a gamma counter. Most modern liquid scintillation systems have configurations like that shown in Fig. 7-5.

There are two PM tubes, one on each side of the sample. Pulses are accepted only if they occur at the same time in both tubes, since most electronic noise is a single event, occurring randomly in the PM tubes. The output from the two PM tubes is summed and passed to amplifiers.

Because of the low energy transferred from each disintegration, only a rather small signal is transmitted to the photocathode tube. The level of the signal is not much higher than electronic noise from the PM tubes. For this reason it was necessary, with older models, to refrigerate these counting systems to reduce noise. Newer improvements in circuits and PM tubes have made refrigeration unnecessary.

SAMPLE COUNTING. A variety of techniques have been employed to accomplish the main goals of having a fully soluble sample that is in as intimate contact as possible with the organic fluor. All this must be done without interfering with the transmission of the light produced during fluorescence to the PM tubes.

The sample for liquid scintillation counting includes a mix, or ''cocktail,'' of at least three components: the specimen containing radioactivity, an organic solvent, and an organic molecule as fluor. Other material may be included to enhance the transfer of energy from the beta particle to the fluor or to increase the solubility of the radioactive sample. Mixing the sample and the detector in this way allows easy detection of radioactive particles of very short range, such as the beta radiation from ^{14}C and ^{3}H.

The *solvent* serves three primary purposes. It dissolves both the organic fluor and the radioactive sample; it transfers energy radiation to the fluor; and it permits ready transmission of the light produced to the PM tubes. The sol-

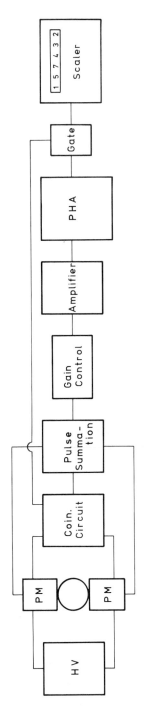

Fig. 7-5. Block diagram of the principal components of a coincidence circuit type of liquid scintillation counter. *HV*, high voltage; *PM*, photomultiplier tube; *PHA*, pulse height analyzer. The two PM tubes record scintillations in the sample located between them. The coincidence circuit registers the scintillations that are recorded by both PM tubes and will open the gate only for them.

vent most frequently used is *toluene*. Toluene transfers the energy readily to the primary fluor and has good solubility for organic samples, such as hydrocarbons and lipids. However, because *dioxane* is freely miscible with water, it is used widely for the counting of aqueous samples. Dioxane gives a lower counting efficiency than toluene, however, because of its less efficient energy transfer from the emitted radiation to the fluor. Naphthalene is frequently added to dioxane-containing cocktails because it frequently improves the energy transfer to the primary fluor.

The *fluor molecule* has the property of releasing light when it receives energy from beta radiation. The most widely used fluor is 2,5-diphenyloxazole (PPO), with fluorescence at the wavelength of 3,800 Å. Frequently, a secondary fluor also is used. The secondary fluor has the property of altering the wavelength of transmitted light to a wavelength that is more suitable for use with a particular PM tube.

Quenching is anything that reduces the amount of light reaching the PM tubes from the primary fluor. Three types of quenching are observed: chemical quenching, color quenching, and optical quenching. *Chemical quenching* occurs when solution components are present that reduce the transfer of energy from solvent to fluor. Examples include strongly acidic solutions and high primary fluor concentrations (self-quenching). *Color quenching* refers to the presence in the cocktail of a colored component that absorbs light photons that have been emitted by the primary and secondary fluors. Addition of a bleaching material, such as H_2O_2, may obviate this problem. *Optical quenching* is the absorption of light photons by a substance, such as condensation or other residue, on the external surface of the vial. Some degree of quenching can be expected in every specimen sample prepared for liquid scintillation counting.

Several techniques have been developed to correct for the quenching effect. Correction is important because the relative sensitivity of detection may be significantly reduced by quenching. In addition, the effect may be variable from sample to sample, as in plasma samples from patients with varying degrees of renal failure, icterus, or hemolysis.

Methods for making such corrections include *internal standardization,* in which a small amount of radioactive standard is added to the sample. By counting before and after addition of the standard, one can determine the sample counting efficiency from the change in count rate. *Channels ratio* is also used to determine counting efficiency of particular samples. This technique relies on the fact that quenching shifts the spectrum of pulse heights observed toward smaller pulse heights. Current liquid scintillation counters have multiple energy channels that record simultaneously. Two channels may be set so that the total spectrum of pulse heights (energies) is counted in one channel, whereas only a fixed fraction (for example, the upper one half to one third) is counted in the other channel. Any shift in the pulse height spectrum, such as would occur with quenching, will be reflected in a change in the ratio between the two channels. The efficiency of counting for unknowns is determined by reference to a standard curve that contains varying amounts of an added quenching agent. *External standardization* is also employed for quench correction. A gamma ray source is placed near the sample. Some of the gamma rays interact within the liquid scintillation cocktail, causing the production of electrons that produce a fluorescence that varies with the degree of quenching. The counting rate in two channels is compared in a manner similar to the channels ratio technique.

In conclusion, the utilization of liquid scintillation counting for samples of biologic material with high protein concentration is significantly more tedious, expensive, and complicated than gamma radiation counting with crystal detectors.

Statistics of radioactive decay

For a particular radioactive nuclide, the probability of decay is not related to the history of the nucleus or to its environment. Thus, within a given population, radioactive decay is essentially a random event for the individual nucleus. However, if the population as a whole is considered, the probability of a given decay follows, and the rate of decay can be predicted. The following formula (Poisson distribution) describes this process:

$$P_n = \frac{r^n}{n!} \, e^{-r}$$

where

P_n = the probability of observing a decay rate in time t
r = the true average decay rate
$n! = n \times (n - 1) \times (n - 2) \times \ldots$
n = number of decays

The Poisson distribution density formula is used to describe the likelihood of occurrence of a rare random event within a population of known characteristics. Its principal application to radioactive decay has been in the calculation of the precision of measurement at a given count rate. It can be shown that for a population that follows a Poisson probability density, the standard deviation of the measurements equals the square root of the mean of the population.

Thus, for a radioactive sample, the total count can be used to determine the precision of radioactivity measurement as simply the square root of the total count rate. Thus, at a total count of 100, a standard deviation of $\pm 10\%$ is to be expected; at 1,000, approximately 3%; at 10,000, about 1%. This approximation is useful only when the background count is negligible compared with the sample count.

Separation devices

A large-sample capacity, general purpose refrigerated centrifuge is basic to the smooth operation of the radioassay laboratory. All assays may be standardized to a particular test tube size, in general 12×75 mm tubes or smaller. A variety of manufacturers make suitable machines of this type. The availability of high-capacity rotor heads, capable of spinning several hundred to 1,000 samples at a time, greatly facilitates high-volume assay work. Interchangeable lower-capacity heads may also be useful.

The usual temperature of operation of the refrigerated centrifuges is around 4° C. At this temperature, no adverse effect on the equilibrium between antibody and antigen is likely to occur.

For most purposes related to separation, high *g* force is not necessary. Most separations require spinning at about 2,000*g*. This is well within the range of most general purpose laboratory centrifuges.

AUTOMATION VERSUS MANUAL PERFORMANCE

Considerations regarding automation usually include *size of individual runs* and *number of reagent steps*.

In general, it is usually not worth automating an assay that has a low-run frequency, such as less than once per week, or a small number of individual tubes in each run. As a rule of thumb, for runs of greater than 100 tubes some degree of automation is usually appropriate.

The number of reagent steps will also influence the desirability of automation. The number of reagent additions will in general not exceed three or four. Automation becomes increasingly desirable as the number of addition steps increases. In some cases, only the radio-active marker and the antibody need to be added to the sample. If the incubation time of the primary reaction is long relative to the time of addition of the reagents, it is usually possible to mix the labeled material and the binder before addition to the sample. This combines the operation into a single step that can be easily performed either by hand or with a simple diluter.

For more complicated assays, more sophisticated radioassay systems have been developed. These include those based on centrifugation flow systems and on systems working with samples in individual tubes. The application of any of these complex systems is a relatively major economical enterprise and should be based on thorough consideration of all aspects of the costs and cost savings involved, that is, not only the instrument price but also reagents, personnel, service, and so forth.

BIBLIOGRAPHY FOR PART I

General

Berson, S. A., and Yalow, R. S., editors: Methods in investigative and diagnostic endocrinology, vols. 2A and 2B, Amsterdam, 1973, North-Holland Publishing Co.

Breuer, H., Hamel, D., and Krüskemper, H. L., editors: Methods of hormone analysis, Stuttgart, 1976, Georg Thieme Verlag.

Cameron, E. H. D., Hillier, S. G., and Griffiths, K.: Steroid immunoassay, Cardiff, U.K., 1975, Alpha Omega Publishing Co.

Diczfalusy, E., editor: Immunoassay of gonadotrophins. Karolinska Symposia No. 1, Acta Endocrinol. (Kbh) **142**(suppl.):1969

Hayes, R. L., Goswitz, F. A., and Pearson Murphy, B. E., editors: Radioisotopes in medicine; in vitro studies. A.E.C. Symposium Series 13, Oak Ridge, Tenn., 1968, U.S. Atomic Energy Commission.

International Atomic Energy Agency: In vitro procedures with radioisotopes in medicine, Vienna, 1970, I.A.E.A.

International Atomic Energy Agency: Radioimmunoassay and related procedures in medicine, Vienna, 1974, I.A.E.A.

Jaffe, B. M., and Behrman, H. R., editors: Methods of hormone radioimmunoassay, New York, 1974, Academic Press, Inc.

Kirkham, K. E., and Hunter, W. M., editors: Radioimmunoassay methods, Edinburgh, 1971, Churchill Livingstone.

Luft, R., and Yalow, R. S., editors: Radioimmunoassay; methodology and applications in physiology and in clinical studies, Stuttgart, 1974, Georg Thieme Verlag.

Odell, W. D., and Daughaday, W. H., editors: Principles of competitive protein-binding assays, Philadelphia, 1971, J. B. Lippincott Co.

Pasternak, C. A., editor: Radioimmunoassay in clinical biochemistry, London, 1975, Heyden & Son Ltd.

Ransom, J. P.: Practical competitive binding assay methods, St. Louis, 1976, The C. V. Mosby Co.

Rothfeld, B., editor: Nuclear medicine in vitro, Philadelphia, 1974, J. B. Lippincott Co.

Sönksen, P. H., editor: Radioimmunoassay and saturation analysis, Br. Med. Bull. **30**(1):1974.

Specific

Bassiri, R. M., and Utiger, R. D.: The preparation and specificity of antibody to thyrotropin releasing hormone, Endocrinology **90**:722, 1972.

Berson, S. A., and Yalow, R. S.: Kinetics of reaction between insulin and insulin binding antibody, J. Clin. Invest. **36**:873, 1957.

Berson, S. A., and Yalow, R. S.: Quantitative aspects of the reaction between insulin and insulin binding antibody, J. Clin. Invest. **38**:1996, 1959.

Berson, S. A., and Yalow, R. S.: Immunoassay of protein hormones; dependence of sensitivity of assay on energy of antigen-antibody reaction. In Pineus, G., Thimann, K. V., and Astwood, E. B., editors: The hormones, vol. IV, II D, New York, London, 1964, Academic Press, Inc., pp. 567-572.

Berson, S. A., and Yalow, R. S.: Iodoinsulin used to determine specific activity of iodine-131, Science **152**:205, 1966.

Berson, S. A., Yalow, R. S., Bauman, A., Rothchild, M. A., and Newerly, K.: Insulin-I[131] metabolism in human subjects; demonstration of insulin binding globulin in the circulation of insulin treated subjects, J. Clin. Invest. **35**:170, 1956.

Bolton, A. E., and Hunter, W. M.: The labelling of proteins to high specific radioactivities by conjugation to a ^{125}I-containing acylating agent, Biochem. J. **133**:529, 1973.

Catt, K., Niall, H. D., and Tregear, G. W.: Solid phase radioimmunoassay of human growth hormone, Biochem. J. **100**:31, 1966.

Catt, K., and Tregear, G. W.: Solid phase radioimmunoassay in antibody-coated tubes, Science **158**:1570, 1967.

Catt, K. J., Tsuruhara, T., and Dufau, M. L.: Radioligand receptor assay of luteinizing hormone, Biochim. Biophys. Acta **279**:194, 1972.

Chard, T., Kitau, M. S., and Landon, J.: The development of a radioimmunoassay for oxytocin; radioiodination, antibody production and separation techniques, J. Endocrinol. **46**:296, 1970.

Dean, P. D. G., Exley, D., and Johnson, M. W.: Preparation of 17β Oestradiol-6-(O-carboxymethyl)-oxime-bovine serum albumin conjugate, Steroids **18**:5, 1971.

den Hollander, F. C., and Schuurs, A. H.: Discussion. In Kirkham, K. E., and Hunter, W. M., editors: Radioimmunoassay methods, Edinburgh, 1971, Churchill Livingstone, p. 419.

Desbuquois, B., and Aurbach, G. D.: Use of polyethylene glycol to separate free and antibody-bound peptide hormones in radioimmunoassays, J. Clin. Endocrinol. Metab. **33**:732, 1971.

Ekins, R. P.: The estimation of thyroxine in human plasma by an electrophoretic technique, Clin. Chim. Acta **5**:463, 1960.

101

Ekins, R. P.: Theoretical aspects of saturation analysis. In International Atomic Energy Agency: In vitro procedures with radioisotopes in medicine, Vienna, 1970, I.A.E.A., p. 325.

Ekins, R. P.: Radioimmunoassay design. In Pasternak, C. A., editor: Radioimmunoassay in clinical biochemistry, London, 1975, Heyden & Son Ltd.

Ekins, R. P., Newman, G. B., and O'Riordan, J. L. H.: Theoretical aspects of saturation and radioimmunoassays. In Hayes, R. L., Goswitz, F. A., and Pearson Murphy, B. E., editors: Radioisotopes in medicine; In vitro studies. A.E.C. Symposium Series 13, Oak Ridge, Tenn., 1968, U.S. Atomic Energy Commission, p. 59.

Ekins, R. P., Newman, G. B., and O'Riordan, J. L. H.: Saturation assays. In McArthur, J. W., and Colton, T., editors: Statistics in endocrinology, Cambridge, Mass., 1970, The MIT Press, p. 345.

England, B. G., Niswender, G. D., and Midgley, A. R., Jr.: Radioimmunoassay of estradiol 17β without chromatography, J. Clin. Endocrinol. Metab. **38:**42, 1974.

Erlanger, B. F., Borek, G., Beiser, S. M., and Lieberman, S.: Steroid-protein conjugates. I. Preparation and characterization of conjugates of bovine serum albumin with testosterone and with cortisone, J. Biol. Chem. **228:**713, 1957.

Erlanger, B. F., Borek, G., Beiser, S. M., and Lieberman, S.: Steroid-protein conjugates. II. Preparation and characterization of conjugates of bovine serum albumin with progesterone, deoxycorticosterone and estrone, J. Biol. Chem. **234:**1090, 1959.

Feinstein, A. R., Bethard, W. F., and McCarthy, J. D.: A new method, using radioiron, for determining the iron binding capacity of human serum, J. Lab. Clin. Med. **42:**907, 1953.

Feldman, H., and Rodbard, D.: Mathematical theory of radioimmunoassay. In Odell, W. D., and Daughaday, W. H., editors: Principles of competitive protein binding assays, Philadelphia, 1971, J. B. Lippincott Co., pp. 158.

Frohman, L. A., Reichlin, H., and Sokal, J. E.: Immunologic and biologic properties of antibodies to glucagon-serum albumin polymer, Endocrinology **87:**1055, 1970.

Garaud, J. C., Moody, A. J., Eloy, R., and Grenier, J. F.: Unusual specificities of antibodies to glucagon-glutaraldehyde-albumin conjugates, Horm. Metab. Res. **8:**241, 1976.

Goodfriend, T. L., Fasman, G., Kemp, D., and Levine, L.: Immunochemical studies of angiotensin, Immunochemistry **3:**223, 1966.

Goodfriend, T. L., Levine, L., and Fasman, G.: Antibodies to bradykinin and angiotensin; a use of carbodiimides in immunology, Science **143:**1344, 1964.

Greenwood, F. C., Hunter, W. M., and Glover, J. S.: The preparation of ^{131}I labelled human growth hormone of high specific activity, Biochem. J. **89:**114, 1963.

Haber, E., Page, L. B., and Jacoby, G. A.: Synthesis of antigenic branch-chain copolymers of angiotensin and poly-L-lysin, Biochemistry **4:**693, 1965.

Haber, E., Page, L. B., and Richards, F. F.: Radioim-

munoassay employing gel filtration, Anal. Biochem. **12:**163, 1965.

Hales, C. N., and Randle, P. S.: Immunoassay of insulin with insulin-antibody precipitate, Biochem. J. **88:**137, 1963.

Hamolsky, M. W., Stein, M., and Freedberg, A. S.: The thyroid hormone–plasma protein complex in man. II. A new in-vitro method for study of uptake of labelled hormonal compounds by human erythrocytes, J. Clin. Endocrinol. Metab. **17:**33, 1957.

Heding, L. G.: A simplified insulin radioimmunoassay method. In Donato, L., Milhaud, G., and Suchis, J., editors: Labelled proteins in tracer studies, Brussels, 1966, Euratom, p. 345.

Heding, L. G.: Determination of total serum insulin (IRI) in insulin treated diabetic patients, Diabetologia **8:**260, 1972.

Helmkamp, R. W., Contresas, M. A., and Bale, W. F.: I-131-labelling of proteins by the iodine monochloride method, Int. J. Appl. Radiat. Isot. **18:**737, 1967.

Herbert, V., Lau, K-S., Gottlieb, C. W., and Bleicher, S. J.: Coated charcoal immunoassay of insulin, J. Clin. Endocrinol. Metab. **25:**1375, 1965.

Hossein, G., Ryan, R. J., Mayberry, W. E., and Hockert, T.: Radioimmunoassay for triiodothyronine (T_3). I. Affinity and specificity of the antibody for T_3, J. Endocrinol. **33:**509, 1971.

Hughes-Jones, N. C.: Nature of the reaction between antigen and antibody, Br. Med. Bull. **19:**171, 1963.

Hunter, W. M., and Greenwood, F. C.: Preparation of iodine-131 labelled human growth hormone of high specific activity, Nature **194:**495, 1962.

Hunter, W. M., and Greenwood, F. C.: A radioimmunoelectrophoretic assay for human hormone, Biochem. J. **91:**43, 1964.

Karush, F.: Immunologic specificity and molecular structure, Adv. Immunol. **2:**1, 1962.

McFarlane, A. S.: Efficient trace-labelling of proteins with iodine, Nature **182:**53, 1958.

Miles, L. E. M., and Hales, C. N.: Labelled antibodies and immunological assay systems, Nature **219:**186, 1968.

Morgan, C. R., and Lazarow, A.: Immunoassay of insulin: two antibody system; plasma insulin levels of normal, subdiabetic, and diabetic rats, Diabetes **12:**115, 1963.

Nars, P. W., and Hunter, W. M.: A method for labelling oestradiol-17β with radioiodine for radioimmunoassays (abstract), J. Endocrinol. **57:**47, 1973.

Orskov, H.: Wick-chromatography for the immunoassay of insulin, Scand. J. Clin. Lab. Invest. **20:**297, 1967.

Peskar, B. A., Peskar, B. M., and Levine, L.: Specificities of antibodies to normetanephrine, Eur. J. Biochem. **26:**191, 1972.

Reichlin, M., Schnur, I. J., and Vance, V. K.: Induction of antibodies to porcine ACTH in rabbits with nonsteroidogenic polymers of BSA and ACTH, Proc. Soc. Exp. Biol. Med. **128:**347, 1968.

Rodbard, D.: Statistical quality control and routine data processing for radioimmunoassays and immunoradiometric assays, Clin. Chem. **20:**1255, 1974.

Rodbard, D., and Cooper, J. A.: A model for the prediction of confidence limits in radioimmunoassays and competitive protein binding assays. In International Atomic Energy Agency: In vitro procedures with radioisotopes in medicine, Vienna, 1970, I.A.E.A., p. 659.

Roitt, I. M., and Torrigiani, G.: Identification and estimation of undegraded thyroglobulin in human serum, Endocrinology **81**:421, 1967.

Rosa, V., Pennisi, F., Bianchi, R., Federighi, G., and Donato, L.: Chemical and biological effects of iodination on human albumin, Biochim. Biophys. Acta **133**: 486, 1967.

Rosselin, G., Assan, R., Yalow, R. S., and Berson, S. A.: Separation of antibody bound and unbound peptide hormones labelled with iodine-131 by talcum powder and precipitated silica, Nature **212**:355, 1966.

Roth, J.: Peptide hormone binding to receptors; a review of direct studies in vitro, Metabolism **22**:1059, 1973.

Scatchard, G.: The attractions of proteins for small molecules and ions, Ann. N.Y. Acad. Sci. **51**:660, 1949.

Scatchard, G., Hughes, W. H., Gurd, F. R. N., and Wilcos, P. E.: In Gurd, F. R. N., editor: Chemical specificity in biological interactions. Memoirs of the University Laboratory Related to Medicine and Public Health, Harvard University, No. 3. New York, 1954, Academic Press, Inc., p. 193.

Sheehan, J. C., Cruickshank, P. A., and Boschart, G. L.: A convenient synthesis of water-soluble carbodiimides, J. Org. Chem. **26**:2525, 1961.

Sheehan, J. C., and Hlavka, J. S.: The use of water-soluble and basic carbodiimides in peptide synthesis, J. Org. Chem. **21**:439, 1956.

Sips, R.: On the structure of a catalyst surface, J. Chem. Phys. **16**:490, 1948.

Spragg, J., Austen, K. F., and Haber, E.: Production of antibodies against bradykinin; demonstration of specificity by complement fixation and radioimmunoassay, J. Immunol. **96**:865, 1966.

Thorell, J. I.: Use of immunosorbent in the preparation of "antigen-free" plasma; an adequate diluent for standards in radioimmunoassay, Clin. Chim. Acta **22**:579, 1968.

Thorell, J. I., and Holmström, B.: Production of antisera against highly purified human follicle-stimulating hormone, luteinizing hormone and thyroid stimulating hormone, J. Endocrinol. **70**:335, 1976.

Thorell, J. I., and Johansson, B. G.: Enzymatic iodination of polypeptides with ^{125}I to high specific activity, Biochim. Biophys. Acta **251**:363, 1971.

Thorell, J. I., and Lanner, Å.: Influence of heparin-plasma, EDTA-plasma, and serum on the determination of insulin with three different radioimmunoassays, Scand. J. Clin. Lab. Invest. **31**:187, 1973.

Thorell, J. I., and Larsson, I.: Lactoperoxidase coupled to polyacrylamide for radio-iodination of proteins to high specific activity, Immunochemistry **11**:203, 1974.

Utiger, R. D., Parker, M. L., and Daughaday, W. H.: Studies on human growth hormone. I. A radioimmunoassay for human growth hormone, J. Clin. Invest. **41**: 254, 1962.

von Schenck, H., and Jeppsson, J-O.: Preparation of mono-iodothyrosine-13-glucagon, Biochim. Biophys. Acta **491**:503, 1977.

von Schenck, H., Larsson, I., and Thorell, J. I.: Improved radioiodination of glucagon with the lactoperoxidase method; influence of pH on iodine substitution, Clin. Chim. Acta **69**:225, 1976.

WHO Expert Committee on Biological Standardization: Twenty-sixth report, Technical Report Series No. 565, Geneva, 1975, World Health Organization.

Wide, L., and Porath, J.: Radioimmunoassay with the use of Sephadex-coupled antibodies, Biochim. Biophys. Acta **130**:257, 1966.

Yalow, R. S.: Radioimmunoassay; practices and pitfalls, Circ. Res. **32**(suppl. 1):116, 1973.

Yalow, R. S., and Berson, S. A.: Immunoassay of endogenous plasma insulin in man. J. Clin. Invest. **39**:1157, 1960.

Yalow, R. S., and Berson, S. A.: General principles of radioimmunoassay. In Hayes, R. L., Goswitz, F. A., and Pearson Murphy, B. E., editors: Radioisotopes in medicine; in vitro studies, AEC Symposium Series 13, Oak Ridge, Tenn., 1968, U.S. Atomic Energy Commission, p. 7.

Yalow, R. S., and Berson, S. A.: Special problems in the radioimmunoassay of small peptides, In Protein and polypeptide hormones, vol. I, 1968, Excerpta Medica Foundation, p. 71.

Yalow, R. S., and Berson, S. A.: Review paper; general aspects of radioimmunoassay procedures. In International Atomic Energy Agency: In vitro procedures with radioisotopes in medicine, Vienna, 1970, I.A.E.A., p. 455.

Yalow, R. S., and Berson, S. A.: Radioimmunoassays. In McArthur, J. W., and Colton, T., editors: Statistics in endocrinology, Cambridge, Mass., 1970, The MIT Press, p. 327.

Young, J. D., Byrnes, D. J., Chisholm, D. J., Griffiths, F. B., and Lazarus, L.: Radioimmunoassay of gastrin in human serum, J. Nucl. Med. **10**:746, 1969.

PART II

Clinical applications

The optimal utilization of the radioligand techniques in clinical practice is dependent not only on high quality performance of the assays, but also on their appropriate application to the clinical situation. There are several aspects that must be considered in every individual case. These include factors such as timing and conditions of sampling in relation to the state of the patient with respect to time of day, diet, therapy, and so forth. The treatment and transportation of the sample may also affect the results. The sample usually consists of venous blood. Capillary blood sometimes gives spurious results, probably related to hemolysis. In fact, hemolysis in a plasma sample may adversely affect any assay. Thus freezing and thawing of whole blood make it unsuitable for assay. Both plasma and serum are usually equally suitable for assay work, although excessive amounts of heparin as an anticoagulant may influence the precipitation step in double-antibody methods. Most proteins are quite stable once blood has been drawn, but generally plasma or serum should be separated rapidly from blood cells. Certain proteins are prone to degradation in vitro; this may be reduced by the addition of enzyme inhibitors, such as Trasylol or benzamidin, and rapid freezing. When plasma or serum has been frozen at $-20°$ C, most proteins are stable for long periods.

Let us next consider the problem of when samples should be drawn from the patient. Both the secretion rate and the turnover rate in plasma of the compound to be assayed must be considered in the light of the function to be measured. Medium-size polypeptides, including most protein hormones, circulate without being bound to any carrier protein, and, as a result,

these substances have a very rapid plasma clearance rate that ranges from a clearance half-time of about 4 minutes for insulin to about 30 minutes for chorionic gonadotropin. When plasma clearance is this rapid, plasma levels will primarily reflect the secretion rate. The secretion pattern of many hormones is characterized by intermittent bursts of secretion separated by long periods of relatively low rates of secretion. In such instances, random samples may not reveal overall functional activity. Plasma or urine sampling must be carefully planned to permit detection of these rapid changes, usually by frequent sampling over extended periods or by use of special sampling devices that allow virtually continuous sampling. Usually it is not practical to continuously sample in this way, and another approach is taken; the gland is stimulated or suppressed to achieve a known functional status at the time of sampling. Generally, stimulation tests are used when hypofunction of the organ is suspected. Inhibition tests are usually used to verify hyperfunction, for example, the autonomous type of secretion observed in certain neoplastic diseases. Since the response to stimulation or inhibition tests is subject to biologic variation, accuracy of such tests is improved by obtaining repeated samples over a period of time instead of simply measuring a single point on the response curve. Baseline samples should also be included. This is particularly important since the between-assay variation of many RIAs is great; changes from baseline levels are often more informative than the absolute values after stimulation or suppression.

It is also important to be assured that stimulation or inhibition has been achieved. If possible, the effect should be monitored by some parameter unrelated to the assay. For example, during an insulin tolerance test performed to induce growth hormone release, the blood glucose should be monitored to be certain that adequate hypoglycemia has been induced. The blood sugar should fall to half the control value. Monitoring is also performed to be sure that hypoglycemia does not become too severe. During prolonged fasting to inhibit insulin secretion, blood glucose levels should be measured to ensure a gradual decrease in the values.

Other examples are given in the sections that follow. In general, it can be stated that viewing the assay in the light of the clinical questions and with careful design of the sampling process will result in more information than simple inspection of laboratory results that have reached the patient's chart by some mysterious procedure unknown to the physician taking care of the patient.

What should a physician do when faced with an unexpected result? He first asks himself whether his initial hypothesis was wrong or if the results could be otherwise explained by the state of the patient. However, he must also be aware of the possibility that the results are related to technical inaccuracies anywhere along the line from the point when he requested a particular study to the report of the assay results. Inaccuracies due to technical errors may yield results that are too high or low, depending on the type of assay. Substances that inhibit the binding of ligand to receptor will increase the free fraction in the assay; this will usually be falsely interpreted as an elevated value. However, if the inhibition of binding is the result of degradation of the radioligand, the type of separation method used in the assay will determine whether a falsely low or high value will result. If the bound fraction is measured after antibody precipitation, the bound activity will be low, and therefore the final assay value reported will be too high. If the free fraction is measured instead, following adsorption to charcoal, degraded radioligand may not absorb to the charcoal. The apparent value will then be too low. Technically, the spurious nature of values that are too low is more easily determined, since this situation often results in some

samples with "negative" values, which obviously will increase the suspicion that something is wrong.

In the clinical chapters that follow we have attempted insofar as possible to maintain a consistent organizational scheme to facilitate use of this text as a ready reference. The following scheme is used in all the chapters.

- A. Chemistry
- B. Physiology
- C. Method
  1. Reagents
  2. Performance
  3. Assay properties
- D. Clinical applications
  1. Pathophysiology
  2. Sampling
  3. Reference values
  4. Interpretation of results

After a variable degree of introductory material to set the stage for the test in the clinical context, we discuss *chemistry,* particularly from a structural viewpoint. The chemistry will determine several important assay parameters, such as the use of the untreated substance as an immunogen, the stability of the substance, and appropriate separation techniques. In a discussion of *physiology,* the normal function that the substance to be assayed performs in the well patient is described. *Method* is a description of the radioassay of the substance, with emphasis on common generally applicable methods for clinical measurement. Typically, this section is subdivided into a discussion of reagents, assay performance, and special assay properties, such as problem areas and sensitivity. We summarize the assays in schematic fashion in boxes in which the information about common methodology is condensed. The abundance of methodologic variants despite the common principles used in most methods has made this condensation necessary. These overviews do not intend to cover all possible variants reported. However, the main procedures presented in the boxes have been performed in our own laboratories in heavy clinical practice over a long period. This implies at least that they have worked well in our hands and should not involve unanticipated problems in actual performance. The sections on *clinical applications* include discus-

---

LEGEND TO BOXES

Principle

R $\quad$ = *Receptor (binding protein)*

R_L $\quad$ = *Subscript* L *indicates the ligand to which R is directed*

R_a $\quad$ = *Receptor added during course of assay*

R_e $\quad$ = *Endogenous receptor*

$\qquad$ *The expressions R_L, R_a, and R_e are used only when some clarification is required regarding which receptor-ligand combination is being discussed*

L $\quad$ = *Ligand*

L* $\quad$ = *Radioligand*

S-R = *Receptor coupled to a solid phase*

S-L = *Ligand coupled to a solid phase*

RL $\quad$ = *Ligand bound to receptor*

Horizontal part of arrow indicates the $\qquad$ *Arrow indicates separation between reactants affected by separation* $\qquad$ *bound and free activity method*

Protocol

| R | | *Receptor preparation of the assay (specific binder)* |

| S-R | | *Receptor coupled to a solid phase* |

| L* | | *Radioligand* |

| L | | *Ligand; alternatively, the preparation and concentrations used for* standard *or the form of* sample *to be assayed* |

| S-L | | *Ligand coupled to a solid phase* |

| I | | *Inhibitor used, for example, to prevent binding to plasma proteins or to other nonspecific binders* |

───────── *Time of primary incubation* ─────────

 $\quad$ *Procedures and reagents used to achieve separation of bound and free activity*

───────── *Time of incubation for separation step* ─────────

Reagents $\qquad$ *More specific description of the reagents with reference to the appendixes where their production and properties are given*

$\qquad$ T = *Total activity and amount of radioligand added to each tube*

Alternatives $\qquad$ *References to alternative reagents and procedures reported*

sions of *pathophysiology* (that is, the abnormalities that occur in concentration of the substance to be assayed in various disease states), and *sampling* (that is, the problems related to obtaining the specimen in the appropriate state for testing). This section also includes the various provocative tests that may be used to improve diagnostic accuracy. *Reference values* are then quoted for the commonly accepted values of the normal range and the normal results of provocative testing. *Interpretation of results* of testing is then discussed, including interpretation of elevated and decreased values relative to the normal range. Provocative test (stimulation and inhibition) outcomes are also discussed. These results are discussed in the context of the principal indications for using the assay in the clinical setting.

8 PITUITARY-THYROID AXIS

Thyroid-stimulating hormone
Thyroxine
Triiodothyronine
T_3-binding capacity

Clinical thyroid testing is becoming more dependent on RIA and similar in vitro methodologies. These techniques have largely supplanted the radioactive iodine–uptake and other in vivo thyroid tests. With increasing availability of the newer RIA tests for thyroid function, this trend is likely to continue.

Current medical practice relies on a measurement of the total thyroxine circulating in the blood, the T_4 (D) or T_4 (RIA),* as the basic screening test for patients suspected on clinical grounds of having thyroid dysfunction. Fre-

---

*Throughout this chapter we use the standard nomenclature proposed by the American Thyroid Association for thyroid testing (Table 8-1).

Table 8-1. Standard abbreviations of thyroid tests

Description	Test abbreviation
^{131}I-thyroid uptake	RAIU
Thyrotropin by RIA	TSH (RIA)
Total serum T_4	
By competitive protein binding (displacement analysis)	T_4 (D)
By radioimmunoassay	T_4 (RIA)
Total serum T_3	T_3 (RIA)
By radioimmunoassay	
Measurements of hormone binding	
Percent free T_4	$\% FT_4$
Free T_4 concentration	FT_4
Resin T_3 uptake in vitro	RT_3U
Free T_4 index	T_4-RT_3 index

quently an estimate of the binding capacity of serum proteins for T_4, such as the resin triiodothyronine (T_3) uptake test (RT_3U), is included as a part of the screening examination. Triiodothyronine by RIA, T_3 (RIA), and thyroid-stimulating hormone by RIA, TSH (RIA) are commonly employed to aid in the differential diagnosis of thyroid problems.

Methods for measuring thyroglobulin, thyroglobulin antibodies, reverse T_3, and thyroid-binding globulin by RIA have recently become available. Thus radioligand assays have been developed for most of the known substances involved in thyroid-pituitary homeostasis.

In this chapter we consider in detail the most widely used of these methods: TSH (RIA), T_4 (RIA), T_3 (RIA), and resin T_3 uptake (RT_3U).

PITUITARY-THYROID HOMEOSTASIS

Normal thyroid status depends on effective function at five levels: (1) the hypothalamus and its release of thyrotropin-releasing hormone, TRH (synonymous terms are thyrotropin-releasing factor, TRF, and thyroliberin); (2) the adenohypophysis and its release of thyroid-stimulating hormone, (TSH or thyrotropin); (3) the thyroid and its secretion of the active thyroid hormones thyroxine (T_4) and triiodothyronine (T_3); (4) the plasma space with its specific thyroid-binding plasma proteins; and (5) the target organ and its specific cell receptors.

TRH is produced in the hypothalamus as a tripeptide amide, pyroglutamyl-histidyl-prolinamide. TRH is transported from the hypothalamus via the portal system of the pituitary to the region of the adenohypophysis where it stimulates basophilic cells to produce and release TSH. The TSH thus produced stimulates the thyroid gland to increase the production and release of the active thyroid hormones T_3 and T_4; therefore, plasma levels of T_3 and T_4 are increased. Increased plasma levels of T_3 and T_4 in turn inhibit the release of TSH and probably also TRH. Conversely, if the plasma levels of T_4 and T_3 fall, TSH secretion is stimulated. Thus TSH is the prime regulator of the rate of function of the thyroid gland and hence of thyroid hormone production and secretion. The secretion of TSH is in turn regulated by the concentration of thyroid hormones in the blood.

In view of the several levels of control of thyroid homeostasis, it is not surprising that the clinical assessment of thyroid function usually requires the combined interpretation of several tests.

THYROID-STIMULATING HORMONE
Chemistry

TSH is a glycoprotein with a molecular weight of approximately 28,000. The protein contains one alpha and one beta polypeptide subunit. The alpha chain is shared with other glycoprotein hormones of the same species, such as human chorionic gonadotropin (hCG), luteinizing hormone (LH), and follicle-stimulating hormone (FSH). It differs between species; thus the native TSH molecule is highly species specific.

It is the beta subunit of TSH that determines the specific physiology of the hormone.

Physiology

TSH is essential to normal thyroid function, and, in the absence of TSH, the thyroid gland undergoes involution. TSH is involved in the

---

hTSH METHOD

Principle

Double antibody

$$R + [L + L^*] = [RL + RL^*] + [L + L^*]$$

Protocol

		Reagent	Volume
DAY 1	R	*Rabbit antiserum to hTSH*	*200 μl*
	L*	*^{125}I-hTSH*	*200 μl*
	L { Standard / Sample }	*hTSH, 1.88, 3.75, 7.5, 15, 30, 60 μU/liter* / *Plasma*	*100 μl*

16 hours, 4° C

		Reagent	Volume
DAY 2	↓	*Normal human plasma to standards*	*100 μl*
		Barbital-BSA to plasma samples	*100 μl*
		Normal rabbit serum (1:250)	*50 μl*
		Goat antiserum to rabbit IgG (1:10)	*50 μl*

16 hours, 4° C

Box 8-1 (see p. 107 for legend to boxes)

---

hTSH METHOD, cont'd

DAY 3	Add diluent	*500 μl*
	Centrifugation, 2,500g, 15 minutes, 4° C	
	Decant supernatant	
	Count precipitate 2 minutes	

Reagents

R — *Antiserum to hTSH absorbed with hCG (Appendix 39); no cross-reaction with hCG, hFSH, or hLH after absorption Avidity:$K_a \approx 1.2 \times 10^{11}$*

L* — *Labeled with ^{125}I by lactoperoxidase (Appendix 17) Specific activity 120μCi-160μCi/μg; separation on Sephadex G-50 (Appendix 19) T = 10,000 cpm ≈ 0.05 ng*

L — *Standards diluted in diluent EDTA-plasma; plasma may be transported unfrozen*

Diluent — *Barbital-BSA (Appendix 34)*

↓ *Appendix 28*

Alternatives

R — *Guinea pig antiserum to hTSH[30]*

L* — *hTSH labeled with ^{131}I[30,46,56] or ^{125}I[1,26,29,57,58,60,76] by the chloramine-T method*

L — *Serum[26,30,46,57,58,60,76]*

I — *hCG added[26,57,58,60]*

Diluent — *Phosphate-BSA,[57,76] phosphate-HSA[1,29,58]*

↓ *Solid phase coupled antibody[26] DA-sheep,[29] DA-rabbit,[46] DA-donkey[1]*

Box 8-1 (see p. 107 for legend to boxes)

regulation of all levels of thyroid endocrine function: (1) the production of hormone is stimulated by increasing the amount of thyroid iodide transported into the gland and by increasing the organic binding of iodide; (2) storage of hormone is affected, since TSH increases the rate of coupling of iodotyrosines into thyroglobulin; (3) release of hormone is stimulated both directly and via an increased proteolysis of thyroglobulin. Accompanying these effects, there is a general increase in glandular intermediary metabolism.

TSH is a part of a sensitive control system that keeps the serum concentration of thyroid hormones within fairly narrow limits. TSH secretion is under direct control of the hypothalamus. The tripeptide amide, pyroglutamyl-histidyl-prolinamide (TRH), is produced in the hypothalamus. TRH is transported from the hypothalamus to the pituitary via the portal system.

TRH stimulates basophilic cells in the adenohypophysis to produce TSH. The TSH produced stimulates the thyroid gland to produce T_4. Increasing blood levels of T_4 inhibit the release of TSH and probably also of TRH. Conversely, in response to a falling concentration of T_4 and T_3 in the blood, TSH secretion is stimulated. In man, the half-time of TSH turnover in plasma is approximately 1 hour, and the daily secretory rate of TSH is about 170 mU. Both the half-time of plasma clearance and the secretory rate of TSH are increased in hypothyroidism. In hyperthyroidism, however, plasma half-time is shortened.

Method

Reagents

The development of highly purified TSH preparations paved the way for subsequent development of an RIA for serum TSH. Even the most highly purified preparations of TSH contain fractions of different chromatographic and electrophoretic behavior. Some of these fractions have equivalent biologic potency; others have lower potencies. The situation has been improved by the development of standards that have been made available by agencies such as the World Health Organization, the Medical Research Council (Great Britain), and the Na-

tional Institutes of Health (United States). The standard preparations of TSH are calibrated by bioassay in international units (IU) of TSH activity. Because of impurities in these preparations, they usually give quite different potencies in immunoassays. In addition, since the standards are impure, the immunologic potency depends to an extent on the specificity of the anti-TSH antibodies used for immunoassay. Different antisera may give different potency estimates. Furthermore, the immunologic potency is usually considerably higher than the biologic potency.

The antisera often show marked cross-reaction with the glycoprotein hormones (LH, FSH, and hCG). This is partly the result of a true cross-reaction against the common antigenic sites in the alpha subunit shared by all of the glycoprotein hormones. Furthermore, a portion of the nonspecificity of the antisera may be caused by the presence of contaminating pituitary material in the immunogen used to produce TSH antisera, so that antibodies to LH and FSH may actually be induced. Regardless of the causes of this nonspecificity, the antisera may be made significantly more specific for TSH by absorbing anti-TSH antisera with hCG before TSH assay. Antibodies directed against the alpha chain, as well as those against the LH subunit, will react against hCG. The more specific antibodies, which are directed against the TSH beta chain, will still be available for binding to TSH. Most assays utilize rabbit anti-TSH as the receptor and ^{125}I-labeled TSH as radioligand.

Performance

With the improvement of antisera avidity, incubation time has been significantly shortened, from 5 to 7 days down to 24 hours or less. Double-antibody precipitation (DA) and solid phase techniques have been the separation methods most widely used; hCG is usually added to absorb out alpha chain–directed antibodies. TSH-free serum, either from hormone-suppressed normal volunteers or from hyperthyroid or hypophysectomized patients, may be added to the standard curve tubes in order to reduce the importance of nonidentity between samples and standards due to nonspecific protein interactions that interfere with the receptor-ligand interaction or separation of bound and free activity.

Assay properties

The development of TSH (RIA) has been complicated by two factors: the variability of reference TSH preparations and the cross-reactivity of TSH antisera with other glycoprotein hormones.

Assay sensitivities of the various RIAs reported are comparable, varying from $0.1\mu U$ to $1.0\mu U/ml$. Despite this fact, most TSH assays do not permit the measurement of decreased values. This is in part related to the fact that there is significant variation in plasma interference between individuals; thus it is particularly difficult to determine a true 0-level for TSH hormone. TSH concentration is usually at or below the limits of assay sensitivity in normal patients. For this reason, extraction procedures have been developed to concentrate TSH. For most clinical problems, however, such sensitivity is not necessary, and TSH is usually measured in unextracted serum.

Clinical applications
Pathophysiology

Hypersecretion of TSH occurs as a consequence of hypofunction of the thyroid due to decreased plasma levels of thyroid hormones. The suspicion of hypothyroid disorders is the main clinical reason for assaying TSH in plasma. This secondary TSH overproduction is not known to have any pathophysiologic effects. Primary TSH overproduction may very rarely give rise to hyperthyroidism. This situation has been reported with pituitary tumors and increased TRH secretion. Also, certain malignancies may produce TSH-like material, particularly hydatidiform mole and choriocarcinoma.

Hyposecretion of TSH occurs in secondary hypothyroidism, which refers to the clinical state in which there is insufficient secretion of TSH to support normal metabolism of the thyroid gland and a fall in thyroid hormone to low levels is observed. Most commonly, a destructive process of the pituitary is the cause. Important clinical states that give rise to pituitary in-

sufficiency are postpartum pituitary necrosis and pituitary tumors (such as chromophobe adenomas or craniopharyngiomas), and following hypophyseal surgery. Usually the TSH abnormality is associated with deficiency of other trophic hormones, such as the gonadotropins and ACTH.

Sampling

TSH is usually collected in serum and is stable at room temperature. If frozen, TSH is stable for years. Random serum sampling is the most common method employed. Serum TSH concentration does not undergo marked diurnal variation, and stimuli that elicit secretion of some pituitary hormones, such as hypoglycemia or other stressful situations, do not affect the release of TSH. In pregnancy, TSH concentrations are unchanged. A TRH stimulation test was recently introduced as a method for study of hyposecretion of TSH. The initial test is done by giving intravenously a dose of $200\mu g$ of synthetic human TRH. In normal patients, a prompt increase in serum TSH concentration is observed to peak at about 30 minutes

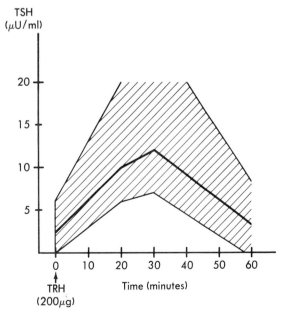

Fig. 8-1. Plasma levels of TSH following intravenous injection of $200\mu g$ TRH (mean and 95% confidence limits).

after injection. The average increase is about $10\mu U/ml$ (Fig. 8-1).

Reference values

Normal: $0\text{-}10\mu U/ml$
Hypothyroidism: $> 15\mu U/ml$

Interpretation of results

ELEVATED TSH CONCENTRATION. Serum TSH levels are greatly elevated in primary myxedema. With replacement of thyroid hormone, there follows a progressive decrease in serum TSH concentration. Levels up to $100\mu U/ml$ are frequently seen in untreated hypothyroidism. Monitoring of TSH levels is a useful guide to the adequacy of replacement therapy.

DECREASED TSH CONCENTRATION. TSH levels are not measurable in hyperthyroidism or hypopituitarism and secondary myxedema. As mentioned previously, most assays do not permit differentiation between normal and decreased TSH levels. In hypothyroidism the response of serum TSH to TRH infusion (see Sampling, above) is greatly increased. In circumstances of increased concentration of thyroid hormone, however, the response of TSH to TRH administration is markedly reduced. In patients with thyrotoxicosis, no effect is observed; thus TRH may be used in the differential diagnosis of thyrotoxicosis. In particular, in patients with coexisting cardiac disease, it may replace T_3 suppression testing in the differential diagnosis. Also, in a manner analogous to the T_3 suppression test, it may be possible to identify autonomous thyroid nodules that have not as yet developed the hyperthyroid state. With increasing age, a blunted TSH response to TRH occurs in a normal population. For this reason, the TSH stimulation test should not be taken as the only indicator of thyroid hyperfunction. However, a normal or supranormal response to TRH injection is good evidence of the absence of hyperthyroidism. As a very rare clinical circumstance, an isolated deficiency of TSH may lead to hypothyroidism. This disorder has been reported in association with pseudohypoparathyroidism and hypothalamic disorders in which TRH secretion is reduced. The diagnosis of isolated TSH deficiency is made when TSH levels are low, bovine TSH causes a definite in-

crease in T_4 and RAIU, and other pituitary functions are normal.

THYROXINE
Chemistry

The chemical structure of L-thyroxine (L-tetraiodothyronine) is shown in Fig. 8-2. The active hormonal form has the same structure in all vertebrates. During storage T_4 is joined by peptide linkage within a storage protein thyroglobulin. Just before secretion of T_4, thyroglobulin is broken into its constituent amino acids.

Physiology

T_4 is produced by the acinar epithelium of the thyroid gland. A large reserve of T_4 is stored in the thyroid gland, within the thyroid follicle. This reserve is sufficient to supply the body's need for thyroid hormone for 2 weeks or more.

Within the bloodstream, T_4 circulates bound to plasma proteins. Over 99.97% of plasma T_4 is bound, principally to the interalpha globulin TBG. Some T_4 is also bound to albumin and thyroid-binding prealbumin (TBPA). Protein-bound thyroid hormone is metabolically inac-

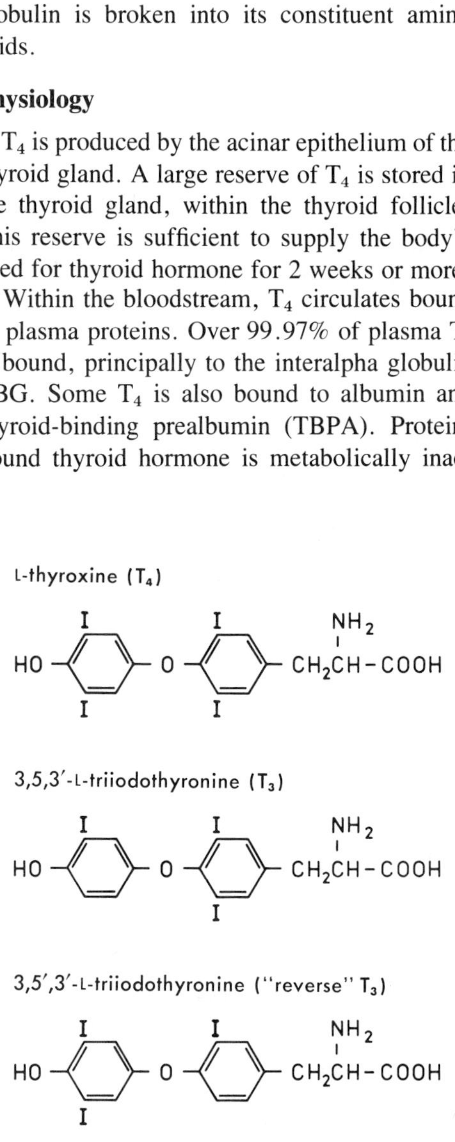

Fig. 8-2. Structure of L-thyroxine (T_4), triiodothyronine (T_3), and "reverse" triiodothyronine ("reverse" T_3).

tive; it is the "free" T_4 that exerts metabolic effects. Within the plasma, T_4 has a half-life of about 8 days. About $60\mu g$ of T_4 are extracted daily from the blood by target tissues.

Specific binding proteins have been found for T_4 and T_3, in the cytoplasm of cells. In addition, there also appear to be nuclear receptor sites that are particularly avid for T_3. A significant proportion of T_4 is metabolized to T_3 circulating in plasma.

Method

Reagents

Measurement of total T_4 was one of the first radioligand assays developed. Development was made easier because the natural iodine constituent of thyroxine facilitated production of the radioactive tracer; in addition, a specific binding protein was readily available in serum. The first decade of measurement of total T_4 was dominated by assays that employed TBG as receptor. The improved methodology for producing antibodies to small molecules permitted the development of antibodies to T_4 coupled to serum albumin. These antibodies are highly specific and are able to distinguish between molecules differing by only one atom, for example, between thyroxine and triiodothyronine.

Most methods use antibodies against a serum albumin–thyroxine conjugate. Thyroglobulin has also been used as an immunogen, since this protein contains thyroxine as part of its structure. Various reagents have been employed to inhibit the binding of thyroxine to plasma proteins in patient samples, since such binding interferes with the primary antibody-antigen reaction. 8-Anilino naphthalene sulfonic acid (ANS) and thimerosal (Merthiolate) are thus presently used for this purpose. Other compounds that have been used include salicylate, tetrachlorothyronine (a halogenated thyroxine derivative), and phenytoin (Dilantin). ^{125}I is by far the most commonly employed tracer, although ^{131}I has been used as well.

Performance

Serum absorbed with charcoal to remove thyroxine (T_4-free serum) is frequently added to standard curve samples. Separation techniques vary, but adsorption of unbound thyroxine to activated charcoal predominates. Time needed to perform the assay ranges from a few hours to several days. Other separation techniques used include double-antibody methods and polyethylene glycol precipitation.

Assay properties

These RIA techniques have the major advantage of being able to measure T_4 in unextracted serum. RIA has now become the dominant assay type for the measurement of total T_4. Sensitivity and specificity claims for the reported methods are comparable. Sensitivity is about 10 to 15 ng/ml.

Thyroid-binding proteins can interfere with the primary antigen-antibody reaction; however, with the use of specific agents to block uptake, this is usually not a major problem.

Method overview for T_4 (RIA) is presented in Box 8-2. A method for measuring T_4 and T_3 together is shown in Box 8-4.

"Free" T_4

Since the free thyroid hormone in blood is the active hormonal form, considerable effort has been directed toward measurement of the concentration of free T_4 (FT_4) present. FT_4 may be estimated indirectly by a dialysis technique. A small quantity of ^{125}I-T_4 or ^{131}I-T_4 is added to serum and allowed to equilibrate with hormone that is bound to thyroid-binding proteins. The tracer rapidly equilibrates between the bound and unbound fractions. The labeled serum is then dialyzed against a buffer. The free hormone readily penetrates the pores of the dialysis membrane, whereas the hormone bound to proteins is retained within the membrane. The fraction of dialyzable ("free") T_4 is measured by counting the radioactivity present. If this test is combined with a measurement of total T_4—T_4 (RIA) or T_4 (D)—the concentration of FT_4 can be calculated. Normal range is 1 to 2 ng/100 ml.

The assay of FT_4 is relatively tedious to perform, since it requires 24 hours of dialysis for best results. The absolute amount of free hormone is only 0.03% of the total hormone concentration; thus great care is required to avoid contamination of the "free" hormone fraction by the total hormone fraction. Because of these

---

T_4 METHOD

Principle

Charcoal adsorption

$$R + [L + L^*] = [RL + RL^*] + [L + L^*]$$

Protocol

	Reagent	Volume
DAY 1 R	*Rabbit antiserum to thyroxine*	*200 μl*
L*	*^{125}I-thyroxine*	*200 μl*
L Standard / Sample	*L-thyroxine, 7, 5, 15, 30, 60, 120, 240 nmol/liter* / *Serum*	*50 μl*
I	*ANS*	

─────── *16 hours, 4° C* ───────

DAY 2 ↓
Dextran-coated charcoal   *1,000 μl*
1 hour, 4° C
Centrifugation, 2,500g, 4° C, 15 minutes
Decant supernatant in another tube
Count supernatant 2 minutes

Reagents

R
Avidity: $K_a \approx 10^9$

L*
Specific activity $\gtrsim 50 \mu Ci/\mu g$
T = 20,000 cpm $\approx$ 0.6 ng

L
Standard diluted in hormone-free normal human serum (Appendix 36)
Serum

I
ANS (8-anilino-naphthalene sulfonic acid sodium salt): 1 mg of ANS per ml, added to ^{125}I-thyroxine reagent

Diluent
Barbital-BSA (Appendix 34)

↓
Appendix 27

Box 8-2

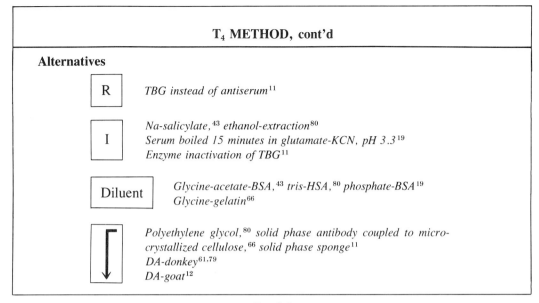

T₄ METHOD, cont'd

Alternatives

R — *TBG instead of antiserum*[11]

I — *Na-salicylate,*[43] *ethanol-extraction*[80]
Serum boiled 15 minutes in glutamate-KCN, pH 3.3[19]
Enzyme inactivation of TBG[11]

Diluent — *Glycine-acetate-BSA,*[43] *tris-HSA,*[80] *phosphate-BSA*[19]
Glycine-gelatin[66]

↓ — *Polyethylene glycol,*[80] *solid phase antibody coupled to micro-crystallized cellulose,*[66] *solid phase sponge*[11]
DA-donkey[61,79]
DA-goat[12]

Box 8-2

requirements, the test has been primarily used for research applications. A simplified estimate of FT₄ is the FT₄ index, which is calculated by multiplying the estimate of total T₄ with the T₃-binding capacity (expressed as a percent of a normal value).

Clinical applications

Pathophysiology

Hyperfunction of the thyroid gland or, more broadly speaking, "thyrotoxicosis" is a clinical state in which an excess amount of thyroid hormone is presented to the peripheral tissues. This excess of thyroid hormone is manifested in virtually every organ system, with the common denominator of accelerated metabolism. Thyrotoxicosis is usually associated with hyperfunction of thyroid glandular tissue with accelerated production and release of thyroid hormone into the bloodstream. Among several disease states that cause hyperthyroidism, diffuse toxic goiter (Graves' disease or Basedow's disease) is the most common. Other causes include toxic multinodular goiter and toxic adenoma. In all of these disorders, the thyroid has lost its normal responsiveness to the inhibition of a falling serum TSH level. The hyperthyroid gland is said to be "nonresponsive," "autonomous," and "nonsuppressible," because it functions

independently of the TSH concentration in the blood. Thyrotoxicosis factitia is a disorder that occurs because of excessive ingestion of thyroid hormone.

Hypofunction occurs when the thyroid tissue fails to provide enough thyroid hormone to the peripheral tissues. There is a widespread reduction in the metabolism and activity of a variety of tissues. The absence of thyroid hormone will lead ultimately to coma, with progressively falling body temperatures and failure of several organ systems, leading to death. Hypothyroidism may be caused by primary failure of the thyroid gland (primary or thyroprival hypothyroidism). Most commonly, this is idiopathic, although it is thought to be a late manifestation of an autoimmune thyroiditis. Hypothyroidism also occurs quite commonly as an end stage of treated hyperthyroidism. Hypothyroidism may occur at birth if the thyroid does not develop normally. This can lead to cretinism, a state of mental and physical retardation that is only partially reversible by replacement of thyroid hormone. Hypothyroidism may also occur because of a low level of circulating TSH (p. 113).

Sampling

T₄ samples are usually serum. T₄ is stable in serum for several days even at room tempera-

Table 8-2. Clinical states that alter thyroid-binding protein concentrations

Protein	Increase	Decrease
TBG	Pregnancy	Hyperthyroidism
	Hypothyroidism	Acromegaly
	Hepatitis	Klinefelter's syndrome
	Cirrhosis	Down's syndrome
	Acute intermittent porphyria	Nephrotic syndrome
		Hyperlipidemia, type III
		Metabolic acidosis
		Major illness
		Major surgery
TBPA	Acromegaly	Pregnancy
		Hyperthyroidism
		Major illness
		Major surgery

Table 8-3. Drugs that alter thyroid-binding protein concentrations

Protein	Increase	Decrease	Competes for binding with T_4
TBG	Estrogens	Androgens	Phenytoin (Dilantin)
	Oral contraceptives	Corticosteroids	T_3
	Perphenazine (Trilafon)	Phenylbutazone	Dicumarol
TBPA	Androgens	Penicillin	Salicylates
	Corticosteroids	(high dose)	Dinitrophenol

ture and for prolonged periods when frozen. There is little diurnal variation, and T_4 concentration is relatively unaffected by fasting or acute febrile illness. Random serum samples give a reliable indication of clinical status.

Reference values

Normal: 45 to 120 ng/ml (60-150 nmol/liter)
Hypothyroid: 5 to 50 ng/ml (<65 nmol/liter)
Hyperthyroid: 120 to 460 ng/ml (> 150 nmol/liter)

Interpretation of results

Elevated levels are observed in patients with hyperthyroidism. In addition, patients who are undergoing replacement therapy with thyroxine may also have elevated immunoreactivity without hypermetabolism. In this case, the elevations are mild, perhaps just above the normal range.

Decreased levels are observed in hypothyroidism of both primary and secondary types.

The differential diagnosis of these disorders is best made using TSH.

A wide variety of clinical conditions can increase or decrease the plasma concentration of T_4 by affecting binding proteins (Table 8-2). This can have important implications for interpretation of the tests of T_4 concentration, since an elevation of T_4 in the blood may be wrongly thought to be due to thyroid overactivity when the real cause is an increase in binding protein concentrations. Certain drugs may interfere with the binding of T_4 (Table 8-3). Thus the T_4 (RIA) is often interpreted along with a test of T_3-binding capacity to give an estimate of expected free hormone concentration (p. 117).

TRIIODOTHYRONINE
Chemistry

The chemical form of T_3 (3,5,3'-L-triiodothyronine) is shown in Fig. 8-2. Like T_4 it is stored within the thyroid as part of the protein thyroglobulin.

Physiology

Like T_4, T_3 is produced within the thyroid gland by the acinar epithelium. The thyroid secretes T_3 in mass amounts that are less than 10% of the T_4 secreted. However, the thyroid secretion of T_3 is only a minor source of the T_3 produced. The majority is produced by mono-deiodination of T_4 in the peripheral tissues. On a mass basis, T_3 is about four times more potent than T_4. Therefore, T_3 may be regarded as the major biologically active thyroid hormone and T_4 essentially as a prohormone. T_3 concentration is influenced by changes in TBG concentration, in a manner similar to T_4. The biologic effects of T_3 are the same as those mentioned for T_4. About 99.9% of T_3 within the bloodstream is protein bound, almost exclusively to TBG. T_3 has a $T_{1/2}$ in plasma of 2.0 days. The daily runover of T_3 is about $30\mu g/day$.

Method

TBG was used as a binder in the earliest assays of total T_3 concentration. These methods required separation of T_3 and T_4 before assay, and the relatively low affinity of T_3 for TBG compromised sensitivity. With the development of T_3 (RIA), measurement of total T_3 concentration on a routine clinical basis became practical for the first time.

Reagents

Specific antisera to T_3 were first produced by Brown and associates, using polylysine conjugate of T_3 as immunogen.

Most methods of RIA employ antibodies directed against an albumin-T_3 conjugate, although antibodies to polylysine conjugates and thyroglobulin have also been used. As in T_4 (RIA), ANS in a barbital buffer is used to block binding of T_3 to serum proteins.

Performance

Charcoal adsorption is the most frequently used separation method. Separation by solid phase methods has also been successfully employed in several "kit" methods.

Several investigators have employed simultaneous RIA for T_3 and T_4 in serum. These methods use two isotopes of iodine, ^{131}I and ^{125}I, and differential gamma spectroscopy to trace the radioligands. The technique has the advantage of saving technician time, since two assays can be performed simultaneously (see Box 8-4).

Assay properties

Thyroid-binding proteins in serum may interfere with the primary antigen-antibody reaction. Since the T_4 concentration is about 80 to 100 times the concentration of T_3 in serum, the close structural similarity of T_3 and T_4 makes some degree of cross-reactivity likely; thus a highly specific antiserum is required for T_3 (RIA).

Assay sensitivity and specificity for most assays reported are comparable, and cross-reactivity of the T_3 antibody with T_4 is less than 1:5,000 of T_3 reactivity on a weight basis. An overview of available methods is shown in Box 8-3.

Clinical applications

Pathophysiology

Hyperproduction of T_3 is always found in hyperthyroidism as far as is now known. Frequently, T_3 levels are much more elevated than T_4 levels, which indicates that T_3 is being produced directly by the thyroid gland in relatively greater abundance than T_4. In addition, the ratio of T_3 to T_4 within the thyroid gland is much increased in hyperthyroidism. In some patients hyperthyroidism may be manifested only by T_3 elevation. This diagnostic entity has been called T_3 thyrotoxicosis. This disorder tends to occur early in the course of thyrotoxicosis, and in the majority of cases it is later associated with T_4 elevations as well. T_3 thyrotoxicosis may not be accompanied by any other laboratory abnormalities of thyroid function. For example, the T_4 may be normal or even low; the radioactive iodine uptake (RAIU) may be high, normal, or low. A T_3 suppression RAIU will be abnormal; however, T_3 thyroxicosis probably makes up less than 5% of hyperthyroidism in most patient series. T_3 thyrotoxicosis is very common in hyperthyroid patients in iodine-deficient areas and may make up the majority of patients in these areas.

Hypoproduction of T_3 accompanies hypothyroidism and may also occur in the euthyroid

T₃ METHOD

Principle

Charcoal adsorption

$$R + [L + L^*] = [RL + RL^*] + [L + L^*]$$

Protocol

		Reagent	Volume
DAY 1	R	Rabbit antiserum to triiodothyronine	200 μl
	L*	¹²⁵I-triiodothyronine	200 μl
			50 μl
	L	Standard / Sample — 3,5,3'-triiodo-L-thyronine (0.38, 0.75, 1.5, 3.0, 6.0, 12.0 nmol/liter) / Serum	
	I	ANS	

―――――――――― 16 hours, 4° C ――――――――――

| DAY 2 | ↓ | Dextran-coated charcoal 1 hour, 4° C Centrifugation 2,500g, 4° C 15 minutes Decant supernatant in another tube Count supernatant 2 minutes | 1,000 μl |

Reagents

R — Antiserum with cross-reaction to L-tetraiodothyronine less than 0.1%; avidity: $K_a \approx 1 \times 10^{10}$

L* — Specific activity = 500 μCi/μg; T = 20,000 cpm ≈ 30 pg

L — Standard diluted in hormone-free normal human serum (Appendix 36); Serum

I — ANS (8-anilino-naphthalene sulfonic acid sodium salt): 1 mg of ANS per ml, added to ¹²⁵I-triiodothyronine reagent

Diluent — Barbital-BSA (Appendix 34)

↓ — Appendix 27

Box 8-3

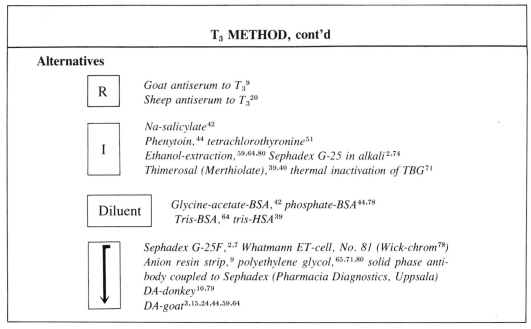

T₃ METHOD, cont'd

Alternatives

| R | *Goat antiserum to T₃*[9]
 Sheep antiserum to T₃[20] |

| I | *Na-salicylate*[42]
 Phenytoin,[44] *tetrachlorothyronine*[51]
 Ethanol-extraction,[59,64,80] *Sephadex G-25 in alkali*[2,74]
 Thimerosal (Merthiolate),[39,40] *thermal inactivation of TBG*[71] |

| Diluent | *Glycine-acetate-BSA,*[42] *phosphate-BSA*[44,78]
 Tris-BSA,[64] *tris-HSA*[39] |

| ↓ | *Sephadex G-25F,*[2,7] *Whatmann ET-cell, No. 81 (Wick-chrom*[78])
 Anion resin strip,[9] *polyethylene glycol,*[65,71,80] *solid phase antibody coupled to Sephadex (Pharmacia Diagnostics, Uppsala)*
 DA-donkey[10,79]
 DA-goat[3,15,24,44,59,64] |

Box 8-3

---

patient during an acute febrile illness. This is apparently due to a change in the normal peripheral conversion of T₄ to T₃; more reverse T₃ is formed instead.

Sampling

T₃ (RIA) methods usually measure T₃ in serum. After drawing the sample, the serum is separated from the clot as soon as is practical and stored in the refrigerator before assay. If more than 24 hours will elapse between sampling and assay, the serum samples are frozen.

Reference values

Normal: 1.5 ± 1 ng/ml
Hyperthyroidism: > 3.0 ng/ml

Interpretation of results

Elevation of T₃ by RIA is probably the single best indicator of hyperthyroidism. In fact, if T₃ (RIA) is normal in what seems to be a hypermetabolic state, the diagnosis should be carefully scrutinized.

Decreased values of T₃ by RIA do not necessarily imply hypothyroidism. T₃ (RIA) may be low in euthyroid patients during acute febrile illness. Although T₃ (RIA) tends to be de-creased in hypothyroidism, normal T₃ (RIA) values are not infrequent in the hypothyroid state. Thus T₃ (RIA) is not particularly helpful in the diagnosis of hypothyroidism.

"REVERSE" T₃

During hormone metabolism the inactive metabolite "reverse" T₃, 3,3′,5′-L-triiodothyronine, is formed (see Fig. 8-2). This metabolite may be measured by a specific RIA. The measurement of reverse T₃ may have clinical usefulness in the evaluation of thyroid function of the fetus. If the fetal thyroid gland is functioning, reverse T₃ levels in amniotic fluid are relatively high and easily measured by RIA. This test provides the best assessment of fetal thyroid function; although maternal thyroid hormones and metabolites pass the placenta, the fetal thyroid produces a relatively large amount of reverse T₃, and thus amniotic reverse T₃ predominantly reflects fetal and not maternal thyroid activity.

**T₃-BINDING CAPACITY
(RESIN T₃ UPTAKE)
Method**

Since most thyroid hormone circulates bound to protein in plasma, changes in the concentra-

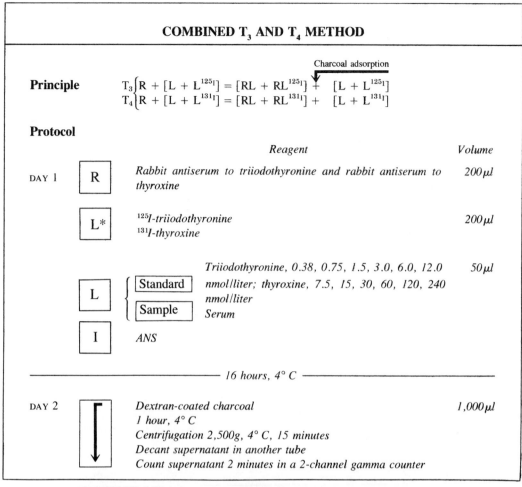

COMBINED T₃ AND T₄ METHOD

Principle

$$T_3 \begin{cases} R + [L + L^{125I}] = [RL + RL^{125I}] + [L + L^{125I}] \\ R + [L + L^{131I}] = [RL + RL^{131I}] + [L + L^{131I}] \end{cases}$$

Charcoal adsorption

Protocol

		Reagent	Volume
DAY 1	R	*Rabbit antiserum to triiodothyronine and rabbit antiserum to thyroxine*	*200 μl*
	L*	*^{125}I-triiodothyronine* *^{131}I-thyroxine*	*200 μl*
	L { Standard	*Triiodothyronine, 0.38, 0.75, 1.5, 3.0, 6.0, 12.0 nmol/liter; thyroxine, 7.5, 15, 30, 60, 120, 240 nmol/liter*	*50 μl*
	Sample	*Serum*	
	I	*ANS*	

——————— *16 hours, 4° C* ———————

| DAY 2 | ↓ | *Dextran-coated charcoal*
1 hour, 4° C
Centrifugation 2,500g, 4° C, 15 minutes
Decant supernatant in another tube
Count supernatant 2 minutes in a 2-channel gamma counter | *1,000 μl* |

Box 8-4

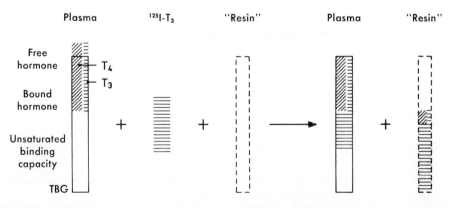

Fig. 8-3. Principle of the T_3 binding capacity test (RT₃U). The added ^{125}I-T_3 is taken up by the free binding sites of TBG and by the resin. If the free binding sites of TBG are decreased (for example, because of a TBG deficiency or because the sites are occupied by an increased T_4 production), the ^{125}I-T_3 will to a greater degree be taken up by the resin. If the free binding capacity of TBG is increased (for example, by low T_4 levels or increased TBG as in pregnancy), the resin will bind less ^{125}I-T_3.

COMBINED T$_3$ and T$_4$ METHOD, cont'd

Reagents

R	*Antiserum to triiodothyronine with less than 0.1% cross-reaction to thyroxine; avidity: $K_a = 1 \times 10^{10}$*
	Antiserum to thyroxine; avidity: $K_a = 1 \times 10^9$

L*	*^{125}I-triiodothyronine, specificity activity $\geqq 500\,\mu Ci/\mu g$*
	$T = 20,000$ cpm ≈ 30 pg
	^{131}I-thyroxine, specific activity $\geqq 50\,\mu Ci/\mu g$
	$T = 20,000$ cpm ≈ 0.6 ng

L	*Standard diluted in hormone-free normal human serum (Appendix 36)*
	Thyroxine standard may not contain more than 0.1% triiodothyronine

I	*ANS: 1 mg ANS contained per ml of radioligand solution*

Diluent	*Barbital-BSA (Appendix 34)*

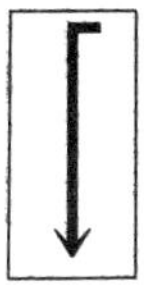

Appendix 27

Box 8-4

---

tion of the binding proteins will markedly influence the thyroid hormone concentration. An indirect estimate of the capacity of plasma proteins to bind thyroid hormones has been developed, the T$_3$ uptake test (RT$_3$U). This test measures the ability of the patient's plasma proteins to compete with a secondary binder, such as a resin bed, red cells, or a rubber sponge matrix, for radiolabeled T$_3$. T$_3$ is used in this test because it is bound less avidly than T$_4$ to the thyroid-binding proteins. This allows more favorable uptake onto the resin bed or other binder, which can be more easily quantitated. The principle of the resin T$_3$ uptake is given in Fig. 8-3. This technique gives an estimate of unoccupied binding sites of transporting proteins, chiefly TBG, that is, the thyroid-binding

capacity of TBG. ^{125}I-triiodothyronine is added to a serum sample. Equilibrium occurs with binding to TBG that is proportional to the number of binding sites available on the proteins. The mixture is passed through a resin column, and any unbound triiodothyronine is absorbed. Radioactivity is then measured, and the results are expressed as the percent of total activity taken up onto the column. The greater the number of binding sites, the lower the uptake on the resin.

Reagents

^{125}I-triiodothyronine is most often used as the radioligand. A variety of secondary binders, such as resin, silicate, sponge, Sephadex, and red cells, have been employed.

T₃-UPTAKE TEST

Nonsoluble phase

Principle $R_e + L^* + R_a = R_eL^* + R_aL^*$ (see Fig. 8-3)

Protocol

	Reagent	Volume

DAY 1 $\boxed{L^*}$ *¹²⁵I-triiodothyronine*   *5.0 ml*

$\boxed{R_e}$ $\left\{\begin{array}{l}\boxed{\text{Standard}} \\ \boxed{\text{Sample}}\end{array}\right.$ *Normal pool serum*
Serum sample   *0.5 ml*

Sephadex G-25 Coarse, powder

——————————— *10 minutes, room temperature* ———————————
(tubes rotated continuously)

$\boxed{R_a}$ *Gel is allowed to settle; aspirate supernatant; add 10 ml diluent, rotate tubes 60 times, aspirate supernatant; repeat washing twice; count the gel; collect at least 6,000 counts*

Reagents

$\boxed{L^*}$ *¹²⁵I-triiodothyronine, specific activity = 50 μCi/μg*

$\boxed{R_a}$ *Sephadex G-25 Coarse (0.5 g added to each tube)*

$\boxed{R_e}$ *Serum; sample expressed in percent binding of normal pool serum, set to 100%*

$\boxed{\text{Diluent}}$ *Barbital-BSA (Appendix 34)*

Alternatives

$\boxed{L^*}$ *¹³¹I-triiodothyronine*[23,25,27,28,32,38]

$\boxed{\text{Diluent}}$ *Saline,*[23,27,32] *saline with HSA*[33]*; tris buffer*[28]*; phosphate buffer*[25]*; acetate-barbiturate buffer*[38]*; Michaels buffer with albumin*[63]

$\boxed{\downarrow}$ *Red blood cells*[27,32]*; Amberlite IRA-400 on sponge*[28] *or on paper disc*[23]*; BSA-coated charcoal*[38]*; hemoglobin-coated charcoal*[33]
Albumin microspheres[63]
Resin sponge (Abbots, Inc., Chicago); molecule sieve (Radiochemical Center, Amersham)

Box 8-5

Performance

Binding to the TBG in patient serum is facilitated by an incubation step in some assays. The labeled serum is then added to the secondary binder, which extracts any unbound T_3 from the mixture. The amount of radioactivity extractable from the plasma is an estimate of the number of unoccupied binding sites available on the TBG. In some procedures, a ''standard'' serum is included for reference, and the results of the T_3 uptake are expressed as a percent of the standard.

Assay properties

The details of a specific method are shown in Box 8-5.

Variations in temperature may interfere with the test, since the binding to resins of T_3 is somewhat temperature dependent. Also, since the binding of T_3 to the resin is somewhat time dependent, it is important that the samples and standards have about the same time of incubation. If these precautions are taken, however, reproducible results are obtained.

Clinical applications
Sampling

Random serum samples are usually employed.

Reference values

Data are presented in terms of the percent of the total that is taken up onto the resin column or secondary binder, that is, that which is *not* bound to TBG. For most assays, values range from 35% to 45%, but the actual value is a function of the particular method used and depends on the specific activity of the tracer T_3 and the avidity of the secondary binder for T_3. A number of approaches have been taken to standardize this number. One method has been to express these results in relationship to a normal plasma pool with uptake set at 100%. In this situation, the usual normal range is 80% to 125%.

Interpretation of results

Decreased uptake. Relatively low T_3-uptake values occur when the number of available binding sites increases. With an increase in con-

centration of TBG, there will be a relatively reduced free fraction of radio-T_3 to bind to the resin; thus the measured uptake will be below the normal range.

Increased uptake. Relatively high values of resin T_3 uptake indicate a relatively lower number of available TBG binding sites. This situation could occur either if there were more binding sites occupied by total T_3 or if there was a reduced concentration of the hormone.

See Tables 8-2 and 8-3 for factors likely to affect thyroid-binding protein concentrations.

Resin T_3 uptake should be interpreted in the light of a total T_4 serum concentration determined either by RIA or by competitive protein binding.

FREE T_4 INDEX. In order to give an estimate of the amount of free thyroxine hormone present in plasma, the values from T_3 uptake and total T_4 have been combined into a free T_4 index. This free T_4 index has been shown to be closely related to the actual concentration of free T_4 in serum as measured by the dialysis technique for free T_4 concentration. The index is the product of total T_4 concentration times the value of the RT_3U test. Since the resin T_3 uptake reflects the number of TBG binding sites present and since total T_4 concentration indicates total hormone, the product should be approximately proportional to free T_4. Some assays combine these measurements into a single value, that is, the effective thyroxine ratio; however, since both total T_4 and TBG binding capacity are important in themselves, we believe that each should be measured separately if possible.

REFERENCES

1. Acebedo, G., Hayek, A., Klegerman, M., and others: A rapid ultramicro radioimmunoassay for human thyrotropin, Biochem. Biophys. Res. Commun. **65**(2): 449, 1975.
2. Alexander, N. M., and Jennings, J. F.: Radioimmunoassay of serum triiodothyronine on small, reusable, Sephadex columns, Clin. Chem. **20**:1353, 1974.
3. Beckers, C., Cornette, C., and Thallaso, M.: Serum L-triiodothyronine in radioimmunoassay; measurements in normal subjects and in thyroid patients, J. Nucl. Biol. Med. **1**:121, 1974.
4. Braverman, L. E., Vagenakis, A. G., Foster, A. E., and others: Evaluation of a simplified technique for the specific measurement of serum thyroxine concentration, J. Clin. Endocrinol. Metab. **32**:497, 1971.

5. Brown, B. L., and Ekins, R. P.: A specific saturation assay technique for serum triiodothyronine. In International Atomic Energy Agency: In-vitro procedures with radioisotopes in medicine, Vienna, 1970, I.A.E.A., p. 569.

6. Brown, B. L., Ekins, R. P., Ellis, S. M., and others: Specific antibodies to triiodothyronine hormone, Nature (Lond.) **226:**359, 1970.

7. Burger, A., Sakaloff, C., Staeheli, V., Vallotton, M. B., and Ingbar, S. H.: Radioimmunoassay of 3,5,3'-triiodothyronine with and without a prior extraction step, Acta Endocrinol. (Kbh.) **80:**58, 1975.

8. Burger, A., Suter, P., Nicod, P., and others: Reduced active thyroid hormone levels in acute illness, Lancet **1:**653, 1976.

9. Burman, K. D., Wright, F. D., Earll, J. M., and Wartofsky, L.: Evaluation of a rapid and simple technique for the radioimmunoassay of triiodothyronine (T_3), J. Nucl. Med. **16:**622, 1975.

10. Challand, G. S., Ratcliffe, W. A., and Ratcliffe, J. G.: Semi-automated radioimmunoassays for total serum thyroxine and triiodothyronine, Clin. Chim. Acta **60:** 25, 1975.

11. Chau, K. H., and Cummins, L. M.: A new extractant for serum thyroxine by enzymatic digestion of thyroxine binding proteins, J. Clin. Endocrinol. Metab. **42:**189, 1976.

12. Chopra, I. J.: A radioimmunoassay for measurement of thyroxine in unextracted serum, J. Clin. Endocrinol. Metab. **34:**938, 1972.

13. Chopra, I. J.: A radioimmunoassay for measurement of 3,3',5'-triiodothyronine (reverse T3), J. Clin. Invest. **54:**583, 1974.

14. Chopra, I. J., and Crandall, B. F.: Thyroid hormones and TSH in amniotic fluid, N. Engl. J. Med. **293:**740, 1975.

15. Chopra, I. J., Ho, R. S., and Lam, R.: An improved radioimmunoassay of triiodothyronine in serum; its application to clinical and physiological studies, J. Lab. Clin. Med. **80:**729, 1972.

16. Chopra, I. J., Solomon, D. H., and Beall, G. N.: Radioimmunoassay for measurement of triiodothyronine in human serum, J. Clin. Invest. **50:**2033, 1971.

17. Clark, F., and Horn, D. B.: Assessment of thyroid function by the combined use of the serum protein-bound iodide and resin uptake of ^{131}I-triiodothyronine, J. Clin. Endocrinol. Metab. **35:**39, 1965.

18. Condliffe, P. G.: Purification of human thyrotropin, Endocrinology **72:**893, 1963.

19. Dunn, R. T., and Foster, L. B.: Radioimmunossay of thyroxine in unextracted serum by a single antibody technique, Clin. Chem. **19**(19): 1063, 1973.

20. Eastman, C. J., Corcoran, J. M., Ekins, R. P., Williams, E. S., and Nabarro, J. D. N.: The radioimmunoassay of triiodothyronine and its clinical application, J. Clin. Pathol. **28:**225, 1975.

21. Ekins, R. P.: The estimation of thyroxine in human plasma by an electrophoretic technique, Clin. Chim. Acta **5:**453, 1960.

22. Emerson, C. H., and Utiger, R. D.: Hyperthyroidism and excessive thyrotropin secretion, N. Engl. J. Med. **287:**328, 1972.

23. Faran, H. E. A., and Evans, K.: The uptake of ^{131}I-triiodothyronine from serum by resin impregnated paper in-vitro, J. Clin. Endocrinol. Metab. **32:**265, 1965.

24. Gharib, H., Mayberry, W. E., and Ryan, R. J.: Radioimmunoassay for triiodothyronine; a preliminary report, J. Clin. Endocrinol. Metab. **31:**709, 1970.

25. Gimlette, T. M. D.: Use of Sephadex column chromatography in the assessment of thyroid status, J. Clin. Pathol. **20:**170, 1967.

26. Gladstein, E., McHardy-Young, S., Brast, and others: Alterations in serum thyrotropin (TSH) and thyroid function following radiotherapy in patients with malignant lymphoma, J. Clin. Endocrinol. Metab. **32:**833, 1971.

27. Golden, A. W. G., Gartside, J. M., Jackson, D. J., and Osario, C.: Uptake of ^{131}I-triiodothyronine by red cells, Lancet **2:**218, 1962.

28. Golden, A. W. G., Gartside, J. M., and Osario, C.: An evaluation of ^{131}I-triiodothyronine resin sponge test, J. Clin. Endocrinol. Metab. **25:**127, 1965.

29. Gordin, A., and Sharinen, P.: Methodological study of the radioimmunoassay of thyrotropin, Acta Endocrinol. (Kbh.) **72:**24, 1972.

30. Hall, R., Amos, J., and Ormston, B. J.: Radioimmunoassay of human serum thyrotrophin, Br. Med. J. **1:**582, 1971.

31. Hamilton, C. R., Adams, L. C., and others: Hyperthyroidism due to thyroglobulin-producing pituitary cromophobe adenoma, N. Engl. J. Med. **283:**1077, 1970.

32. Hamolsky, M. W., Stein, M., and Freedberg, A. S.: The thyroid hormone–plasma protein complex in man. II. A new in-vitro method for study of uptake of labelled hormonal components by human erythrocytes, J. Clin. Endocrinol. Metab. **17:**33, 1957.

33. Herbert, V., Gottlieb, C. W., Lau, K. S., and others: Adsorption of I-131-triiodothyronine (T3) from serum by charcoal as an in vitro test of thyroid function, J. Lab. Clin. Med. **66:**814, 1965.

34. Herrmann, J., Rusche, H. J., and Krüskemper, H. L.: Rapid radioimmunoassay for the evaluation of thyroxine in unextracted serum, Clin. Chim. Acta **54**(1): 69, 1974.

35. Hershman, J. M., and Pittman, J. A.: Utility of the radioimmunoassay of serum thyrotropin in man, Ann. Intern. Med. **74:**481, 1971.

36. Hollander, C. S., and Shenkman, L.: Radioimmunoassay of triiodothyronine and thyroxine. In Rothfeld, B.: Nuclear medicine in-vitro, Philadelphia, 1974, J. B. Lippincott Co., p. 136.

37. Ingbar, S. H., Braverman, L. E., Dawber, N. A., and others: A new method for measuring the free thyroid hormone in human serum and an analysis of the factors that influence its concentration, J. Clin. Invest. **44:**1679, 1965.

38. Irvine, W. J., and Stenderer, R. M.: Serum triiodothyronine uptake using coated charcoal in the assessment

of thyroid function, J. Clin. Endocrinol. Metab. **41:** 31, 1968.

39. Kanagasabapathy, A. S., Wellby, M. L.: The use of merthiolate for TBG-blocking in the radioimmunoassay of triiodothyronine, Clin. Chim. Acta **55:**267, 1974.

40. Kirkegaard, C., Friis, T., and Siersbaek-Nielsen, K.: Measurements of serum triiodothyronine by radioimmunoassay, Acta Endocrinol. (Kbh.) **77:**71, 1974.

41. Kourides, I. A., Weintraub, B. D., Levko, M. A., and others: Alpha and beta subunits of human thyrotropin; purification and development of specific radioimmunoassays, Endocrinology **94:**1411, 1974.

42. Larsen, P. R.: Direct immunoassay of triiodothyronine in human serum, J. Clin. Invest. **51:**1939, 1972.

43. Larsen, P. R., Dockalova, J., Sipula, D., and others: Immunoassay of thyroxine in unextracted human serum, J. Clin. Endocrinol. Metab. **37:**177, 1973.

44. Lieblich, J., and Utiger, R. D.: Triiodothyronine radioimmunoassay, J. Clin. Invest. **51:**157, 1972.

45. Ljunggren, J. G., Persson, B., and Tryselius, M.: Rapid simultaneous radioimmunoassay for the measurement of triiodothyronine and thyroxine in unextracted human serum, Acta Endocrinol. (Kbh.) **81:** 487, 1976.

46. Mayberry, W. E., Bilstad, J. M., and Sizemore, G. W.: Radioimmunoassay for human thyrotropin, Ann. Intern. Med. **74:**471, 1971.

47. Meinhold, H., and Wenzel, K. W.: Radioimmunoassay for triiodothyronine and thyroxine in unextracted sera; methodological aspects and clinical application. In International Atomic Energy Agency: Radioimmunoassay and related procedures in medicine, vol. 2, Vienna, 1974, I.A.E.A., pp. 127-160.

48. Michell, J. L., Harden, A. B., and O'Rourke, M. F.: The in-vitro resin sponge uptake of triiodothyronine-^{131}I from serum in thyroid disease and pregnancy, J. Clin. Endocrinol. Metab. **20:**1474, 1960.

49. Mincey, E. K., Thorson, S. C., Brown, J. L., and others: A new parameter of thyroid function, the effective thyroxine ratio, J. Nucl. Med. **13:**165, 1972.

50. Mitsuma, T., Colucci, J., Shenkman, L., and others: Rapid simultaneous radioimmunoassay for triiodothyronine and thyroxine in unextracted serum, Biochem. Biophys. Res. Commun. **46:**2107, 1972.

51. Mitsuma, T., Gershengorn, M., Colucci, J., and others: Radioimmunoassay of triiodothyronine in unextracted human serum, J. Clin. Endocrinol. Metab. **33:** 364, 1971.

52. Murphy, B. E. P., and Pattee, C. J.: Determination of thyroxine utilizing the property of protein-binding, J. Clin. Endocrinol. Metab. **24:**187, 1964.

53. Nauman, J. A., Nauman, A., and Werner, S. C.: Total and free triiodothyronine in human serum, J. Clin. Invest. **46:**1346, 1967.

54. Nelson, J. C., Johnson, D. E., and Odell, W. D.: Serum TSH levels and thyroidal response to TSH stimulation in patients with thyroid disease, Ann. Intern. Med. **76:**47, 1972.

55. Nosslin, B.: A simplified technique for the triiodothy-

ronine uptake test with Sephadex, Scand. J. Clin. Lab. Invest. **17**(Suppl. 86):177, 1965.

56. Odell, W. D., Wilber, J. F., and Paul, W. E.: Radioimmunoassay of thyrotropin in human serum, J. Clin. Endocrinol. Metab. **25:**1179, 1965.

57. Odell, W. D., Wilber, J. F., and Utiger, R. D.: Studies of thyrotropin physiology by means of radioimmunoassay, Recent Prog. Horm. Res. **23:**47, 1967.

58. Patel, Y. C., Benger, H. G., and Hudson, B.: Radioimmunoassay of serum thyrotropin; sensitivity and specificity, J. Clin. Endocrinol. Metab. **33:**768, 1971.

59. Patel, Y. C., and Burger, H. G.: A simplified radioimmunoassay for triiodothyronine, J. Clin. Endocrinol. Metab. **36:**187, 1973.

60. Pekry, A. E., Hershman, J. M., and Parlow, A. F.: A sensitive and precise radioimmunoassay for human thyroid stimulating hormone, J. Clin. Endocrinol. Metab. **41:**676, 1975.

61. Ratcliffe, W. A., Ratcliffe, J. G., McBride, A. D., and others: The radioimmunoassay of thyroxine in unextracted human serum, Clin. Endocrinol. (Oxf.) **3**(4): 481, 1974.

62. Ridgeway, E. C., Weintraub, B. D., Cevallos, J. L., and others: Suppression of pituitary TSH secretion in the patient with a hyperfunctioning thyroid nodule, J. Clin. Invest. **52:**2783, 1973.

63. Rolleri, E., Buzzigoli, G., and Palssio, G.: Serum triiodothyronine (T_3) uptake using albumin microspheres in the assessment of thyroid function, J. Nucl. Med. **13:**893, 1972.

64. Rubenstein, H. A., Butler, J. V. P., and Werner, S. C.: Progressive decrease in serum triiodothyronine concentrations with human aging; radioimmunoassay following extraction of serum, J. Clin. Endocrinol. Metab. **37:**247, 1973.

65. Sekadde, C. B., Slaunwhite, R. W., and Aeltour, T.: Rapid radioimmunoassay of triiodothyronine, Clin. Chem. **19:**1016, 1973.

66. Seth, J., Rutherford, F. J., and McKenzie, I.: Solid phase radioimmunoassay of thyroxine in untreated serum, Clin. Chem. **21**(10):1406, 1975.

67. Solomon, D. H., Bennotti, J., and others: A nomenclature for tests of thyroid hormones in serum; report of a committee of the American Thyroid Association, J. Clin. Endocrinol. Metab. **34:**884, 1972.

68. Sterling, K., Bellabarba, D., Newman, E. S., and others: Determination of triiodothyronine concentration in human serum, J. Clin. Invest. **48:**1150, 1969.

69. Sterling, K., and Brenner, M. F.: Free thyroxine in human serum; simplified measurement with the aid of magnesium precipitation, J. Clin. Invest. **45:**153, 1966.

70. Sterling, K., Brenner, M. A., and others: The significance of triiodothyronine (T_3) in maintenance of euthyroid status after treatment of hyperthyroidism, J. Clin. Endocrinol. Metab. **33:**729, 1971.

71. Sterling, K., and Milch, P. O.: Thermal inactivation of thyroxine-binding globulin for direct radioimmunoassay of triiodothyronine in serum, J. Clin. Endocrinol. **38:**866, 1974.

72. Sterling, K., Refellof, S., and others: T_3 thyrotoxicosis; thyrotoxicosis due to elevated serum triiodothyronine levels, J.A.M.A. **213:**571, 1970.
73. Sterling, R., and Tabachnik, M.: Resin uptake of I-131-triiodothyronine as a test of thyroid function, J. Clin. Endocrinol. Metab. **21:**456, 1961.
74. Surks, M. I., Schadlow, A. R., and Oppenheimer, J. H.: A new radioimmunoassay for plasma L-triiodothyronine; measurements in thyroid disease and in patients maintained on hormonal replacement, J. Clin. Invest. **51:**3104, 1972.
75. Utiger, R. D.: Radioimmunoassay of human plasma thyrotropin, J. Clin. Invest. **44:**1277, 1965.
76. Utiger, R. D.: Thyrotropin radioimmunoassay. In Jaffe, B. M., and Behrman, H. R., editors: Methods of hormone radioimmunoassay, New York, 1974, Academic Press, Inc., pp. 161-171.
77. Vaitukaitis, J. L., Ross, G. T., Reichert, L. E., Jr., and others: Immunologic basis for within and between species cross-reactivity of luteinizing hormone, Endocrinology **91:**1337, 1972.
78. Weeke, J., and Örskoy, H.: Ultrasensitive radioimmunoassay for direct determination of free triiodothyronine concentration in serum, Scand. J. Clin. Lab. Invest. **35:**237, 1975.
79. Wenzel, K. W., and Meinhold, H.: Radioimmunoassay for T_3 and T_4 in unextracted sera. In International Atomic Energy Agency: Radioimmunoassay and related procedures in medicine, Vienna, 1974, I.A.E.A., p. 127.
80. Werner, S. C., Acebedo, G., and Radichewich, I.: Rapid radioimmunoassay for T4 and T3 in the same sample of human serum, J. Clin. Endocrinol. Metab. **38**(3):493, 1974.

9 PITUITARY-ADRENAL AXIS

ACTH
Cortisol

The pituitary-adrenal axis is involved in the regulation of only one aspect of adrenal function, the secretion of glucocorticoids. The main participants in this system are adrenocorticotropic hormone (ACTH) of the anterior pituitary and cortisol of the adrenal cortex.

ADRENOCORTICOTROPIC HORMONE
Chemistry

ACTH is a single-chain polypeptide with a molecular weight of 4,500; it consists of 39 amino acids. The part containing the first 24 N-terminal amino acids is essential for its biologic effect and is identical in many mammalian species. Species differences are principally located in the 25-39 portion, the function of which is unknown. Synthetic ACTH containing the 1-24 amino acids is used for clinical purposes.

Several other polypeptides with varying degrees of homology with ACTH are produced in the anterior pituitary. These include melanocyte-stimulating hormones (α-MSH and β-MSH) and lipotropin. Their state and biologic effects are still a matter of debate. A peptide that shares immunoreactivity with ACTH has been isolated. This polypeptide has been named "big ACTH," since it has a much larger molecular weight than ACTH. Big ACTH has about 2% of the biologic activity of ACTH.

Physiology

ACTH is released intermittently from the anterior pituitary (adenohypophysis). ACTH circulates in plasma without any obvious binding to transporting proteins and, like other small protein hormones, disappears rapidly from blood with a half-life of 5 to 10 minutes in vivo.

The production of ACTH by the pituitary is primarily under the influence of three factors: the level of cortisollike steroids, a biologic clock, and stress. When the cortisol level goes up, the production of ACTH goes down. If cortisol is maintained at high serum levels, the ACTH will fall to unmeasurable levels. Similarly, when cortisol levels fall, ACTH levels rise.

There is a natural rhythm to ACTH secretion, and the secretion of cortisol (Fig. 9-1) parallels

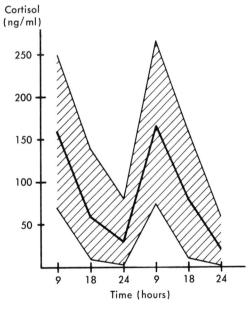

Fig. 9-1. Serum concentration of cortisol versus time of day. There is a marked diurnal variation in serum cortisol concentration, with a peak in the early morning and a low point after midnight.

Cortisol

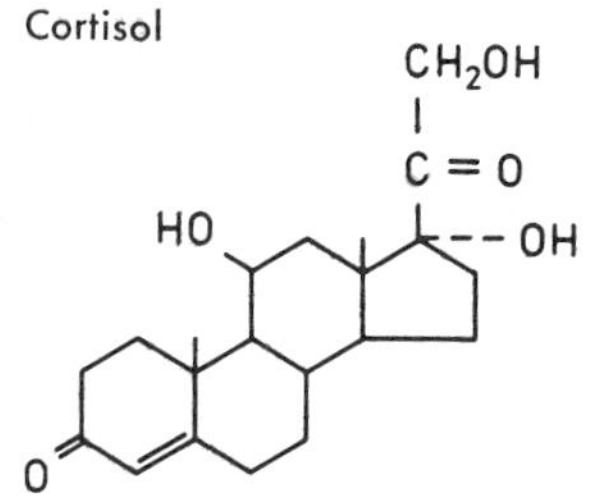

Fig. 9-2. Chemical structure of cortisol.

this very closely. The low point in this cycle occurs shortly after beginning sleep; there is a gradual rise throughout the sleeping period until a peak occurs just after awakening from sleep. In response to stressful situations, such as insulin injection, pyrogens, fright, or excitement, there is a marked and rapid increase in ACTH secretion with a concomitant rise in cortisol production. Both the diurnal response and the response of ACTH to stress are mediated by corticotropin-releasing factor (CRF), apparently via stimulation from higher cortical centers.

The main biologic action of ACTH is to promote the synthesis of steroids in the adrenal cortex. ACTH also causes an increase in adrenal blood flow and adrenal weight. ACTH receptors have been identified in adrenal tissue. ACTH has several extraadrenal effects in experimental animals, but the clinical significance of these effects are unknown. Increased pigmentation is frequently seen in association with excessive ACTH levels, but this may be an effect of the β-MSH released together with the ACTH. In plasma, there is heterogeneity of ACTH immunoreactivity with some of the ACTH circulating in the "big" form. Because this substance occurs in higher proportion in the pituitary extracts, the possibility exists that big ACTH may be a prohormone.

Method

Reagents

The antibodies produced have shown varying degrees of specificity, which are possible to map out in great detail because of the availability of a great number of different synthetic ACTH and MSH analogues. If synthetic $^{1-24}$ACTH (1 through 24 amino acid sequence

of ACTH) is used as immunogen, the antiserum necessarily contains binding sites against the biologically active part of ACTH. However, the antisera so produced may still vary in specificity, particularly in regard to their cross-reaction with β-MSH, which (in contrast to α-MSH) occurs in the circulation, and may affect the results of serum assays.

If ACTH conjugated to a protein such as serum albumin or thyroglobulin is used as immunogen, the likelihood of producing a high-avidity, high-titer antiserum is much greater than with ACTH alone in adjuvant. The instability of labeled ACTH makes it necessary to use freshly iodinated or repurified preparations of ^{125}I-labeled ACTH.

Performance

Most of the early assays involved an initial extraction step for plasma samples with adsorption of ACTH to a solid material. This was done because labeled as well as unlabeled ACTH is liable to degradation in the presence of plasma, and the physiologic concentrations in blood are lower than those of many other polypeptide hormones. Extraction methods that have been utilized are cation exchangers or silicates. Assay methods not requiring an extraction step have also been reported.

Trasylol may be added to decrease the degradation of ACTH during incubation. In addition, temperature control with careful maintenance of 4° C is critical to decrease damage. Most methods have used long incubation times to achieve sufficient sensitivity. Methods used for separation of antibody-bound and free radioactivity have included chromatoelectrophoresis; adsorption on talc, dextran, and coated charcoal; and polyethylene glycol precipitation.

Assay properties

ACTH radioimmunoassays (RIAs) are technically difficult. ACTH is a relatively poor immunogen, is degraded by enzymes in blood and plasma, and occurs in relatively low concentrations physiologically. Its high content of cylic amino acids makes ACTH highly adsorptive to solid material but also makes it liable to losses on tube walls and so forth when handled in low concentrations.

Clinical applications
Pathophysiology

Hypersecretion of ACTH is associated with primary adrenal insufficiency. In this situation very high levels have been observed, 10 to 20 times the upper limit of normal. In addition, when hyperadrenocorticism is associated with overproduction of ACTH, as in the case of a pituitary tumor (Cushing's syndrome) or ectopic ACTH production by tumors, high levels are seen.

Hyposecretion of ACTH accompanies treatment with exogenous steroids. Adrenal tumors, either adenomas or carcinomas, suppress ACTH to subnormal levels.

Sampling

ACTH levels are influenced by a number of factors, including prior administration of corticosteroids (decreases ACTH levels), stress (increases ACTH levels), and the time of day (maximum between 6 AM and 8 AM, with a low point at 12 midnight). In addition, ACTH is highly adsorbed to glass surfaces and undergoes rapid proteolysis in plasma. Accordingly, samples for RIA should be drawn at a set time of day, usually in the early morning, with plastic syringes, and the samples should be kept cold. In patients with Cushing's syndrome, drawing of samples late in the evening (10 PM to midnight) may be useful to distinguish primary from secondary hyperadrenocorticism.

Reference values

The normal basal ACTH levels reported by most laboratories are 10 to 70 pg/ml in the morning.

Interpretation of results

Elevated levels of basal ACTH occur in primary adrenal insufficiency, with serum concentrations that reach several thousand picograms per milliliter. ACTH levels are usually elevated in adrenal hyperplasia secondary to ACTH overproduction, but levels may also be normal in this condition. However, almost universally in this situation there is a loss of the normal circadian rhythm, and levels are relatively constant throughout the day. Ectopic ACTH production is frequently associated with very high

plasma levels. ACTH determinations have also been reported to be helpful in the follow-up of treatment effects in Cushing's syndrome and for measurement of ACTH secretion following adrenalectomy. High ACTH levels are assumed to be associated with high β-MSH secretion and therefore are associated with a higher risk of hyperpigmentation after removal of the adrenals. The low secretion of cortisol in adrenal hyperplasia caused by congenital defects in the steroid-metabolizing enzymes also induces a marked increase of ACTH levels.

Decreased levels of ACTH are noted when insufficiency is due to a pituitary or hypothalamic defect. The levels are low irrespective of the cause of pituitary deficiency (for example, organic lesions in this region or functional disorders, such as long-standing corticosteroid therapy).

When the steroids are produced by an adrenal tumor, the ACTH secretion is inhibited. ACTH determinations have yet to find wide clinical application. They are most useful in differentiating between primary and secondary adrenocortical insufficiency. The assay is valuable as an adjunct for separating Cushing's syndrome from adrenal tumor and ectopic ACTH production.

CORTISOL
Chemistry

Like all glucocorticoids, cortisol is a C_{21}-steroid with a typical configuration at the C_{17}-C_{20}-C_{21} chain and a C_{11}-hydroxyl group (see Fig. 9-2). Like most corticosteroids, whether androgen, mineralocorticoid, or glucocorticoid, the A ring contains a double bond, and there is a ketone group at C_3. Cortisol is secreted in large amounts, approximately 25 mg/day. Like all steroids, it circulates bound to plasma proteins, such as transcortin and albumin. Its half-life in plasma is 1 to 2 hours. About 1% of the secreted cortisol appears unaltered in the urine, whereas the remainder is metabolized in the liver. Cortisol clearance is influenced by liver function as well as by drugs that alter liver enzymatic activity.

Physiology

The secretion of cortisol follows a marked circadian rhythm. It is highest in the early

CORTISOL METHOD

Principle

Charcoal adsorption

$$R + [L + L^*] = [RL + RL^*] \downarrow + [L + L^*]$$

Protocol

		Reagent	Volume
DAY 1	R	Rabbit antiserum to cortisol-3-carboxymethyloxime-BSA	100 μl
	L*	Cortisol-3-carboxymethyloxime-^{125}I-labeled TME	100 μl
	L	Standard 15.6, 31.3, 62.5, 125, 250, 500, 1,000 ng/ml	100 μl
		Sample EDTA-plasma diluted in buffer	
	I	100 μl plasma and 9.9 ml diluent are incubated 30 min at 72° C	100 μl

—————————————— 18 hours, 4° C ——————————————

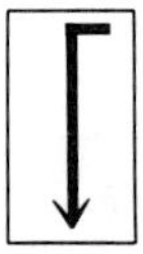

⬇	Dextran-charcoal at 4° C, 10 minutes Centrifugation, 2,500g, 15 minutes, 4° C Decant supernatant in another tube Count supernatant for 2 minutes	500 μl

Reagents

R	Rabbit antiserum to cortisol-3-carboxymethyloxime-BSA Avidity: $K_a = 2 \times 10^{10}$ (Appendix 5)
L*	Cortisol-3-carboxymethyloxime-TME labeled with ^{125}I by lacto-peroxidase; separation on TLC (Appendixes 12 and 13)
L	EDTA-plasma
I	100 μl sample or standard in 9.9 ml diluent is placed in 72° C water bath for 30 minutes; cover tubes with Parafilm
Diluent	Phosphate-gelatin (Appendix 34)
⬇	Appendix 27

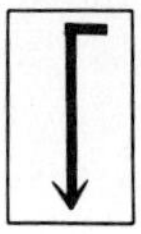

Box 9-1

CORTISOL METHOD, cont'd

Alternatives

R	*Rabbit antiserum to cortisol-21-succinyl-BSA*[1,7,17-19] *Rabbit antiserum to prednisolone-3-BSA*[5]
L*	*(1,2-³H)*[1,5,10,17-19] *or (1,2,6,7,-³H)*[7,8]*-labeled cortisol* *Cortisol-21-succinyl-TME labeled with* ¹²⁵*I by chloramine-T method*[9]
L	*Separation on TLC; chromatography on Lipidex-5000*[1] *Separation on Sephadex LH-20*[18]
I	*Extraction with methylene chloride,*[18] *ethanol*[5,19] *Ether-ethylacetate (1:1)*[1] *Enzyme denaturation of transcortin*[9]*; low-pH incubation (pH 3.5)*[17]
Diluent	*Phosphate-BSA (0.01%)*[8] *PBS,*[1,5] *PBS–gamma globulin (0.05%)*[7] *Borate-lysozyme (0.1%)*[19] *Citrate-phosphate-lysozyme (0.25%), pH 3.5*[17]
⬇	*Charcoal coated with hemoglobin*[8] *DA-goat;*[5] *ammonium sulfate precipitation*[10] *Solid phase; antiserum coupled to cellulose*[17] *Antibody preprecipitated with second antibody*[9]

Box 9-1

---

morning hours and falls during the day to reach its lowest concentration in early evening. This rhythm is controlled by the ACTH secretion. As in many of the other hormone systems stimulated by pituitary tropic hormones, there is a negative feedback from plasma cortisol levels, which, via the pituitary or the hypothalamus, inhibit the secretion of ACTH. The release of cortisol is also greatly stimulated by any stressful situation, an effect that may disrupt the circadian rhythm.

Once secreted into the bloodstream, cortisol is bound to transcortin, a plasma glycoprotein with a high affinity for most steroids. About 75% of cortisol in plasma is bound to transcortin. About 15% of cortisol is bound to albumin, and the remaining 10% is free in the serum.

Analogous to thyroid hormone, it is the free form of the hormone that is metabolically active. In normal subjects, plasma-binding capacity for cortisol is about $20\mu g/ml$. In pregnancy, however, the concentration of transcortin increases greatly, and, accordingly, serum cortisol concentrations may be increased two to three times. On the other hand, in clinical conditions associated with low serum protein concentrations, the serum cortisol concentration may be correspondingly reduced.

The glucocorticoids influence a large number of biologic processes, many of which are mediated by the liver. Glucocorticoids have a profound influence on carbohydrate metabolism, with increased production of glucose by different pathways, particularly from proteins (gluconeogenesis). They also affect diuresis and promote excretion of free water. Gluco-corticoids suppress the inflammatory response and decrease the number of circulating lympho-cytes and antibody production. Glucocorticoids also affect the intermediate metabolism of pro-teins and fats.

Method

The first radioligand assays for cortisol uti-lized transcortin as binding protein. Although these methods are still quite widely used, they are being gradually substituted by RIAs because of the higher specificity and sensitivity of the latter.

Reagents

Cortisol antisera with high specificity have been produced against cortisol 21-hemisucci-nate-BSA. These show varying degrees of specificity and frequently have marked cross-reaction with compound S or 17-OH-proges-terone. Higher specificity may be achieved after immunization with cortisol-6 conjugates, and many antisera reported have been quite specific. Furthermore, the high concentrations of cortisol in plasma reduce the importance of many cross-reactions.

Until recently, ^{3}H-cortisol was the most com-monly used radioligand. Lately, both selenium 75–labeled cortisol (^{75}Se is a gamma emitter with principal gamma energies of 140 keV, 54%; and 270 to 280 keV, 79%) and ^{125}I-labeled cortisol have been used.

Performance

Earlier methods usually involved extraction of plasma (for example, with methylene chlo-ride or ethanol). Improved binders, such as high-avidity antibodies, have made it possible to use methods without extraction, where the binding proteins are denatured by heating or treatment with proteolytic enzymes.

Because of the high concentrations of corti-sol in plasma, the antigen-antibody reaction reaches equilibrium quite rapidly; thus the in-cubation time used is in the order of hours. Methods used for separation of bound and free radioactivity have included dextran- or hemo-globin-coated charcoal and double-antibody and ammonium sulfate precipitation. A detailed

method for corticosteroid assay is shown in Box 9-1.

Clinical applications
Pathophysiology

HYPERFUNCTION. Patients with Cushing's syndrome may have elevated or normal morn-ing levels of cortisol, but they typically lack the normal circadian rhythm. In combination with a suppression test (dexamethasone suppression test), cortisol determinations may be used to differentiate between hyperadrenocorticism due to adrenal hyperplasia and adrenal tumors. Cushing's syndrome is primarily a defect of pituitary hyperfunction, and in this situation, cortisol secretion is usually suppressible to some degree. However, no suppression is ob-served in the case of tumors of the adrenal cortex. Hyperadrenocorticism due to ectopic ACTH production is frequently associated with high cortisol levels that are not suppressible.

HYPOFUNCTION. The basal cortisol levels are frequently low in adrenocortical insufficiency whether due to a primary organic adrenal dis-order (Addison's disease) or secondary to pi-tuitary insufficiency. Occasionally, however, values within the normal range and the circa-dian rhythm may be maintained. The diagnosis can be established with an ACTH stimulation test, which, if positive, excludes the diagnosis of Addison's disease. However, the response may be blunted in ACTH deficiency or as a con-sequence of long-term steroid therapy because of secondary adrenal atrophy. In such cases, more prolonged stimulation may be used; this usually will induce some cortisol response in patients with secondary adrenal atrophy.

Cortisol secretion may be decreased in asso-ciation with congenital adrenal hyperplasia due to associated enzymatic defects, such as 21-hydroxylase deficiency. Excessive stimulation of adrenal activity associated with elevated ACTH levels may be required to maintain a normal basal cortisol production. These patients characteristically have high ACTH or 17-OH-progesterone levels.

Sampling

Since there is a marked circadian rhythm in cortisol levels in plasma, it is important to sample at a fixed time of day, usually early morning (9 AM).

In situations in which the serum cortisol is taken to evaluate hyperfunctional states, it is frequently important to determine the circadian rhythm of cortisol excretion, since this is frequently lost in Cushing's syndrome. Sequential blood samples are taken, for example, at 9 AM, 6 PM, and possibly 12 midnight for a period of 48 hours. The midnight sample should be drawn while the patient is asleep, with a minimum of prior warning, to minimize patient stress.

Dexamethasone suppression tests are useful for evaluating adrenal hyperfunction. Several protocols have been suggested. In the overnight suppression test, one or more control blood samples are drawn at 9 AM. The patient is then given 1.0 mg dexamethasone by mouth between 11 PM and 12 midnight, and a repeat cortisol determination is performed at 9 AM the following morning. In the normal unstressed patient, plasma cortisol levels will be near zero at 9 AM. When the degree of suppression is equivocal, a 72-hour dexamethasone suppression test may be performed. After a 9 AM blood sample is obtained, dexamethasone is given orally in doses of 0.5 mg every 6 hours for the first 24-hour period. A 9 AM blood sample is then drawn, and the patient is treated with an increased dose of 1.0 mg four times a day for the second 24-hour period. Another 9 AM blood sample is then drawn, and the dose is increased to 2.0 mg four times a day for the next 24 hours. In normal subjects, in the absence of stress, plasma cortisol values should fall to less than 60 ng/ml by 48 hours. By 72 hours these levels should be close to zero.

ACTH stimulation tests are also used on occasion, particularly to evaluate the functional status of the adrenals in suspected adrenocortical insufficiency. As a screening test, $250\mu g$ (25 units) of synthetic [1-24]ACTH may be given intravenously. Thirty- and 60-minute plasma samples are then obtained. Normally, plasma cortisol levels should double and/or increase by 100 ng/ml at 1 hour. If an inadequate response is seen, more prolonged stimulation by ACTH is required. A 1-mg injection of depot ACTH, daily for 2 days, will result in at least a doubling

of plasma cortisol levels in normal subjects. These tests may be performed on a patient who is receiving replacement doses of dexamethasone.

Reference values

Plasma cortisol: 9 AM, 50 to 250 ng/ml
6 PM,   0 to 150 ng/ml
12 midnight, 0 to 70 ng/ml

These values should be considered a general guide only, and a normal range should be determined for each individual assay.

Interpretation of results

Elevated values found in Cushing's syndrome are in the range of 250 ng/ml up to more than 500 ng/ml of plasma. The plasma level correlates with the degree of severity of the disorder. In mild Cushing's syndrome, screen level may be within the normal range. Characteristically, there is a loss of the normal circadian rhythm when an adenoma or a carcinoma causes the disorder, and levels greater than 90 ng/ml are seen at the midnight sampling. On the other hand, bilateral adrenal hyperplasia due to an oversecretion of ACTH may show an exaggerated diurnal variation. As mentioned above under Pathophysiology, these two forms of hyperadrenocorticism can sometimes be differentiated by a dexamethasone suppression test. ACTH assay is also helpful in this case. With the overnight dexamethasone suppression test, normal subjects show values below the normal range at the 9 AM sampling (see Sampling above). Such a normal response is very good evidence that the patient does not have Cushing's syndrome. However, females with increased plasma cortisol levels due to oral contraceptives or stressed subjects may not suppress. More prolonged suppression is therefore indicated. Patients with Cushing's syndrome due to adrenal tumors will not suppress, whereas patients with ACTH overproduction may suppress slightly.

Decreased values for serum cortisol are often observed in patients with primary adrenocortical insufficiency. The most reliable way to make the diagnosis, however, is with an ACTH stimulation test (see Sampling above).

REFERENCES

1. Apter, D., Janne, O., and Vihko, R.: Lipidex chromatography in the radioimmunoassay of serum and urinary cortisol, Clin. Chim. Acta **63:**139, 1975.
2. Berson, S. A., and Yalow, R. S.: Radioimmunoassay of ACTH in plasma, J. Clin. Invest. **47:**2725, 1968.
3. Berson, S. A., and Yalow, R. S.: Radioimmunoassay of ACTH. In Berson, S. A., and Yalow, R. S.: editors: Methods in investigative and diagnostic endocrinology, vol. 2, New York, 1973, American Elsevier Publishing Co., Inc., pp. 371-375.
4. Besser, G. M., and Edwards, C. R. W.: Cushing's syndrome, Clin. Endocrinol. metab. **1:**451, 1972.
5. Colburn, W. A.: Radioimmunoassay for cortisol using antibodies against prednisolone conjugated at the 3-position, J. Clin. Endocrinol. Metab. **41:**868, 1975.
6. Croughs, R. J., Tops, C. F., and de Jong, F. H.: Radioimmunoassay of plasma adrenocorticotrophin in Cushing's syndrome, J. Endocrinol. **59:**439, 1973.
7. Donohue, J., and Sgoutas, D.: Improved radioimmunoassay of plasma cortisol, Clin. Chem. **21:**770, 1975.
8. Foster, L. B., and Dunn, R. T.: Single-antibody technique for radioimmunoassay of cortisol in unextracted serum or plasma, Clin. Chem. **20:**365, 1974.
9. Hasler, M. J., Pointer, R., and Niswender, G. D.: An ^{125}I-labeled cortisol radioimmunoassay in which serum binding proteins are enzymatically denatured, Clin. Chem. **22:**1850, 1976.
10. Kao, M., Voina, S., Nichols, A., and Horton, R.: Parallel radioimmunoassay for plasma cortisol and 11-deoxycortisol, Clin. Chem. **21:**1644, 1975.
11. Landon, D. N., and Greenwood, F. C.: Homologous radioimmunoassay for plasma levels of corticotrophin in man, Lancet **1:**273, 1968.
12. Murphy, B. E. P., Engelberg, W., and Poter, C. J.: Method for determinations of corticoids in plasma, J. Clin. Endocrinol. Metab. **23:**293, 1963.
13. Murphy, B. E. P., Engelberg, W., and Poter, C. J.: Modification of a method for determining cortisol in plasma, J. Clin. Endocrinol. Metab. **24:**919, 1964.
14. Nugent, C. A., Nichols, T., and Tyler, F. H.: Diagnosis of Cushing's syndrome; single dose dexamethasone stimulation tests, Arch. Intern. Med. **116:**172, 1965.
15. Orth, D. N.: ACTH radioimmunoassay. In Jaffe, B. M., and Behrman, H. R., editors: Methods of hormone radioimmunoassay, New York, 1974, Academic Press, Inc., pp. 125-159.
16. Ratcliffe, J. G., and Edwards, C. R. W.: Adrenocorticotropin. In Kirkham, K. E., and Hunter, W. M., editors: Radioimmunoassay methods, Edinburgh, 1971, Churchill Livingstone, p. 502.
17. Rolleri, E., Zannino, M., Orlandini, S., and Malvana, R.: Direct radioimmunoassay of plasma cortisol, Clin. Chim. Acta **66:**319, 1976.
18. Ruder, H. J., Guy, R. L., and Lipsett, M. B.: A radioimmunoassay for cortisol in plasma and urine, J. Clin. Endocrinol. Metab. **35:**219, 1972.
19. Vecsei, P.: Glucocorticoids: cortisol, corticosterone and compound S. In Jaffe, B. M., and Behrman, H. R., editors: Methods of hormone radioimmunoassay, New York, 1974, Academic Press, Inc., pp. 393-415.

10 PITUITARY-GONADAL AXIS

Pituitary gonadotropins
   Follicle-stimulating hormone
   Luteinizing hormone
Sex steroids
   Estradiol
   Progesterone
   Testosterone
Prolactin

The reproductive system is regulated by three distinct classes of hormones: (1) the *hypothalamic releasing hormones;* (2) the *gonadotropins,* which exert no target organ effect except to stimulate release of other hormones, such as the anterior pituitary hormones, follicle-stimulating hormone (FSH) and luteinizing hormone (LH), and the placental hormone, human chorionic gonadotropin (hCG); and (3) the *gonadal steroids.* Several other hormones are also loosely related to this system, such as human chorionic somatomammotropin (hCS, sometimes called human placental lactogen, hPL), pituitary prolactin, steroids of adrenal or fetal origin, as well as the peptide hormones of the posterior pituitary. Some of these are discussed in other sections.

The hypothalamic releasing hormone known to be of importance in reproductive physiology is gonadotropin-releasing hormone (gon RH or LH-RH). LH-RH is a decapeptide (10 amino acids) with the following structure: Glu-His-Trp-Ser-Try-Gly-Leu-Arg-Pro-Gly-NH$_2$. LH-RH is produced by the hypothalamus and migrates within the portal venous system to the pituitary, where it stimulates production of LH and FSH. Synthetic LH-RH is available for testing the capacity of the anterior pituitary to release LH and FSH. LH in the male is sometimes designated interstitial cell–stimulating hormone (ICSH). FSH and LH stimulate the gonads to produce a number of sex steroids, principally estradiol and progesterone from the ovaries and testosterone from the testes.

The complex interrelationships between the gonadotropins and the sex steroids that produce the cyclic changes of the ovary, such as maturation of the follicle, ovulation, and formation of the corpus luteum, are only partially understood. Estrogen and testosterone exert an inhibiting feedback on the secretion of FSH and LH. Increased plasma levels of these sex steroids will inhibit the release of gonadotropins, and decreased plasma levels will stimulate the release of the gonadotropins. Accordingly, castration, oophorectomy, and the menopause are followed by a marked increase of the release of gonadotropins.

The feedback of estradiol is always negative as far as FSH secretion is concerned. The higher the levels of estradiol, the less the secretion of FSH. However, for LH both low levels and very high levels of estradiol appear to be inhibitory, but at intermediate estradiol levels, such as occur just prior to midcycle, the secretion of LH is actually stimulated. It is this midcycle peak of estradiol that causes the LH response in midcycle that promotes ovulation. At higher levels of estradiol, the inhibitory effects predominate again, and LH (and hence ovulation) is suppressed. Progesterone does not directly inhibit FSH-LH in itself. However, progesterone appears to enhance the effects of estradiol in plasma.

During pregnancy, hCG intervenes in this regulatory system, and the secretion of FSH and LH is suppressed. This feedback inhibition is probably directed against the anterior pituitary, since the administration of LH-RH during pregnancy will not induce any increased release of pituitary gonadotropins.

Radioimmunoassays (RIAs) are available for the gonadotropins and the sex steroids. An RIA for LH-RH has been recently described, but its clinical usefulness has yet to be established.

PITUITARY GONADOTROPINS: FOLLICLE-STIMULATING HORMONE AND LUTEINIZING HORMONE
Chemistry

The gonadotropic hormones FSH, LH, and hCG are all glycoproteins. Thyroid-stimulating hormone (TSH) also belongs to this group. Structurally, they are made up of two subunits associated by noncovalent bonds, the alpha and beta subunits, of which the alpha subunit is identical for all four hormones. The beta subunit differs among these hormones, and the

specificity of the biologic action resides in this part. The isolated subunit has no biologic action. The glycoprotein hormones have molecular weights of 26,000 to 30,000 daltons, except for hCG, which has a molecular weight of 36,000 to 46,000. The main carbohydrate residue is sialic acid. The biologic potency of the gonadotropins is dependent on the carbohydrate content. This may be due in part to variations in turnover rate, since turnover is accelerated by removal of sialic residues. The hormones show high species specificity, and between-species differences in structure are located mainly within the alpha subunit.

The identity of the alpha subunits of the various hormones and, to an extent, similarities within the beta subunits account for the considerable cross-reactions between these hormones in RIAs. LH and hCG show extensive similarities in the beta subunit with large regions of homology. In most assays LH and hCG show complete cross-reaction. This has been utilized in LH assays, since hCG has been available in relatively pure form much longer than LH. The beta subunits of LH and FSH are much less

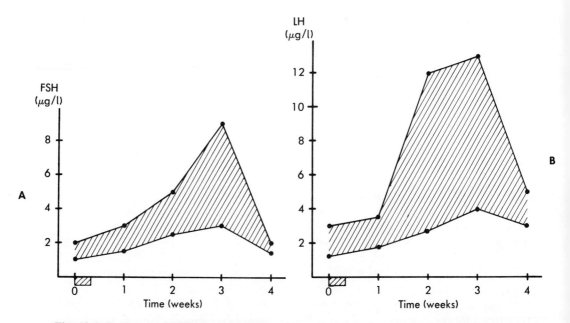

Fig. 10-1. Responses of FSH, **A,** and LH, **B,** to intravenous injection of 25µg LH-RH during the menstrual cycle. Time is counted from the onset of menses. Duration of menses is shown as a rectangle on the time axis. The upper line shows mean peak value and the lower line mean basal value. Accordingly, the response is the difference between the upper and lower lines (hatched area).

similar, so there is much less and frequently no cross-reaction between them. Furthermore, the gonadotropins may cross-react with TSH assays.

Physiology

FSH stimulates the development of the primordial follicles of the ovary. A surge in the secretion of LH and FSH initiates ovulation, and the corpus luteum is then essentially maintained by LH. This function of LH is taken over by hCG produced by the placental trophoblasts if pregnancy occurs.

In males, the gonadotropins maintain spermatogenesis and testosterone secretion; FSH acts mainly on spermatogenesis, and LH (ICSH) stimulates interstitial cell activity.

The pituitary glycoprotein hormones are all produced and released from cells with basophilic tinctorial characteristics in the anterior pituitary. More recent studies have indicated that among the basophilic cells there is one group of thyrotropic and another group of gonadotropic cells. These cells may be distinguished by immunologic and ultrastructural characteristics. Like the other anterior pituitary hormones, the release of gonadotropin is

intermittent with short-term fluctuations in the secretion rate (the fluctuation is smaller for FSH than for LH). These fluctuations are relatively minor in comparison with those of growth hormone or adrenocorticotropic hormone (ACTH). For most clinical purposes, the levels can be regarded as stable within any given day during the ovulatory phase. Gonadotropin release is acutely stimulated by the administration of LH-RH (Fig. 10-1); the effect is more prominent for LH than for FSH. Low levels of estrogen or testosterone enhance the response to LH-RH.

Both FSH and LH show variation with age and during the menstrual cycle (Figs. 10-2 and 10-3). FSH and LH levels are low in childhood. During puberty they increase to adult levels in males and females. In fertile women, they show a characteristic pattern during the menstrual cycle, with slightly higher values during the follicular phase than during the luteal phase. In the middle of the cycle, there is a marked surge in LH secretion, with a peak in the plasma concentration 5 to 20 times higher than the basal level. This peak has a duration of about 1 day. There is a corresponding FSH peak but of much lower height. The peak occurs about a day after

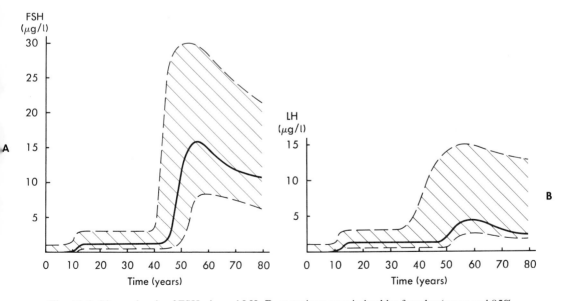

Fig. 10-2. Plasma levels of FSH, **A,** and LH, **B,** at various ages in healthy females (mean and 95% range).

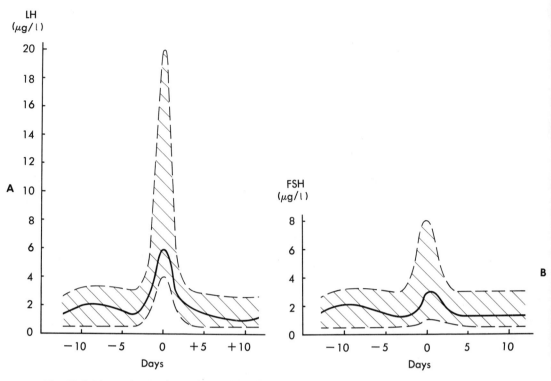

Fig. 10-3. Plasma levels of LH, **A,** and FSH, **B,** during the menstrual cycle in fertile women (mean and 95% range). Days are counted at ovulation.

the maximal level of estradiol occurs and causes ovulation. No cyclic changes have been recorded in males.

At the beginning of the menopause FSH and LH increase markedly, FSH more than LH. They then gradually tend to fall with advancing age, although FSH never reaches premenopausal levels. In males there are no corresponding changes of FSH and LH with age, except that the levels tend to decrease with age. The glycoprotein hormones are predominantly secreted as native hormones, but a small fraction is probably released in the form of isolated alpha or beta subunits. The hormones are not bound to any transporting protein and have relatively rapid disappearance rates from plasma. $T_{1/2}$'s reported have been on the order of ½ hour to 4 hours. The disappearance rate is slightly slower for hCG. The gonadotropins are excreted in the urine, but the urinary gonadotropins differ immunologically from the hormones that occur in plasma.

Method

Reagents

The gonadotropin assays have mainly utilized native hormone preparations as ligand and immunogen, although isolated beta subunits with improved specificity have been introduced more recently. Such beta-chain assays avoid cross-reactions between the common alpha chains. However, some of the cross-reactions recorded previously are probably effects of impure preparations of pituitary hormones rather than true cross-reactions between related antigenic sites. It seems possible to achieve a degree of specificity in assays against native hormones that is sufficiently high for clinical purposes.

Antisera against hCG are used in many LH assays, but there are antisera against LH available. However, because they usually cross-react almost completely with hCG, there is no real advantage in using an LH antiserum instead of an hCG antiserum.

The gonadotropins available are not absolutely pure. The biologic potencies of pure preparations are still a subject of debate but are assumed to be on the order of 18,000 to 20,000 units/mg for hCG, 12,000 to 16,000 units/mg for LH, and about 12,000 to 14,000 units/mg for FSH. The purest hCG preparations available have a potency of 12,000 units/mg, whereas most FSH and LH material available have potencies only on the order of 5,000 units/mg.

The International WHO reference preparation for bioassay of gonadotropins (2 IRP-HMG-Human Menopausal Gonadotropin) is the basis for the potency estimates of the gonadotropins. This preparation is not suitable as standard in most RIAs. It is highly impure, and, since the active material is extracted from urine, it is probably immunologically different from the hormones circulating in plasma. It does not give parallel inhibition lines in most assays when compared with pituitary material. The Division of Biological Standards in London has adopted temporary standards for FSH (MRC 68/39) and LH (MRC 68/40). These have bioassay potencies of about 6,000 IU/mg and 35,000 IU/mg, respectively. However, their potencies in immunoassays still remain to be established. A corresponding standard distributed by the National Pituitary Agency of NIH (Bethesda, Md.) is LER 907. These standards are available to qualified researchers. The impurity of the available standards has caused significant problems in standardization of the assays. Apparent potency of standards may vary with specificity of the antiserum. For this reason, adequate standardization of the assay in absolute terms, such that it could be directly compared with other assays, is virtually impossible. The absolute levels of the reference values quoted here, therefore, must be regarded as arbitrary. Hormones of adequate purity for radioiodination are available from commercial and other sources and have also been produced by several research laboratories. Radioiodinated LH and FSH have been reported to be unstable, with a relatively short shelf life of the labeled material, which occasionally necessitates repurification of the labeled material every week. In our experience with lactoperoxidase labeling, we have not found this to be true, and we regularly use the labeled material for 4 to 6 weeks after iodination without any subsequent repurification.

Reagents for assay of gonadotropins of some other species are available from the National Pituitary Agency.

Performance

In our experience, the nonspecific influence of plasma is low in the primary antigen-antibody reaction. Therefore we do not include any "hormone free" serum in the standards. However, other antisera may be more sensitive in this respect. Since there is a slight plasma effect in our double-antibody step, we add pool plasma with low gonadotropin concentration to the standard tubes just before this step (and buffer sample tubes to compensate for this increase in volume). Double-antibody techniques are most widely used for separation of bound and free activity. In gonadotropin assays other methods used are solid phase coupled antibodies, chromatoelectrophoresis, and dioxane and polyethylene glycol precipitation.

Assay properties

There have been a number of problems associated with the assay of the gonadotropins. These have been related to cross-reactions due to their structural similarity, to problems related to impure preparations, and to difficulties associated with their radioiodination.

RIA methods for FSH are shown in Box 10-1. An RIA for LH is shown in Box 10-2. RIA for hCG is presented in Chapter 11.

Clinical applications
Pathophysiology

Abnormalities may occur in the production and release of the gonadotropins because of disorders at different levels of the hypothalamic pituitary-gonadal axis. The clinical effects of such disorders and the changes in the secretion of the gonadotropins they cause depend on the functional stage at which they occur: infancy, fertile male or female, or advanced age.

PREPUBERTAL. The development of reproductive capacity and secondary sexual characteristics during normal puberty is associated with a rise of both FSH and LH from the low in-

hFSH METHOD

Principle

Double antibody

$$R + [L + L^*] = [RL + RL^*] + [L + L^*]$$

Protocol

		Reagent	Volume
DAY 1	R	Rabbit antiserum to hFSH	200 μl
	L*	^{125}I-hFSH	200 μl
	L	Standard 0.83, 1.67, 3.13, 6.25, 12.5, 25 μg/l	
		Sample EDTA-plasma	100 μl

──────── 72 hours, 4° C ────────

DAY 4	Normal human plasma to standards	100 μl
	Barbital-BSA to plasma samples	100 μl
	Normal rabbit serum (1:250)	50 μl
	Goat antiserum to rabbit IgG (1:10)	50 μl

──────── 18 hours, 4° C ────────

DAY 5	Add diluent	500 μl
	Centrifugation 2,500g, 15 minutes 4° C	
	Decant supernatant	
	Count precipitate for 2 minutes	

Reagents

R — Rabbit antiserum to hFSH absorbed with hCG (so that final concentration is 0.1 μg hCG per tube)
No cross-reaction with hLH or hCG after absorption
Avidity: $K_a = 1.8 \times 10^{11}$

L* — Labeled with ^{125}I by lactoperoxidase
Specific activity: 120-160 μCi/μg; separation on Sephadex G-50
(Appendix 17) T = 10,000 cpm ≈ 0.05 ng

L — EDTA-plasma

Diluent — Barbital-BSA (Appendix 34)

Double antibody (Appendix 28)

Box 10-1

---

hFSH METHOD, cont'd

Alternatives

| R | *Guinea pig antiserum to hFSH*[19]
 Rabbit antiserum to ovine FSH[29] |

| L* | *hFSH labeled with* [131]*I*[19,22,29,34,41] *or* [125]*I*[35] *by chloramine-T method* |

| L | *Serum*[19,29,35] |

| I | *hCG added*[19,34] |

| Diluent | *Phosphate-BSA,*[22,34,35] *barbital-HSA*[41]
 Phosphate-egg albumin[29] |

| 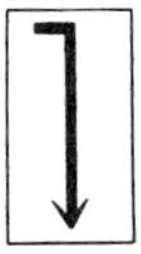 ↓ | *DA-rabbit,*[19] *sheep*[29,34]
 DA coupled to solid phase (BioRIA, Montreal)
 Solid phase antiserum[35,47] |

Box 10-1

---

fantile value to the levels found in fertile adults (Fig. 10-2). The occurrence of true premature puberty (precocious puberty) causes the same increase in the FSH and LH levels. In pseudo-precocious puberty, which is associated with the development of secondary sexual characteristics but no maturation of the gonads, gonadotropin secretion remains low. In constitutionally delayed puberty, the rise in gonadotropin levels is delayed as well. In the normal situation, the FSH increase occurs at an early stage of puberty, 2 to 4 years before LH reaches the same level. Therefore, the plasma FSH level may be a valuable indicator of the difference between delayed puberty and primary amenorrhea. However, if delayed puberty is only a part of another abnormality, various patterns of gonadotropin secretion may be found.

In the rare cases of gonadotropin-secreting malignant tumors, such as primary ovarian or testicular teratocarcinomas, hCG-like material may be secreted, which may be discovered by hCH assays or with LH assays that cross-react with hCG.

REPRODUCTIVE MATURITY. Primary alterations of hypothalamic and pituitary function may cause abnormal secretion of gonadotropin. Defects of the hypothalamic regulation of the pituitary function with decreased gonadotropin release cause hypogonadotropic hypogonadism. This may rarely be a primary defect of the hypothalamus. Both FSH and LH levels are usually decreased, but isolated LH insufficiency occasionally occurs. Some of these cases are genetically defined; others are sporadic without evident organic lesions and appear to be an extended gonadal infancy in which puberty does not occur. Moreover, many types of secondary amenorrhea are due to hypothalamic dysfunction, with loss of the cyclic stimulation of gonadotropin release during the menstrual cycle. The disorders may be associated with low, nor-

hLH METHOD

Principle

Double antibody

$$R + [L + L^*] = [RL + RL^*] + [L + L^*]$$

Protocol

		Reagent	Volume
DAY 1	R	Rabbit antiserum to hLH	200 μl
	L*	${}^{125}I$-hLH	200 μl
	L	Standard 0.83, 1.67, 3.13, 6.25, 12.5, 25 μg/liter	100 μl
		Sample EDTA-plasma	

——————————————— 72 hours, 4° C ———————————————

DAY 4	↓	Normal human plasma to standards	100 μl
		Barbital-BSA to plasma samples	100 μl
		Normal rabbit serum (1:250)	50 μl
		Goat antiserum to rabbit IgG (1:10)	50 μl

——————————————— 18 hours, 4° C ———————————————

DAY 5	↓	Add diluent	500 μl
		Centrifugation, 2,500g, 15 minutes, 4° C	
		Decant supernatant	
		Count precipitate for 2 minutes	

Reagents

R Rabbit antiserum to hLH
Avidity: $K_a \approx 1.4 \times 10^{11}$

L* hLH labeled with ${}^{125}I$ by lactoperoxidase (Appendix 17)
Specific activity: 120-160 μCi/μg; separation on cellulose (Appendix 20)
T = 10,000 cpm ≈ 0.05 ng

L EDTA-plasma

Diluent Barbital-BSA (Appendix 34)

↓ Appendix 28

Box 10-2

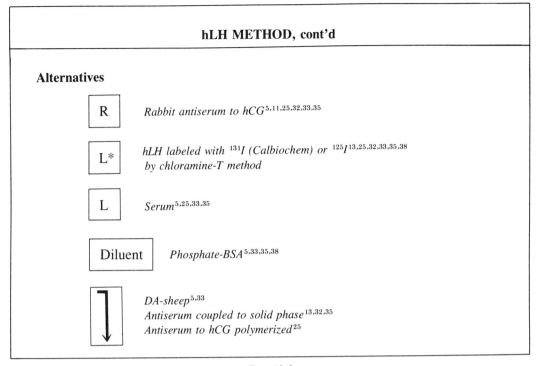

Box 10-2

mal, or slightly elevated levels of FSH and LH. Characteristically, the midcycle LH peak is missing. Although this group of disorders is still relatively poorly defined it probably includes conditions such as anorexia nervosa (which frequently have low LH and normal FSH values), postcontraceptive amenorrhea, polycystic ovary syndrome, psychogenic functional amenorrhea, and certain types of hypopituitarism.

Insufficient gonadotropin secretion is associated with many diseases. It is usually secondary to organic processes in or around the pituitary sella. These disorders may be caused either by interruption of the connection between the hypothalamus and the pituitary or by direct interference with the gonadotropic cells of the anterior pituitary. Such lesions may be the effect of surgical or radiation ablation, non-hormone-producing tumors, such as craniopharyngioma, chromophobe adenoma, metastases, or expansive processes in the adjacent bone, such as histiocytosis. Other causes include pituitary infarction (Sheehan's syndrome)

and the so-called "empty sella" syndrome. Gonadotropin secretion is usually the pituitary function that is impaired first during progress to a general hypopituitarism.

Several extra-hypothalmic-pituitary diseases are associated with altered gonadal function and amenorrhea. Some of these are endocrine states, such as congenital adrenal hyperplasia, that directly inhibit pituitary gonadotropin secretion. Some diseases cause such disorders indirectly. Debilitating diseases, such as tumors and severe infections, and several endocrine disorders, such as hyper- and hypothyroidism, are examples of conditions that probably interfere in the delicate cooperation between the hypothalamus and the pituitary.

A decreased production of pituitary gonadotropins can be caused by treatment with high doses of estrogen and occurs in estrogen- and hCG-producing tumors, both in males and females.

The high gonadotropin secretion of the normal menopause is also found in association with decreased gonadal function in younger adults.

Accordingly, gonadotropin secretion, particularly the FSH level, is a sensitive indicator of decreased ovarian or testicular hormone production.

Increased levels of FSH (and to a lesser extent of LH) are found in various forms of male or female gonadal dysgenesis, such as Klinefelter's and Turner's syndromes. The increased gonadotropin production of these conditions is only found at postpuberty ages and cannot be used as an indicator of gonadal function in infancy. If the deficiency of estrogen or testosterone production is compensated for, the elevated gonadotropin levels will be normalized.

Moderately elevated LH levels with a tendency to low FSH values are frequently seen in polycystic ovary syndrome (Stein-Leventhal syndrome).

POSTMENOPAUSAL PERIOD. Essentially, the same disorders that occur in fertile life may cause a marked decrease of the gonadotropin secretion in the postmenopausal period. Moreover, the normal high basal levels, particularly of FSH, make the gonadotropin levels more sensitive indicators of hypopituitarism than in previous periods of life.

The lack of estrogen inhibition of FSH release in the normal postmenopausal woman makes it possible to detect abnormal estrogen production, such as that associated with an ovarian tumor, from its inhibition of the FSH secretion.

Sampling

Serum samples are principally used for LH and FSH. FSH and LH are relatively stable in serum. Samples kept more than 24 hours before assay should be stored frozen.

Reference values

LH
   males, 1-3 ng/ml
   females
      prepubertal, 1-3 ng/ml
      fertile, basal, 1-3 ng/ml; midcycle peak,
        5×-20× basal
      menopausal, 2-8 ng/ml
FSH
   males, 1-3 ng/ml
   females

      prepubertal, 1-3 ng/ml
      fertile, basal, 1-3 ng/ml; midcycle peak,
        2× basal
      menopausal, 5-29 ng/ml

These concentrations are expressed in terms of the pure hormone preparations available and correspond to potencies of about 8,000 IU/mg of FSH and 6,000 IU/mg of LH.

Interpretation of results

Elevated LH levels are found in postmenopausal and castrated women and are typically in the range of about four to five times the normal basal values. This elevation is actually less than that which normally occurs during the midcycle peak. The LH surge usually occurs at the fourteenth day of a 28-day menstrual cycle in normal fertile women. In males, LH values are significantly elevated with castration. LH levels are also usually increased during pregnancy and in association with trophoblastic tumors. This is not due to increased LH itself but is because LH and hCG cross-react in almost all assays.

Decreased LH levels are associated with a variety of destructive disorders of the hypothalamus and pituitary. In several types of secondary amenorrhea, the levels of LH in the serum are normal, but the normal midcycle peak is decreased or absent.

Elevated FSH levels are observed in the same general situations as elevated LH: castration and the postmenopausal state are probably the most common causes. (See Comparative levels, below.)

Decreased FSH levels are observed with disorders of the hypothalamus-pituitary axis. Go-

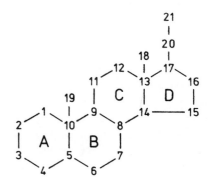

Fig. 10-4. Nomenclature of the steroid structure.

nadotropins are very sensitive to pituitary destruction and are frequently the first trophic hormones to show decreased levels.

COMPARATIVE LEVELS OF FSH AND LH. Castration gives high levels of both, but FSH values are markedly higher; 5 to 12 times the basal levels are observed. During the midcycle, LH values are greater than FSH values. During hCG production, FSH levels are markedly inhibited, but measured LH values will be greatly increased because of the cross-reactivity of LH and hCG in almost all assays. In early puberty FSH is elevated, whereas LH is still low. This may aid in dating the onset of puberty.

SEX STEROIDS

There are three main groups of sex steroids when classified according to function: estrogens, progestins, and androgens. The details of chemistry, biosynthesis, and metabolism of the various hormones are not covered here, but the reader is referred to standard texts on endocrinology. To facilitate the understanding of this reputedly difficult subject, the notation of the steroid structure is given in Fig. 10-4.

ESTRADIOL
Chemistry

Estrogens are characterized by the benzene structure of the A ring with a hydroxyl group

in position 3 (Fig. 10-5). 17 β-Estradiol (often abbreviated E_2) and estrone (E_1) are the main estrogens produced by the ovary. Their concentration and secretion rate are approximately the same, but estradiol is considerably more potent and is therefore the main component. Estradiol and estrone are interconvertible, and the enzymes that cause these alterations are found in many tissues. A third form, estriol (E_3), is an irreversible metabolite of estradiol, with much less potency. Estriol occurs in high concentrations during pregnancy.

Circulating estradiol is primarily secreted by the ovaries, whereas other estrogens are also derived from extraovarian sources, such as the adrenals. The estrogens circulate in blood bound to transporting plasma proteins, and only a very small fraction is in an unbound form. Sex hormone–binding globulin is a transporting protein that specifically binds estradiol and testosterone. Like all steroids, estrogens are excreted after conjugation with glucuronic or sulfuric acid in the liver.

Physiology

The ovarian estrogens are produced by the granulosa cells of the theca interna of the follicles. Estradiol, as the main estrogen produced by the ovary, is the one that most closely reflects ovarian function. The plasma concen-

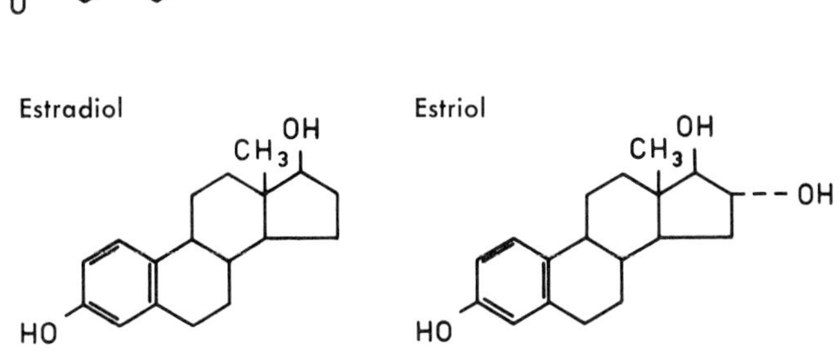

Fig. 10-5. Chemical structure of major sex steroids.

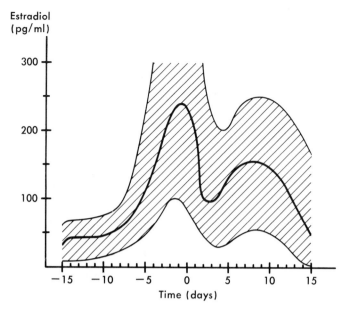

Fig. 10-6. Plasma levels of estradiol during the menstrual cycle in fertile women (mean and 95% range). Days are counted at ovulation.

tration of estradiol shows a cyclic pattern during the menstrual cycle (Fig. 10-6). The secretion rate is controlled by the pituitary gonadotrophins, but the exact relationship between the various hormonal factors that regulate the cyclic maturation of the ovarian follicles is only partially known. The development of the follicles and the gradual increase in the secretion of estradiol during the follicular phase are influenced by both FSH and LH. Estradiol reaches a peak value at the midcycle and is involved in triggering the FSH and LH peaks that cause ovulation. Following ovulation, estradiol will drop initially but will then increase gradually to a broad second peak with the development of the corpus luteum. Like progesterone, the estradiol level will then decline to the low menstrual levels when the corpus luteum undergoes regression. The production of estradiol is low in childhood and after the menopause, when the ovaries do not contain any maturating follicles.

Method

Reagents

Diethyl ether is usually used for extraction of estradiol from serum samples. It should be used fresh or as newly distilled solution. Stor-

age in containers that have been opened may cause explosion. Benzene has also been employed. When the extract must be further purified, chromatography on Sephadex LH-20 columns has been most widely used in recent methods.

Antisera have been produced against estradiol conjugated to serum albumin via the 3, 6, 11, or 17 carbon. Since the hydroxyl group in the 3 position is characteristic for the estrogens, coupling from the other end of the molecule could be assumed to produce the most suitable immunogen. However, antisera against such 17-conjugated steroids seem to give too low a specificity in terms of their ability to distinguish between various estrogens and between precursors, such as dehydroepiandrosterone. Antisera against 6- and 11-conjugated estradiol have been reported to have the highest specificity. Early methods utilized ^{3}H-estradiol as radioligand, but more recently ^{125}I has become the most commonly used tracer. To accomplish iodination of the estradiol, the organic compounds tyrosine methyl ester, histamine, tyramine, or human serum albumin (HSA) are conjugated to the estradiol. These substances are readily radioiodinated (see Chapter 3).

Performance

The time required for reported assays varies from 1 hour to 24 hours. Most methods require overnight incubation. Separation of bound and free activity is generally performed with dextran-coated charcoal methods. A solid phase coupled antibody and double-antibody precipitation have also been reported for this step.

Assay properties

Reported assays have sensitivities that vary from 1 to 10 pg/ml. Most methods still involve both extraction of plasma and chromatographic separation of the extract. With highly specific antisera, it is possible to perform the assay after extraction only. An example of such a method is described in Box 10-3.

Clinical applications

Of the various estrogens, estradiol is the one that most closely reflects ovarian function. Assays for estradiol in plasma have not been generally available until recently. The experience in clinical application is therefore relatively restricted as yet; information that is available is partly based on older methodology.

Pathophysiology

HYPOFUNCTION. Decreased ovarian production of estradiol may be due to primary ovarian failure or defects at the hypothalamic-pituitary level. Primary ovarian insufficiency after puberty is associated with increased gonadotropin secretion. For example, the menopause is characterized by a low estradiol value and markedly elevated FSH, and to a certain extent, LH levels. Low estradiol values in combination with low gonadotropins occur before puberty. Female hypogonadism in the normally fertile age range is usually associated with amenorrhea and clinically classified as secondary or primary, dependent on whether sexual function had been established before the abnormal state occurred. Primary as well as secondary hypogonadism of ovarian origin may be due to castration, radiation damage, or disease in the pelvic region, such as pelvic inflammatory diseases and pelvic tumors. A primary absence or hypoplasia of the ovaries occurs as a genetic defect in gonadal dysgenesis (Turner's syndrome and its many variants). Because of the low estradiol production despite increasing gonadotropins at puberty, FSH and LH levels will continue to rise after puberty and reach menopausal levels during adolescence. There are also some cases of primary ovarian hypofunction without obvious genetic aberrations, in which the ovaries do not develop normally despite adequate gonadotropin stimulation at the time of puberty.

A failure of the ovaries to function normally at puberty may also be due to a delayed or insufficient stimulation from the pituitary. This group of disorders is discussed in the gonadotropin section.

Decreased ovarian function of the secondary amenorrhea type, which results in markedly diminished estrogen production (and high gonadotropin levels), usually depends on a reduced hormonal production by the follicles, as does the normal menopause. The cause of premature menopause has not been established.

In addition, inhibition of gonadotropin secretion may be caused by diseases in organs other than the ovaries. Thus ovarian hypofunction may be associated with many pathologic states, such as thyrotoxicosis, hypothyroidism, congenital adrenal hyperplasia, Cushing's syndrome, Addison's disease, undernutrition (including anorexia nervosa), chronic debilitating diseases such as malignancy, major infections, and renal insufficiency, and localized diseases of the brain and the pituitary. The reduction of gonadotropin in these disorders is apparently related to subtle alterations of the hypothalamic-pituitary axis. In polycystic ovary disease (Stein-Leventhal syndrome) the secretion of estradiol is low, but the production of large quantities of androstenedione, a precursor of estrogens, causes a conversion of this compound to estrone (as well as to testosterone; for this reason this condition is frequently associated with hirsutism). Therefore, plasma may contain abnormally high levels of estrone despite low concentrations of estradiol.

HYPERFUNCTION. Overproduction of ovarian estradiol may be seen in ovarian tumors, primarily granulosa-theca cell tumors. Other ovarian tumors, such as arrhenoblastoma and lipoid cell tumors, may also produce increased amounts of estrogens, in addition to the greater production of androgens (virilizing tumors). Increased estradiol secretion may also be caused

ESTRADIOL METHOD

Principle   Extraction of plasma estradiol with ether

Charcoal adsorption

$$R + [L + L^*] = [RL + RL^*] + [L + L^*]$$

Protocol

		Reagent	*Volume*
DAY 1	R	*Sheep antiserum to estradiol-6-carboxymethyloxime-BSA*	*200 μl*
	L*	*Estradiol-6-carboxymethyloxime-^{125}I-histamine*	*200 μl*
	L	Standard *9.8, 19.5, 39, 78, 156, 313, 625, 1,250 pg/ml* Sample *EDTA-plasma extracted with ether and dissolved in diluent*	*100 μl*

——————————— *18 hours, 4° C* ———————————

DAY 2

Dextran-coated charcoal   *500 μl*
10 minutes, 4° C
Centrifugation, 2,500g, 15 minutes, 4° C
Decant supernatant in another tube
Count supernatant for 2 minutes

Reagents

R   *Sheep antiserum to estradiol-6-carboxymethyloxime-BSA*
      Avidity: $K_a \approx 2 \times 10^{11}$

L*   *Histamine labeled with ^{125}I by chloramine-T and coupled to*
      estradiol-6-carboxymethyloxime
      Separation on TLC (Appendix 15)

L   *0.5 ml EDTA-plasma extracted with 2.5 ml diethyl ether.*
      The ether phase is evaporated and the residue is dissolved in
      diluent

I   *Diethyl ether extraction*

Diluent   *Phosphate-gelatin (Appendix 34)*

Appendix 27

Box 10-3

ESTRADIOL METHOD, cont'd

Alternatives

R	*Rabbit antiserum to estradiol-17β-succinyl-BSA*[1,16] *Sheep antiserum to estradiol-17β-succinyl-BSA*[36] *Rabbit antiserum to estradiol-11β-succinyl-BSA*[18] *Guinea pig antiserum to estradiol-6-carboxymethyloxime-HSA*[17,27] *Rabbit antiserum to estradiol-6-carboxymethyloxime-BSA*[28]
L*	*(6,7-³H)*[1,28] *or (2,4,6,7,-³H)*[16,36] *labeled estradiol* *Estradiol-6-carboxymethyloxime-histamine,*[17] *estradiol-6-carboxymethyloxime-tyramine*[30]; *estradiol-6-carboxymethyloxime-HSA*[27] *or estradiol-11β-succinyl-TME*[18] *labeled with* ¹²⁵*I by chloramine-T method*
L	*Sample separated on Sephadex LH-20*[16,36]
I	*Extraction with benzene*[18]; *incubation with 1 μg testosterone to displace estradiol from binding proteins*[28]
Diluent	*Phosphate-HSA*[17] *(0.1%), phosphate-BSA*[27] *(0.1%)*
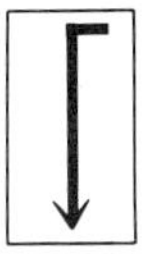 ⌐↓	*DA-sheep*[18] *Antisera-coated tubes*[1,17,27]

Box 10-3

---

by ovarian hyperfunction induced by gonadotropin-producing tumors.

Reference values

Estradiol
  childhood, 2-20 pg/ml
  males, 10-60 pg/ml
  females
    follicular phase, 20-100 pg/ml
    preovulatory peak, 200-600 pg/ml
    midluteal phase, 100-300 pg/ml
    postmenopause, 5-50 pg/ml

PROGESTERONE
Chemistry

The progestins are dominated by one compound, progesterone, which is responsible for the main progestin effect in humans. Progesterone is a product of an early stage in the steroid synthetic pathways and also serves as a precursor for other steroids, among them several of the adrenocortical hormones. Therefore, it is also produced in the adrenal cortex and the testes. Its configuration is relatively similar to the adrenocortical steroids but quite different in comparison with the estrogens (see Fig. 10-5).

Physiology

The main source for circulating progesterone is the corpus luteum, which develops from the ovarian follicle after ovulation. Like other steroids, it circulates bound to transporting proteins. Its principle action is to promote the development of the uterine endometrium. Progesterone causes the secretory changes necessary for implantation of the ovum. If the ovum is not fertilized, the corpus luteum degenerates at the end of the menstrual cycle. Accordingly, the plasma levels of progesterone in the nonfertilized menstrual cycle are characterized by low levels during its first (follicular) half and a broad peak from ovulation to the beginning of the menstruation, with maximum values between days 20 and 25 (Fig. 10-7). If pregnancy occurs, the corpus luteum function is maintained by the rapidly increasing levels of hCG. Later during pregnancy the placenta becomes the main source of progesterone, and the plasma concentration will continue to rise to reach its highest level at the end of gestation, a maximum that is 20 times higher than the peak value of a menstrual cycle.

Method

Reagents

Several RIA methods with or without a chromatographic step have been reported for progesterone. Alumina and Celite columns have been used for chromatography. Extraction of plasma with petroleum ether has the advantage of removing progesterone rather selec-

tively and will therefore reduce the need for subsequent purifications.

Antisera have been produced by conjugation of progesterone to albumin via carbon 3, 6, 11, 20, or 21. Antisera to 11-conjugates have shown the highest specificity and are generally used in nonchromatographic assays.

Radioligands with ^{3}H-progesterone are still used, although ^{125}I-labeled progesterone conjugates are now being more generally applied. The range of physiologic concentrations of progesterone is much higher than that of the estrogens; thus the demand for sensitivity and thereby for specific activity of the radioligand is lower in comparison with the estradiol assays. ^{125}I-labeled progesterone has been produced with tyrosine methyl ester (TME) and histamine as progesterone-11 conjugates.

Dextran-coated charcoal is most widely used for separation of bound and free radioactivity, but solid phase coupled antibodies and ammonium sulfate precipitation have also been utilized.

Performance

Incubation times range from 1 to 24 hours. Most assays use petroleum ether–extracted se-

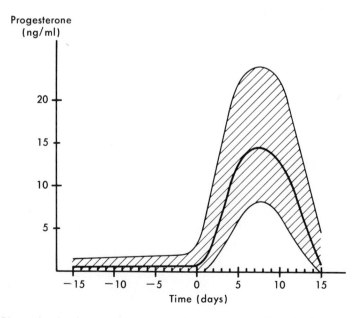

Fig. 10-7. Plasma levels of progesterone during the menstrual cycle in fertile women (mean and 95% range). Days are counted at ovulation.

rum in the standards to ensure identity of samples and standards.

Assay properties

Sensitivity for the various assays has been reported to range from 10 to 200 pg/vial. Most assays still require both plasma extraction with petroleum ether and separation on a chromatographic column. This is done because of the cross-reaction of progesterone with other steroids in RIAs. An RIA for progesterone is shown in Box 10-4.

Clinical applications

Pathophysiology

Hypersecretion of progesterone is seen in granulosa-theca cell tumors and lipoid cell tumors of the ovary. Progesterone levels are also markedly elevated in congenital adrenal hyperplasia.

Hyposecretion of progesterone is seen with disorders of corpus luteum formation. Abnormalities in progesterone production occur in disorders of the corpus luteum function as well as in certain adrenal diseases. During anovulation, no corpus luteum develops; thus anovulatory menstrual cycles will not produce any luteal progesterone peak. Ovulation induced by treatment with hCG, clomiphene citrate, or LHR is followed by a normal progesterone peak if a corpus luteum develops. The normal steady increase of progesterone levels during pregnancy may be interrupted by functional disorders of the placenta or fetus. Low plasma progesterone values have been reported both during placental insufficiency and fetal death, but this has not been a constant finding; thus plasma progesterone levels serve as a relatively poor indicator of such disorders.

Sampling

Serum samples are obtained. By noting the day after onset of menses at the time of sampling, interpretation will be facilitated (see Fig. 10-7).

Reference values

Fertile women: follicular phase, 0.2-1 ng/ml; midluteal phase, 5-20 ng/ml
Pregnancy: first trimester, 20-50 ng/ml, rising to 150 ng/ml at term

TESTOSTERONE
Chemistry

The major androgen is testosterone. Its structure is relatively similar to that of progesterone, from which it differs only in that C_{20}-C_{21} is substituted by a hydroxyl group (see Fig. 10-5). Its immediate precursor is androstenedione. In the target cells, testosterone is converted to dihydrotestosterone, which is much more potent than testosterone and therefore is regarded as the main active androgenic principle.

Physiology

Testosterone is principally produced by the Leydig cells of the testis, but it is also produced in the adrenal cortex and in the ovary. Testosterone is transported in blood bound to plasma proteins. Like estradiol, it is predominantly bound to a specific binder called sex hormone–binding globulin. Testosterone production is stimulated by a pituitary gonadotropin in the male called interstitial cell–stimulating hormone (ICSH), which is presumably identical to LH. For this reason LH is also used to refer to the male hormone. Administration of LH or hCG (2,000-5,000 IU/day) causes a marked increase in plasma testosterone in the male but not in the female. Injection of LH-RH will induce a rise in testosterone levels within 4 hours; this procedure has been suggested as a test for Leydig cell function. Diurnal variation of the plasma testosterone levels has been investigated, and, as in many of the hormones regulated by the pituitary, there seems to be a certain rhythm, with somewhat higher values during the morning than during the evening and early night hours. The day-to-day variation is relatively great, and a certain cyclicity has been reported from many longitudinal studies. However, there is no marked regular variation corresponding to the female menstrual cycle.

The hormonal effects of testosterone are the development and maintenance of the male sex characteristics. It also has general anabolic effects: it stimulates cell growth, increases nitrogen retention, and accelerates bone maturation.

Method

RIAs for testosterone have been developed during the 1970s and are now replacing assays

PROGESTERONE METHOD

Principle

Extraction of plasma progesterone with ether

Charcoal adsorption

$$R + [L + L^*] = [RL + RL^*] + [L + L^*]$$

Protocol

		Reagent	Volume
DAY 1	R	*Rabbit antiserum to progesterone-11α-hemisuccinate-BSA*	*200 μl*
	L*	*Progesterone-11α-hemisuccinate ^{125}I-TME*	*200 μl*
	L	Standard *0.08, 0.16, 0.31, 0.63, 1.25, 2.50, 5.00 ng/ml*	*100 μl*
		Sample *EDTA-plasma extracted with ether and dissolved in diluent*	

─────────────────── *18 hours, 4° C* ───────────────────

DAY 2

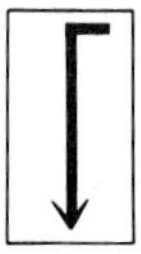

Dextran-coated charcoal, 10 minutes, 4° C *500 μl*
Centrifugation, 2,500g, 15 minutes, 4° C
Decant supernatant in another tube
Count supernatant for 2 minutes

Reagents

R *Rabbit antiserum to progesterone-11α-hemisuccinate-BSA*
Avidity: $K_a \approx 4 \times 10^{10}$

L* *Progesterone-11α-hemisuccinate-tyrosine methyl ester labeled with ^{125}I by lactoperoxidase; separation on TLC (Appendixes 12 and 13)*

L *0.5 ml EDTA-plasma extracted with 2.5 ml diethyl ether; the ether phase is evaporated, and the residue is dissolved in diluent*

I *Diethyl ether*

Diluent *Phosphate-gelatin (Appendix 34)*

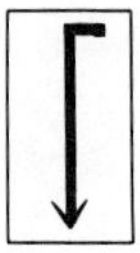

Appendix 27

Box 10-4

PROGESTERONE METHOD, cont'd

Alternatives

| R | *Sheep antiserum to progesterone-11-succinyl-BSA[9,14] or to 11-desoxycortisol-21-succinyl-HSA[2]*
Rabbit antiserum to progesterone-6-BSA[8] |

| L* | *(7-³H),[9] (1,2-³H),[2,37] or (1,2,6,7-³H)[14,15] labeled progesterone*
Progesterone-11α-succinyl-histamine[42] or progesterone-11α-succinyl-TME labeled with ¹²⁵I by chloramine-T method (Micromedic) |

| L | *Sample separated on Celite column[2] or on Sephadex LH-20 (New England Nuclear)* |

| I | *Extraction with petroleum ether[8,9,14,37,42] or petroleum ether-ethanol (9:1)[15]* |

| Diluent | *Tris-normal rabbit serum[8]* |

⌐↓ *Solid phase coupled antiserum[9,15]*
   DA-sheep (Micromedic)

Box 10-4

---

that utilized sex hormone–binding globulin as a receptor.

Reagents

Testosterone has to be extracted from plasma to avoid the influence of the endogenous binding proteins. Diethyl ether, benzene–petroleum ether, hexane-toluene, hexane ether, and methylene chloride have been used for the extraction of testosterone from serum.

Antisera with improved specificity have been developed recently, permitting assay without any purification of the extract. Of related steroids, there is usually a significant cross-reaction with dihydrotestosterone. Since the plasma concentration of this compound is less than 20% of the testosterone concentration, its influence is clinically negligible. Methods using a purification step have employed paper chromatography, column chromatography on Celite, Sephadex LH-20, or alumina, and thin-layer chromatography.

The radioligand most frequently used has been 1,2- or 1,2,6,7-³H-testosterone. Iodinated tyrosine or tyramine methyl ester conjugates have been developed recently and are likely to be used more widely.

Performance

Incubation times vary from 30 minutes up to 24 hours. Typically, serum extracts are added to the standard curve to ensure identity between standards and samples.

Assay properties

Assays have reported sensitivities ranging from 10 to 300 pg/ml. An RIA for testosterone is given in Box 10-5.

TESTOSTERONE METHOD

Principle

Extraction of plasma testosterone with ether

Charcoal adsorption

$$R + [L + L^*] = [RL + RL^*] + [L + L^*]$$

Protocol

		Reagent	*Volume*
DAY 1	R	*Rabbit antiserum to testosterone-3-carboxymethyloxime-BSA*	*200 μl*
	L*	*Testosterone-3-carboxymethyloxime-^{125}I-histamine*	*200 μl*
	L	Standard — *0, 39, 78, 156, 313, 625, 1,250, 2,500 pg/ml*	*100 μl*
		Sample — *EDTA-plasma extracted with ether and dissolved in diluent*	

———————————— *18 hours, 4° C* ————————————

DAY 2 ↓ *Dextran-coated charcoal*   *500 μl*
10 minutes, 4° C
Centrifugation, 2,500g, 15 minutes, 4° C
Decant supernatant in another tube
Count supernatant for 2 minutes

Reagents

R — *Rabbit antiserum to testosterone-3-carboxymethyloxime-BSA*
Avidity: $K_a \approx 9 \times 10^{10}$ (Appendixes 4 and 5)

L* — *Histamine labeled with ^{125}I by chloramine-T and coupled to testosterone-3-carboxymethyloxime*
Separation on TLC (Appendix 15)

L — *0.5 ml EDTA-plasma extracted with 2.5 ml diethyl ether*
The ether phase is evaporated, and the residue is dissolved in diluent

I — *Diethyl ether*

Diluent — *Phosphate-gelatin (Appendix 34)*

↓ *Appendix 27*

Box 10-5

TESTOSTERONE METHOD, cont'd

Alternatives

R — *Rabbit antiserum to testosterone-11-succinyl-BSA[11]*
Sheep antiserum to 15β-carboxyethylmercaptotestosterone-BSA[40]

L* — *$(1,2,-^3H)^{[4,7,12,31,48]}$ or $(1,2,6,7-^3H)^{[20,21,39,46,49]}$ labeled testosterone; testosterone-3-carboxymethyloxime-TME labeled with ^{125}I by chloramine-T method[24]*

L — *Sample separated on Sephadex LH-20,[7,46] Celite column,[4,20] or paper chromatography[21]*

I — *Extraction of sample with methylene chloride[4,21,46]*
Hexane-ethanol (98:2),[12] hexane-ether (6:4),[12] ether-chloroform[40]
Precipitation with ammonium sulfate and extraction with hexane-toluene (4:1),[48] hexane-ethylacetate (9:1),[49] or benzene-petroleum ether (2:5)[24]
Estradiol added (1 μg) to displace testosterone from binding protein[39]

Diluent — *Phosphate–gamma globulin (0.1%),[7] Borate-BSA,[12] Tris-BSA–gamma globulin[21]*
Tris-BSA (0.1%),[39,46,48] Borate-gelatin (0.1%)[49]

⌐↓ — *Ammonium sulfate precipitation[12,21]*
Free testosterone extracted with toluene scintillation solution[46,48]
Polyethylene glycol precipitation[4]
DA-sheep[24]

Box 10-5

Clinical applications

Pathophysiology

HYPOFUNCTION. Low levels of testosterone are found during testicular agenesis and after bilateral ablation, radiation damage, severe orchitis, or torsion with extensive necrosis. There are several types of genetic aberration with decreased Leydig cell function, including Klinefelter's and Reifenstein's syndromes. Low testosterone levels have been reported in myotonic dystrophy.

Secondary testicular failure may also be due to decreased gonadotropin production following disorders of the pituitary-hypothalamic level. A number of drugs may decrease testosterone secretion; such compounds may have their effects on varying levels. These include synthetic androgens, estrogens, progesterone, chlorpromazine, and metyrapone. Testosterone levels reported for impotent men have been conflicting: both normal and lowered values have been found.

HYPERFUNCTION. Overproduction of testosterone in the male is rare, but it may occur in gonadotropin-producing tumors and adrenocortical tumors. In boys with idiopathic sexual precocity and congenital adrenal hyperplasia, testosterone levels are much above those normal for age although no higher than in the normal adult male.

In women, hyperandrogenic conditions, primarily manifested as hirsutism, form a large clinical group. The etiology of the hirsutism remains unexplained in most cases, although organic reasons for hyperandrogenism, such as Cushing's syndrome, congenital adrenal hyperplasia, adrenal tumors, ovarian tumors, polycystic ovaries, and testicular feminization, must be ruled out. Virilizing tumors, such as arrhenoblastoma and lipoid cell tumor, may produce highly elevated testosterone levels. In idiopathic hirsutism, most investigators found that a significant number of the women (but not all) had increased plasma testosterone.

Sampling

Serum samples are normally collected.

Reference values

Normal males: 3-12 ng/ml
Prepubertal boys: < 0.5 ng/ml
Fertile women: 0.2-1.5 ng/ml

Interpretation of results

Elevated levels are uncommonly found in males except in the rare cases of gonadotropin-producing tumors and adrenal tumors. In females with virilizing ovarian or adrenal tumors and testicular feminization, markedly elevated levels are found. In patients with trophoblastic disease or during pregnancy, testosterone levels may be elevated.

Decreased levels in males are associated with gonadal failure. This may be either primary, due to organ damage, or secondary, due to failure of gonadotropin production.

PROLACTIN
Chemistry

Prolactin is a polypeptide of about 200 amino acids, with a molecular weight of 22,000. Prolactin has strong structural similarities to growth hormone (GH) and hCS. Human prolactin is similar to prolactins of other species, particularly ovine prolactin. Ovine prolactin has been completely characterized; this molecule contains 198 amino acids and three disulfide bridges without carbohydrate residues.

Physiology

Prolactin serves to stimulate and maintain lactation. Prolactin itself has little direct effect on the mammary gland but is essential to the initiation of lactation from a gland that has already been primed by the action of estrogen and progesterone. Prolactin has no known function in males. Prolactin is produced and stored by the anterior pituitary. Prolactin is released in response to tactile stimulation of the breast in women but not in men. This effect is apparently mediated by the hypothalamus, which normally secretes factor inhibitory of prolactin secretion, prolactin inhibitory factor (PIF). Under influences that promote prolactin excretion, PIF secretion is correspondingly depressed. PIF is probably identical to dopamine.

During lactation, prolactin levels increase up to 10 times basal levels, with a peak at about 30 minutes after onset of suckling. Thereafter the levels decline gradually and return to baseline levels by 90 to 120 minutes.

There appears to be a certain circadian rhythm to prolactin secretion, with peak values of about twice the basal levels occurring during sleep 2 to 3 hours before awakening. The low point occurs about 12 noon.

During pregnancy, prolactin levels progressively increase so that by term they are about ten times the concentrations at conception. Early in pregnancy, the normal circardian rhythm is lost. After delivery the levels in lactating and nonlactating mothers are similar, except that after nursing there is an abrupt increase in prolactin as noted above. Prolactin secretion may be stimulated by a variety of drugs and other compounds. Estrogen stimulates prolactin secretion, and the use of oral contraceptives with an estrogenic component is associated with elevated prolactin levels. Insulin-induced hypoglycemia, amino acid infusion, reserpine, α-methyldopa, phenothiazine derivatives, amphetamine, heroin, and antidepressants have all been associated with increased levels of prolactin. These agents are thought to act via the hypothalamus. Synthetic thyrotropin-releasing hormone (TRH) causes a significant increase in prolactin levels within 5 minutes after intravenous injection. Peak concentrations are noted by 20 to 30 minutes after injection, at about two to three times the normal basal levels. There is a return to normal baseline values by 4 hours after injection. This effect of TRH has been used as the basis for a test of the integrity of the hypothalamus.

Prolactin secretion may be inhibited by several drugs. In the normal adult, a dose of 500 mg of L-dopa suppresses prolactin release within 30 to 90 minutes. Decreased prolactin secretion has also been noted with apomorphine. The most effective depressant is the ergotamine compound bromocriptine; it is effective therapy for hyperprolactinemia of various causes.

Method
Reagents

Prolactin can be used as immunogen to produce antibody of reasonably high avidity. One of the major early problems was the isolation of human prolactin for use as immunogen. In some of the early assays, ovine prolactin was used, and because of its close similarity to human prolactin, the heterologous antisera were useful in the early assays. More recently, antisera have been made available by the National Institutes of Health that are directed against human prolactin. These antisera are also available from commercial sources. Human prolactin for standards is available to qualified researchers from National Institutes of Health. These reagents are also available commercially. ^{125}I has been the label of choice for prolactin. Lactoperoxidase labeling appears to result in a radioligand that is less degraded and more stable.

Performance

A variety of separation methods have been employed: sheep double antibody, antibody coupled to solid phase, ethanol–ammonium acetate precipitation, and so forth. Incubation time for most assays is on the order of 1 to 2 days.

Assay properties

The correlation of prolactin serum levels measured by antisera to ovine and human prolactin has been relatively poor. In addition, the radioligand has been relatively unstable. With the use of antisera to human prolactin and care in iodination, assays are becoming increasingly reliable. An RIA for prolactin is shown in Box 10-6.

Clinical applications
Pathophysiology

Hyperproduction of prolactin has been reported in nonendocrine neoplasms, particularly in carcinoma of the lung and hypernephroma. In addition, with the advent of improved methodology it has been discovered that oversecretion of prolactin by pituitary tumors is relatively common and occurs in about 30% of cases. This may be a more common cause of infertility and menstrual abnormalities, since high levels of prolactin may interfere with the interaction of FSH, LH, and the ovary. Hyperprolactinemia has been reported to occur in as many as 15% of patients with secondary amenorrhea. Hyperproduction is also associated with hypothalamic disorders, probably due to a decrease in the normal inhibition of prolactin by PIF. With prolonged stimulation, galactorrhea is observed; elevations of prolactin are frequently but not always associated with galactorrhea-amenorrhea syndromes. These conditions may respond to treatment with bromocriptine, and the associated hyperprolactinemia correspondingly declines. A significant proportion (20%-40%) of patients with acromegaly have elevation of prolactin secretion in addition to elevation of GH. However, most of these patients have a blunted response to TRH. Marked elevations may be noted with psychotropic drug therapy.

Hypoproduction of prolactin has been noted in a few cases of the empty-sella syndrome. Although basal prolactin levels are normal in this state, the prolactin response to TRH may be subnormal.

Sampling

Samples are usually obtained for basal levels of prolactin between 10 AM and 12 noon, since this corresponds to the low point in the circardin swing of prolactin concentration. Because the stress of a poor venipuncture can induce a surge of prolactin, care should be taken in obtaining serum.

To test the integrity of the anterior pituitary in its response to stimulators of prolactin, a TRH stimulation test may be performed. The test is performed as described in the section on TSH.

PROLACTIN METHOD

Principle

Double antibody

$$R + [L + L^*] = [RL + RL^*] + [L + L^*]$$

Protocol

		Reagent	Volume
DAY 1	R	Rabbit antiserum to human prolactin	200 μl
	L*	^{125}I-prolactin	200 μl
	L	Standard 6.25, 12.5, 25, 50, 100 μg/liter	100 μl
		Sample EDTA-plasma	

──────── 18 hours, 4° C ────────

DAY 2		Normal human plasma to standards	100 μl
		Barbital-BSA to plasma samples	100 μl
		Normal rabbit serum (1:250)	50 μl
		Goat antiserum to rabbit IgG (1:10)	50 μl

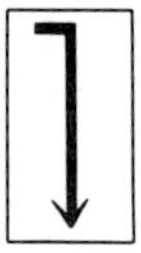

──────── 18 hours, 4° C ────────

DAY 3	Add diluent	500 μl
	Centrifugation, 2,500g, 15 minutes 4° C	
	Decant supernatant	
	Count precipitate for 2 minutes	

Reagents

R — Antiserum to human prolactin
Avidity: $K_a \approx 1.5 \times 10^{10}$

L* — Human prolactin labeled with ^{125}I by lactoperoxidase
(Appendix 17)
Specific activity: 100 μCi/μg; separation on Sephadex G-100
$T = 20,000$ cpm ≈ 0.1 ng

L — EDTA-plasma

Diluent — Barbital-BSA (Appendix 34)

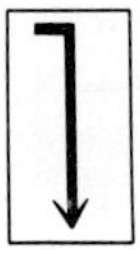

Appendix 28

Box 10-6

PROLACTIN METHOD, cont'd

Alternatives

| R | *Rabbit antiserum to ovine prolactin*[26]
 Guinea pig antiserum to ovine prolactin[6] |

| L* | [125]*I-prolactin labeled by chloramine-T method*[26,40,43,44]
 Heterologous assay using porcine[6] *or ovine*[3] *prolactin labeled by*
 chloramine-T method |

| L | *Serum samples*[3,26,40] |

| Diluent | *Phosphate-BSA,*[6,26,44] *phosphate-gelatin*[3] |

| ↓ | *DA-sheep*[6]
 Ethanol–ammonium acetate precipitation[43] |

Box 10-6

Reference values

Basal prolactin: 10 AM to 12 PM, 0-30 ng/ml

Interpretation of results

Elevated prolactin levels are found in patients who habitually take psychotropic drugs. In addition, elevated prolactin levels may occur during withdrawal from chronic use of oral contraceptives. When an obvious associated cause is not present, hyperprolactinemia should lead one to suspect a pituitary or hypothalamic tumor, since prolactin increase may be noted long before radiographic changes are present. If the prolactin concentration is greater than 500 ng/ml, a prolactin-secreting tumor is probable. Associated testing may be of help in confirming the diagnosis in equivocal cases. This includes the L-dopa inhibition test. L-Dopa will not inhibit prolactinemia from psychotropic agents, however; thus the value of this test is somewhat limited. Stimulation with TRH may be helpful. Tumors will not be stimulated by TRH to a value greater than two times basal values.

In patients undergoing hypophysectomy, prolactin secretion should be elevated if complete transection of the stalk has been achieved. This is a useful way to monitor the adequacy of surgical therapy.

Decreased prolactin values are not commonly of clinical importance. However, there is some evidence to suggest that some breast tumors may be dependent on prolactin secretion for growth. If this finding is substantiated by further work, a decreased prolactin level in serum may become an important indicator of the adequacy of drug therapy.

REFERENCES

1. Abraham, G. E.: Solid-phase radioimmunoassay of estradiol-17β, J. Clin. Endocrinol. Metab. **29**:866, 1969.
2. Abraham, G. E., Swerdloff, R., Tulchinsky, D., and Odell, W. D.: Radioimmunoassay of plasma progesterone, J. Clin. Endocrinol. Metab. **32**:619, 1971.
3. Akbar, A. M., Cannan, C. R., and Burke, G.: The clinical utility of a heterologous radioimmunoassay for human prolactin, Clin. Chim. Acta **61**:391, 1975.
4. Anderson, P., Fukoshima, K., and Schiller, H. S.: Ra-

dioimmunoassay of plasma testosterone with use of polyethylene glycol to separate antibody bound and free hormone, Clin. Chem. **21:**708, 1975.

5. Aono, T., Goldstein, D. P., Taymor, M. L., and Dolch, K.: A radioimmunoassay method for human pituitary luteinizing hormone (HCG) using ^{125}I-labeled LH, Am. J. Obstet. Gynecol. **98:**966, 1967.

6. Aubert, M. L., Grumbach, M. M., and Kaplan, S. L.: Heterologous radioimmunoassay for plasma human prolactin (hPRL); values in normal subjects, puberty, pregnancy and in pituitary disorders, Acta Endocrinol. (Kbh.) **77:**460, 1974.

7. Auletta, F. J., Caldwell, B. V., and Hamilton, G. L.: Androgens; testosterone and dihydrotestosterone. In Jaffe, B. M., and Behrman, H. R., editors: Methods of hormone radioimmunoassay, New York, 1974, Academic Press, Inc.

8. Bauminger, S., Cordova, T., Ayalon, D., and others: Serum levels in progesterone and chorionic somatomammotrophin in human pregnancy determined by radioimmunological methods. In International Atomic Energy Agency: Radioimmunoassay and related procedures in medicine, vol. 2, Vienna, 1974, I.A.E.A, pp. 67-77.

9. Bodley, F. H., Chapdelaine, A., Flickinger, G., Mikhail, G., Yaverbaum, S., and Roberts, K. D.: A highly specific radioimmunoassay for progesterone using antibodies covalently linked to arylamine glass, Steroids **21:**1, 1973.

10. Bolton, A. E., and Hunter, W. M.: The labelling of proteins to high specific radioactivities by conjugation to a ^{125}I-containing acylating agent, Biochem. J. **133:**529, 1973.

11. Bosch, A. M., Den Hollander, F. C., and Woods, G. F.: Specificity of antisera against testosterone linked to albumin at different positions (C3, C11, C17), Steroids **23:**699, 1974.

12. Castro, A., Shih, H., and Chung, A.: A direct plasma testosterone radioimmunoassay, Experientia **29:**1447, 1973.

13. Catt, K. J., Niall, H. D., Tregear, G. W., and Burger, H. G.: Disc solid phase radioimmunoassay of human luteinizing hormone, J. Clin. Endocrinol. Metab. **28:**121, 1968.

14. Devilla, G. O., Roberts, K., Weist, W. G., Mikhail, G., and Flickinger, G.: A specific radioimmunoassay of plasma progesterone, J. Clin. Endocrinol. Metab. **35:**458, 1972.

15. Dighe, K. K., and Hunter, W. M.: A solid phase radioimmunoassay for plasma progesterone, Biochem. J. **143:**219, 1974.

16. Edqvist, L. E., and Johansson, E. D.: Radioimmunoassay of oestrone and oestradiol in human and bovine peripheral plasma, Acta Endocrinol. (Kbh.) **71:**716, 1972.

17. Edwards, R., Gilby, E. D., and Jeffcoate, S. L.: Iodine-125 tracers in steroid radioimmunoassay. In International Atomic Energy Agency: Radioimmunoassay and related procedures in medicine, vol. 2, Vienna, 1974, I.A.E.A., pp. 31-40.

18. England, B. G., Niswender, G. D., and Midgley, A. R., Jr.: Radioimmunoassay of estradiol-17beta without chromatography, J. Clin. Endocrinol. Metab. **38:**42, 1974.

19. Fairman, C., and Ryan, R.: Radioimmunoassay for human follicle-stimulating hormone, J. Clin. Endocrinol. Metab. **27:**444, 1967.

20. Forest, M. G., Cahtiard, A. M., and Bertrand, J. A.: Total and unbound testosterone levels in the newborn and in normal and hypogonadal children, use of a sensitive radioimmunoassay for testosterone, J. Clin. Endocrinol. Metab. **36:**1132, 1973.

21. Forti, G., Pazzagli, M., Calabres, E., Fiorelli, G., and Serio, M.: Radioimmunoassay of plasma testosterone, Clin. Endocrinol. (Oxf.) **3**(1):5, 1974.

22. Franchimont, P.: Radioimmunoassay; FSH and LH. In Berson, S. A., and Yalow, R. S., editors: Methods in investigative and diagnostic endocrinology, vol. 2, New York, 1974, Elsevier North-Holland, Inc., pp. 518-536.

23. Greenwood, F. C., Hunter, W. M., and Glover, J. S.: The preparation of ^{125}I-labelled human growth hormone of high specific radioactivity, Biochem. J. **89:**144, 1963.

24. Ismail, A. A., Niswender, G. D., and Midgley, A. R., Jr.: Radioimmunoassay of testosterone without chromatography, J. Clin. Endocrinol. Metab. **34:**177, 1972.

25. Isozima, S., Naka, O., Koyama, K., and Adachi, H.: Rapid radioimmunoassay of human luteinizing hormone using polymerized anti-human chorionic gonadotropin as immunosorbent, J. Clin. Endocrinol. Metab. **31:**693, 1970.

26. Jacobs, L. S.: Prolactin. In Jaffe, B. M., and Behrman, H. R., editors: Methods of hormone radioimmunoassay, New York, 1974, Academic Press, Inc., pp. 87-102.

27. Jeffcoate, S. L., Gilby, E. D., and Edwards, S. R.: The preparation and use of ^{125}I steroid-albumin conjugates as tracers in steroid radioimmunoassays, Clin. Chim. Acta. **43:**343, 1973.

28. Jurjens, H., Pratt, J. J., and Woldring, M. G.: Radioimmunoassay of plasma estradiol without extraction and chromatography, J. Clin. Endocrinol. Metab. **40:**19, 1975.

29. L'Hermite, M., and Midgley, A. R., Jr.: Radioimmunoassay of human follicle-stimulating hormone with antisera to the ovine hormone, J. Clin. Endocrinol. Metab. **33:**68, 1971.

30. Lindberg, P., and Edqvist, L. E.: The use of 17beta-oestradiol-6-(O-carboxymethyl)oxime-(^{125}I) tyramine as tracer for the radioimmunoassay of 17beta-oestradiol, Clin. Chim. Acta **53:**169, 1974.

31. Lox, L. D., Christian, C. O., and Heine, M. W.: A simple radioimmunoassay for testosterone, Am. J. Obstet. Gynecol. **118:**114, 1974.

32. Maudgal, N. R., and Madhwa, R.: Pituitary gonadotrophins. In Jaffe, B. M., and Behrman, H. R., editors: Methods of hormone radioimmunoassay, New York, 1974, Academic Press, Inc., pp. 57-85.

33. Midgley, A. R., Jr.: Radioimmunoassay; a method for

human chorionic gonadotrophin and human luteinizing hormone, Endocrinology **79**:10, 1966.

34. Midgley, A. R., Jr.: Radioimmunoassay for human follicle-stimulating hormone, J. Clin. Endocrinol. Metab. **27**:295, 1967.

35. Nagata, Y., Nakamura, R. M., Osborne, C. E., Naftalin, F., and Mishell, D. R., Jr.: The effect of pH on radioimmunoassay of LH and FSH, J. Lab. Clin. Med. **85**:515, 1975.

36. Orczyk, G. P., Caldwell, B. V., and Behrman, H. R.: Estrogens; estradiol, estrone, and estriol. In Jaffe, B. M., and Behrman, H. R., editors: Methods of hormone radioimmunoassay, New York, 1974, Academic Press, Inc., pp. 333-346.

37. Orczyk, G. P., Hichens, M., Arth, G., and Behrman, H. R.: Progesterone. In Jaffe, B. M., and Behrman, H. R., editors: Methods of hormone radioimmunoassay, New York, 1974, Academic Press, Inc., pp. 347-358.

38. Pinto, H., Wajchenberg, B. L., Higa, O. Z., Schmidt, R. W., and Ribeiro, R.: Preparation of high-quality iodine-labelled pituitary luteinizing hormone for radioimmunoassay, Clin. Chim. Acta **60**:125, 1975.

39. Pratt, J. J., Wiegman, T., Lappöhn-a, R. E., and Woldring, M. G.: Estimation of plasma testosterone without extraction and chromatography, Clin. Chim. Acta **59**:337, 1975.

40. Rao, P. N., Perry, H., and Moore, P. H., Jr.: Synthesis of new steroid haptens for radioimmunoassay. I. 15β-carboxyethylmercaptotestosterone–bovine serum albumin conjugate; measurement of testosterone in male plasma without chromatography, Steroids **28**:101, 1976.

41. Saxena, B. B., Demura, H., Gandy, H. M., and Peterson, R. E.: Radioimmunoassay of human follicle stimulating and luteinizing hormones in plasma, J. Clin. Endocrinol. Metab. **28**:519, 1968.

42. Scarisbrick, J. J., and Cameron, E. H. D.: Radioimmunoassay of progesterone; comparison of (1,2,6,7-3-H4)-progesterone and progesterone-(^{125}I)-iodohistamine radioligands, J. Steroid Biochem. **6**:61, 1975.

43. Schmidt-Gollwitzer, M., and Saxena, B. B.: Radioimmunoassay of human prolactin (PRL), Acta Endocrinol. (Kbh.) **80**:262, 1975.

44. Sinha, Y. N., Selby, F., Lewis, U. J., and Vanderlaan, V. P.: A homologous radioimmunoassay for human prolactin, J. Clin. Endocrinol. Metab. **36**:509, 1973.

45. Torjesen, P. A., and Sand, T.: Dextran-coated charcoal used in the radioimmunoassay of human pituitary luteinizing hormone, Acta Endocrinol. (Kbh.) **73**:444, 1973.

46. Watson, M. J., and Fleetwood, J. A.: A reliable method for the specific determination of testosterone in plasma, Clin. Chim. Acta **57**:337, 1975.

47. Wide, L., Nillius, S. J., Gemzell, C., and Roos, P.: Radioimmunosorbent assay of follicle stimulating hormone and luteinizing hormone in serum and urine from men and women, Acta Endocrinol. (Kbh.) **73**(suppl.): 1, 1973.

48. Williams, B. M., Horth, C. E., and Palmer, R. F.: The measurement of testosterone in plasma, Clin. Endocrinol. (Oxf.) **3**:397, 1974.

49. Wong, P. Y., Wood, D. E., and Johnson, T.: Routine radioimmunoassay of plasma testosterone, and results for various endocrine disorders. Clin. Chem. **21**:206, 1975.

11 PLACENTA AND FETUS

Human chorionic gonadotropin
Human placental lactogen
Estriol

Methods for monitoring fetal health and development have played an increasingly important role in obstetrics, parallel to the trend for a generally more active approach to the care of the pregnant woman and fetus. Ultrasound measurement of fetal size, fetal electrocardiogram (ECG) recording, and studies of fetal excretion products through amniocentesis are methods that contribute to such management decisions. In this chapter methods are described for evaluation of the state of the fetus and placenta by monitoring of the production of hormones. The concentration of fetal or placental hormones in fetal or maternal fluids is dependent on: (1) the functional status of the hormone-producing organs, (2) the size of the hormone-producing organ, and (3) the ability of the substance to pass the placental barrier. The hormones that have been most often used as indicators in clinical obstetrics and gynecology are human chorionic gonadotrophin (hCG), human placental lactogen (hPL, or human somatomammotropin), and estriol.

HUMAN CHORIONIC GONADOTROPIN
Chemistry

Human chorionic gonadotropin is a glycoprotein with close structural similarities to the pituitary glycoprotein hormones follicle-stimulating hormone (FSH), luteinizing hormone (LH), and thyroid-stimulating hormone (TSH). The carbohydrates that constitute about 30% of the molecule have made molecular weight estimations uncertain; more recent estimates of molecular weight range from 37,000 to 59,000. Like the pituitary gonadotropins, hCG consists of an alpha subunit and a beta subunit, of which the alpha unit is almost identical to the alpha subunit of FSH, LH, and TSH. The beta subunit of hCG is larger than that of the other glycoprotein hormones; it contains about 145 residues. There is also a certain degree of homology between the beta subunits. The pituitary hormone LH is most closely related to hCG. For this reason most antisera to hCG show complete cross-reactivity with LH. The carbohydrate content of hCG is necessary for its biologic activity.

Physiology

Human chorionic gonadotropin is produced by the placental trophoblasts. No control mechanisms for regulating its release have been identified. The concentration of hCG in maternal plasma is 400 to 800 times higher than in fetal plasma. In the amniotic fluid the concentration is higher than in fetal plasma and about 1/50 of the concentration in maternal plasma. The turnover rate of hCG in plasma is somewhat slower than that of the pituitary gonadotropins. $T_{1/2}$ has been estimated to have an initial component of 5 hours and a slow component of 24 hours.

The major role of hCG is to maintain the corpus luteum function in early pregnancy. It is likely that it also exerts a trophic action on the ovaries and the adrenals.

In pregnancy, hCG may be detected in maternal blood 9 to 10 days after conception by utilizing the most sensitive radioimmunoassays (RIAs). Its concentration then increases almost exponentially to a peak value of 20 to 100 IU/ml (which is 1,000 times higher than the basal concentration of any protein hormone in a non-

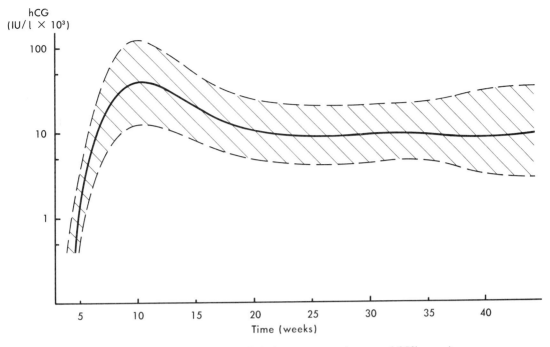

Fig. 11-1. Plasma levels of hCG during pregnancy (mean and 95% range).

pregnant individual and approximately corresponds to 1μg to 10μg/ml) around the tenth week. It then gradually decreases to one tenth to one fifth of this height where it remains for the second half of pregnancy (Fig. 11-1).

Method

Reagents

Human chorionic gonadotropin may be measured specifically either with an hCG method or with an hCG-LH method. Specific hCG assays have utilized antisera raised against isolated hCG beta subunits. Because of the close structural similarity between the LH beta and hCG beta subunits, many antisera discriminate poorly between LH beta and hCG beta subunits. However, it has been possible to find antisera with which LH cross-reacts insignificantly when present in physiologic concentrations. The radioligand used may also influence the specificity, since it has been shown that the use of ^{125}I-labeled hCG may give better discrimination between LH and hCG with some antisera, whereas ^{125}I-labeled hCG beta may have the same effect with other antisera.

The hCG-LH method utilizes antisera that do not discriminate between LH and hCG. The antisera may have been raised against LH or hCG; the methods are essentially identical to the methods described for LH. However, optimal accuracy requires the use of hCG standards instead of LH standards if the standard curves do not show complete coincidence.

Human chorionic gonadotropin of high purity for immunization and for labeling is more generally available than the other glycoprotein hormones. For standardization, there is an international reference preparation (Second International Standard, 1963). However, this consists of relatively impure material (2,600 IU/mg) extracted from urine. This material is somewhat less appropriate for a serum RIA standard; thus it is usually better to use highly purified material (10,000 IU/mg) that has been standardized in bioassays as provisional standards until new international standards for immunoassay become generally available.

Performance

Much of the general methodology for the pituitary gonadotropins applies to hCG as well. Most assays use overnight incubation of the pri-

hCG METHOD

Principle

Double antibody

$$R + [L + L^*] = [RL + RL^*] + [L + L^*]$$

Protocol

		Reagent	Volume
DAY 1	R	*Rabbit antiserum to hCG*	*200 μl*
	L*	*¹²⁵I-hCG*	*200 μl*
	L	Standard *0, 0.78, 1.57, 3.13, 6.25, 12.5, 25, 50 μg/liter* Sample *EDTA-plasma*	*100 μl*

——————————— *16 hours, 4° C* ———————————

DAY 2	↓	*Normal human plasma to standards*	*100 μl*
		Diluent to samples	*100 μl*
		Normal rabbit serum (1:250)	*50 μl*
		Goat antiserum to rabbit IgG (1:10)	*50 μl*

——————————— *4 hours, 4° C* ———————————

Diluent *500 μl*
Centrifugation, 2,500g, 15 minutes, 4° C
Decant supernatant
Count precipitate for 2 minutes

Reagents

R *Rabbit antiserum to hCG*

L* *hCG labeled with ¹²⁵I by lactoperoxidase (Appendix 17)*
Separated on Sephadex G-50 (Appendix 19); specific activity:
120-160 μCi/μg

L *EDTA-plasma*
Highly purified hCG, 10,000 IU/mg

Diluent *Barbital-BSA (Appendix 34)*

↓ *Double antibody (Appendix 28)*

Box 11-1

---

hCG METHOD, cont'd

Alternatives

R — *Rabbit antiserum to hCG[9,11,19]*

L* — *hCG labeled with [125]I[8,9,19,20] or [131]I[11,19] by chloramine-T method*

L — *Sample extracted with concanavallin coupled to Sepharose[11]*

Diluent — *Phosphate-normal rabbit serum[8,11,19,20]*
Phosphate-BSA–normal rabbit serum (Calbiochem)
Phosphate-BSA (BioRIA, Montreal)

↓ — *DA-sheep[8,11,19,20]*
Antiserum coupled to Sepharose[9]

Box 11-1

---

mary antibody step, although shorter periods may be used as well. Separation methods reported are dominated by double-antibody technique. Solid phase coupled antibodies, either of the primary antibody or of the double antibody type, are alternatives used. It has usually not been necessary to add serum to the standard curve.

Assay properties

Many assays cross-react relatively completely with LH; however, assays are available that permit measurement of hCG independent of LH when LH is present in physiologic concentrations. Sensitivities of reported assays have been in the range of 1 to 5 mU/ml. At these sensitivities, hCG is usually detectable by the ninth day after conception. An RIA for hCG is shown in Box 11-1.

Clinical applications

The sensitivity of an RIA is not needed to measure hCG during pregnancy after 19 to 20 days after conception. Clinical application of hCG RIAs has therefore mainly been restricted to abnormalities in early pregnancy and the detection and follow-up of hCG-producing tumors, such as hydatidiform mole.

Pathophysiology

HYPERSECRETION. After a normal delivery or after termination at an earlier occasion, the plasma hCG level declines, with $T_{1/2}$ (in the late, slow phase) of about 24 hours. Dependent on the height of the hCG level at the time of determination and the sensitivity of the assay, hCG is normally found in blood for up to 2 to 4 weeks. Most patients with untreated hydatidiform mole show abnormal hCG production after delivery; that is, hCG is still detectable about 1 month after term. Determinations of hCG levels are invaluable in the observation of these patients as well as those who have developed choriocarcinoma, to evaluate both the need for therapy and the effect of various treatments. In most cases, hCG-LH assays will give sufficient information, but it seems likely that specific hCG assays will make it possible to detect relapses earlier and thereby improve therapeutic results. However, these methods have not been in general use long enough for a final evaluation of their effect on the prognosis of patients with this disease.

In addition, in both men and women, hCG is produced by certain gonadal tumors, such as teratomas, dysgerminomas, and chorioepitheliomas.

HYPOSECRETION. In ectopic pregnancy, the hCG secretion is often so low that common pregnancy tests are negative. An hCG assay usually reveals values well above normal luteal phase levels. A specific hCG method may give even more reliable information.

In other kinds of abnormal pregnancies, hCG determination at low concentrations has not proved to be of much clinical value. Ectopic production of hCG in nonendocrine tumors has been reported to occur with varying incidence, normally in about 10% of cases, including carcinomas of the lung, stomach, pancreas, and breast and melanomas.

Sampling

Serum samples are most commonly used. Human chorionic gonadotropin is relatively stable in serum. Urine samples may also be used. Five milliliters of urine containing 100 mg of thimerosal (Merthiolate) are adequate for RIA.

Reference values

Normal, nonpregnant: nondetectable
Postpartum: nondetectable by 1 month postpartum

Interpretation of results

Human chorionic gonadotropin should not be present in the normal nonpregnant state. Elevated values are noted in hydatidiform mole, choriocarcinomas, and in some gonadal hormone–secreting neoplasms (see Chapter 21 and Pathophysiology, above). In choriocarcinoma there is a close correspondence between the hCG concentration and the amount of tumor present. Teratomatous tumors in testes and ovaries may give rise to choriocarcinomas that

frequently produce hCG and thus cause high plasma levels. In trophoblastic neoplasia, the hCG determination is the most sensitive test for evaluating remaining trophoblastic tissue following the end of pregnancy.

After a normal delivery, hCG concentrations should fall to undetectable levels within 1 month. Most patients with untreated hydatidiform mole have persistently elevated serum concentrations of hCG. Since the risk of choriocarcinoma following molar pregnancy is over 1,000 times the risk following a normal pregnancy, follow-up with hCG determinations is valuable. Somewhat longer persistence of hCG levels after a molar pregnancy are usual; however, elevated levels should not be noted beyond 6 months.

Increasing levels of hCG at any time during this period also require prompt follow-up, since invasive mole or choriocarcinoma may have developed.

Normally, cerebrospinal fluid (CSF) values for hCG are relatively low with a plasma:CSF ratio of more than 60:2. However, in the case of central nervous system (CNS) metastases, higher levels have been noted. These methods have been suggested as a way to follow the course of CNS metastases. Normally, the ratio of plasma hCG to CSF hCG should be less than 60:1. It should be remembered that the follow-up of therapeutic effects with combined hCG-LH assays may be invalidated by the presence of high levels of pituitary LH due to castration effects of surgery or radiation.

When a combined hCG-LH method is used for determination of hCG concentrations, an additional aid in the determination of hCG and LH effects may be found in the FSH values. When LH values are high during the menstrual cycle or as an effect of hypogonadism, FSH values are usually high as well. In pregnancy or hCG production from tumors, the FSH values are low because of inhibition of the pituitary function.

HUMAN PLACENTAL LACTOGEN
Chemistry

Human placental lactogen (somatomammotropin) is a single-chain polypeptide with marked similarity to human growth hormone

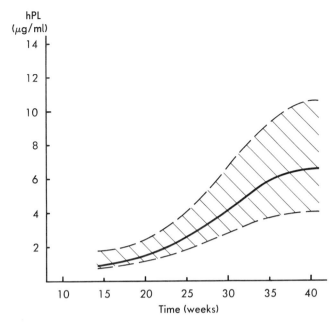

hPL
(μg/ml)

Time (weeks)

Fig. 11-2. Plasma levels of hPL during pregnancy (mean and 95% range).

(hGH). Of its 191 amino acid residues, 161 are identical in hPL and hGH. It also shows large regions of homology with human prolactin.

Physiology

Much of the function of this relatively recently discovered hormone is still unknown. Human placental lactogen is produced in the placental trophoblast. It is present in the maternal circulation, where it, like hCG, reaches high levels (microgram concentrations per milliliter). In the fetal circulation the levels are much lower. Its half-life in maternal circulation is about 20 minutes.

Human placental lactogen influences carbohydrate metabolism and is believed to possibly be the factor causing the diabetogenic tendency of pregnancy. There are reports that plasma levels of hPL are influenced by blood glucose somewhat in the same way as hGH, where hyperglycemia inhibits secretion and hypoglycemia stimulates secretion. Like hGH, hPL increases nitrogen storage and favors amino acid transfer across the placenta.

Human placental lactogen appears in maternal circulation early in pregnancy, and the level rises continuously to reach a plateau during the last month of pregnancy (Fig. 11-2). The daily production of hPL at this stage has been calculated to be as large as 1 to 10 g.

Method
Reagents

The abundance of hPL in the placenta and the easy availability of human placentas have made it possible to prepare highly purified hPL. Such material is commercially available and has been used for production of specific antisera. Human placental lactogen itself is a relatively good immunogen, and antisera have been prepared in rabbits and guinea pigs. Some antisera may cross-react with hGH, but most antisera show high specificity without detectable influence from hGH. When the hPL assay is used on maternal samples collected in late pregnancy, the concentration of hPL is 100- to 10,000-fold higher than the concentration of hGH or prolactin; thus a possible cross-reaction from either of these can be ignored.

Labeling of hPL with ^{125}I does not seem to cause much difficulty irrespective of the method used.

---

hPL METHOD

Ethanol precipitation

Principle $R + [L + L^*] = [RL + RL^*] + [L + L^*]$

Protocol

		Reagent	Volume
DAY 1	R	Rabbit antiserum to hPL	200 μl
	L*	^{125}I-hPL	200 μl
	L	Standard: 1.25, 2.5, 5.0, 10.0, 20.0 mg/liter in male plasma	100 μl
		Sample: EDTA-plasma	

———————— *1 hour, 25°C* ————————

Ethanol 99.5%   1,000 μl

Centrifugation, 2,500g, 15 minutes, 25° C
Decant supernatant
Count precipitate for 30 seconds

Reagents

R Rabbit antiserum to hPL
   Avidity: $K_a \approx 4 \times 10^{10}$

L* hPL labeled with ^{125}I by lactoperoxidase (Appendix 17)
    Specific activity: 30-40 μCi/μg; separation on Sephadex G-50
    (Appendix 19)
    $T = 100,000$ cpm ≈ 2 ng

L EDTA-plasma

Diluent Barbital-BSA (Appendix 34)

Appendix 24

Box 11-2

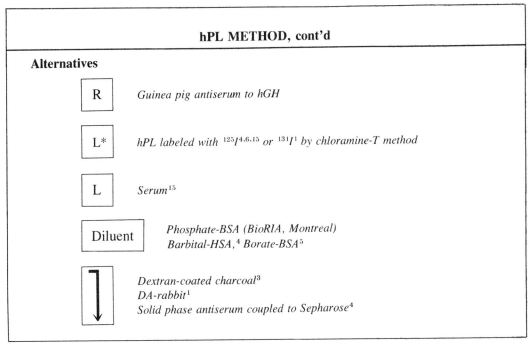

Box 11-2

Performance

The assays generally used have been of the direct competitive type and have essentially differed in the method used for separation of bound and free activity.

A variety of methods have been applied for this purpose, including double antibody, chromatoelectrophoresis, ethanol, dextran-coated charcoal, dixoane, and solid phase coupled antibodies. Since hPL assays usually are applied for semiacute situations, a procedure that does not require a second incubation period is most suitable. Of those mentioned, ethanol precipitation seems the most easy and reliable.

Assay properties

Because of the high concentrations of the reactants, the reaction comes to equilibrium rapidly, requiring incubation times of a few hours at the most. It is even possible to reduce incubation time to minutes rather than hours. The need for sensitivity is not great for most purposes. However, assays capable of detecting 0.05 ng/ml have been developed. In early preg-

nancy a sensitive variant of the assay with a working range of $0.01 \mu g$ to $1.0 \mu g$/ml has been used. An RIA method for hPL is shown in Box 11-2.

Clinical applications

Pathophysiology

The secretion of hPL shows a correlation with the mass and function of total trophoblast tissue. Therefore, plasma levels are correlated with the condition of the placenta as well as with the total placental weight, which in turn correlates with the weight and state of the fetus.

Hyposecretion of hPL carries a poor prognosis in association with threatened abortion by vaginal bleeding at 5 to 20 weeks of gestation. Abnormally low levels have been reported to occur in women in whom the bleeding progressed to abortion. This has been an aid in deciding whether to evacuate the uterus or not. Also, in severe intrauterine growth retardation, significantly reduced hPL levels are seen.

Hypersecretion of hPL occurs in twin pregnancies. If the duration of pregnancy can be appropriately defined (which is important because of the progressive increase of the concentration during gestation), hPL determination has been used as a relatively early screening test for multiple fetuses in the period from the twenty-eighth to the thirty-fourth week of gestation.

Sampling

Serum or plasma samples are usually obtained.

Reference values

Human placental lactogen is not normally detectable in the nonpregnant state. The progressive change during pregnancy is shown in Fig. 11-2. The absolute level may differ slightly for different laboratories. During the last weeks of pregnancy, a value less than 4 μg/ml suggests placental insufficiency.

Interpretation of results

DECREASED hPL CONCENTRATION. From the thirtieth week onward, the hPL levels have been used as an indicator of placental viability. These levels are a relatively poor direct indicator of fetal distress if this condition is not secondary to insufficiency of the placenta. The inter-

individual variation is rather wide, whereas the level remains more constant within each individual. The prognostic utility of the test is significantly improved if the patient can be followed by repeated samples, whereby the trends in the levels are evaluated rather than the absolute level itself. Falling values from the thirtieth week onward are, therefore, a grave sign of placental insufficiency. A patient who has three or more serum measurements less than 4 μg/ml has a 70% chance for fetal complications.

In toxemia of pregnancy, the association of maternal hypertension with low hPL values indicates a markedly increased risk for the fetus.

ELEVATED hPL CONCENTRATIONS. These may occur in twin pregnancies, diabetes mellitus, and rhesus isoimmunization. Trophoblastic tumors also produce hPL, and very high levels may be found.

ESTRIOL
Chemistry

A great number of estrogens are produced in the placenta. Of these, estriol (E_3) dominates. The chemical structure of estriol is shown in Fig. 10-5 (p. 147). In contrast to the estriol in nonpregnant women, which is primarily a me-

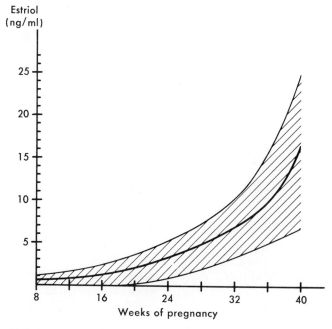

Fig. 11-3. Plasma levels of estriol during pregnancy (mean and 95% range).

tabolite of estradiol, the precursor for estriol in the placenta is 16-hydroxydehydroepiandrosterone.

Physiology

The secretion of placental estriol increases almost 1,000-fold continuously during pregnancy and reaches its highest values at term (Fig. 11-3). There is an accelerated increase during the last weeks of gestation, which is believed to be involved in the mechanisms that initiate the delivery. In blood, the estrogens occur in both conjugated and unconjugated form, whereas in urine they are almost completely conjugated to glucuronic and sulfuric acid. There is a slight circadian rhythm of estriol in plasma, with lowest values in the afternoon, although this is a matter of some debate. The placenta and the fetus serve as one unit in the synthesis of the estrogens. In the quantitatively dominating pathway, the first and final steps of estriol production take place in the placenta, but some intermediate steps are performed in the fetal adrenals and liver.

The high levels of estrogens in pregnancy promote the protein synthesis and the growth of the uterus and placenta and alter the structure of connecting tissue, making it looser and facilitating delivery. Estrogens promote breast development; increase the synthesis of certain plasma proteins, including some coagulation factors; and increase the levels of some hormone-transporting proteins, such as thyroxine-binding globulin.

Method

Assays have been reported both for conjugated and unconjugated plasma estriol. There are reports of relatively good correlation between unconjugated estriol in plasma and the excretion of estriol in urine, but the between-day variations in the unconjugated estriol levels are wider for the urine determinations.

Reagents

Various solvents have been used for extraction of estriol; in a comparative study, ethyl acetate/hexane (3:2 v/v) showed the highest extraction, with a recovery close to 100%. Ether has also been used, but the recoveries reported have varied between 60% and 90%. Following extraction, the solvent is evaporated and the residue taken into a buffer. Because of the high concentration of estriol in relation to the sensitivity of the methods now available, only a small amount of plasma needs to be included in the extraction procedure. This means that the amount of contaminating material is comparatively low; thus the extract usually does not need any further purification. Estriol can be measured by use of antisera raised against estradiol-17β hemisuccinate coupled to BSA. More recently, however, specific estriol antisera have been used.

Most assays reported have utilized ^{3}H-estriol, but recent experience with ^{125}I-labeled materials is promising, and these will probably be the radioligands of choice (see Chapter 3).

Performance

The incubation times are relatively short (1 to 3 hours) in most methods. Technically, it is usually easier to measure unconjugated steroids in blood; some tests convert conjugated estriol to unconjugated estriol by the use of enzymatic methods.

Separation methods have included dextran-coated charcoal, ammonium sulfate precipitation, and solid phase coupled antibody.

Assay properties

All methods require a step that removes or denatures estrogen-binding proteins that otherwise interfere in the assay. In addition, the total estriol assay includes a hydrolysis step. More recently, the assay of unconjugated estriol has become the most widely accepted method, since it avoids the complication of the hydrolysis.

Clinical applications

Pathophysiology

The interaction of the fetus and placenta in estriol synthesis makes estriol quite vulnerable to alterations in the well-being of the fetoplacental unit. Determination of urinary estrogen excretion has been used extensively in clinical practice. Assays on plasma have not been widely applied until recently with the advent of steroid RIAs. Clinical experience with these assays is, therefore, still relatively restricted, and much of our knowledge is extrapolated from determinations of urinary estrogens. It is generally agreed that estriol plasma levels parallel closely the gradual development and growth of the fetus and placenta. Levels are higher in larger fetuses than in smaller ones and normally increase with time until parturition. In contrast, any clinical entity that interferes with the normal development of the fetus or placenta results in either low plasma levels or a subnormal increase with time during gestation. Examples of such disorders include preeclampsia, diabetes, placental insufficiency, molar pregnancy, and fetal death. Like hPL determinations, the evaluation of assay results is facilitated by serial determinations, in which levels are followed longitudinally. Accordingly, a drop in the concentration or failure to increase with time gives more information than a single low value.

Sampling

Serum or plasma may be used. Serum samples should be frozen if collected more than 24 hours before assay. Samples should be collected at a fixed time of day, if possible.

Reference values

Estriol concentration in plasma: 7-25 ng/ml at term

Interpretation of results

Decreased levels of estriol (or a delayed rise during pregnancy) occur in cases of intrauterine growth retardation, preeclampsia, rhesus incompatibility, maternal diabetes, hydatidiform mole, and severe neurologic malformations of the fetus. Low values in these groups indicate a marked increase in the risk for fetal loss, although the correlation is not absolute. In any of these conditions the fetus may die in utero despite normal estriol values. During the last 6 weeks of pregnancy, values considerably less than 7 ng/ml are indicative of fetal distress.

REFERENCES

1. Beck, P., Parker, M. L., and Daughaday, W. H.: Radioimmunologic measurements of human placental lactogen in plasma by a double antibody method during normal and diabetic pregnancies, J. Clin. Endocrinol. Metab. 25:1457, 1965.
2. Cleary, R. E., and Young, P. C. M.: Serum unconjugated estriol in normal and abnormal pregnancy, Am. J. Obstet. Gynecol. 118:18, 1974.
3. De Hertogh, R., Thomas, K., Bietlot, Y., Von der Heyden, and Ferin, I.: Plasma levels of unconjugated estrone, estradiol and estriol and of HCS throughout pregnancy in normal women, J. Clin. Endocrinol. Metab. 40:93, 1975.
4. Gardner, J., Bailey, G., and Chard, T.: Observations on the use of solid phase coupled antibodies in the radioimmunoassay of human placental lactogen, Biochem. J. 137:469, 1974.
5. Gurpide, E., Giebenhain, M. E., Tseng, L., and Kelly, W.: Radioimmunoassay for estrogens in human pregnancy urine, plasma, and amniotic fluid, Am. J. Obstet. Gynecol. 109:897, 1971.
6. Handwerger, S., and Sherwood, L. M.: Human placental lactogen (HPL). In Jaffe B. M., and Behrman, H. R., editors: Methods of hormone radioimmunoassay, New York, 1974, Academic Press, Inc., p. 417.
7. Kao, M., Braunstein, G., Rasor, J., and Horton, R.: A simple radioimmunoassay for unconjugated estriol in pregnancy plasma, J. Lab. Clin. Med. 86:513, 1975.
8. Kosasa, T., Levesque, L., and Goldstein, D. P.: Early detection of implantation using a radioimmunoassay specific for human chorionic gonadotropin, J. Clin. Endocrinol. Metab. 36:622, 1973.
9. Kosasa, T. S., Pion, R. J., Hale, R. W., Goldstein, D. P., Taymor, M. L., Levesque, L. A., and Kobara, T. Y.: Rapid hCG-specific radioimmunoassay for menstrual aspiration, Obstet. Gynecol. 45:566, 1975.
10. Lindberg, B. S., Lindberg, P., Martinsson, K., and Johansson, E. D. B.: Oestrogens during pregnancy, Acta Obstet. Gynecol. Scand. (Suppl.) 32:1, 1974.
11. Louvet, J.-P., Nisula, B. C., and Ross, G. T.: Method for extraction of glycoprotein hormones from plasma for use in radioimmunoassays, J. Lab. Clin. Med. 86:883, 1975.
12. Macrae, D. I., and Mohamedally, S. M.: Comparison between plasma estriol and urinary estriol levels in pregnancy, J. Obstet. Gynecol. Br. Commonw. 77:1088, 1970.
13. Orczyk, G. P., Caldwell, V. V., and Behrman, H. R.: Estrogens; estradiol, estrone, and estriol. In Jaffe, B. M., and Behrman, H. R., editors: Methods of hormone radioimmunoassay, New York, 1974, Academic Press, Inc., p. 333.
14. Saxena, B. N., Emerson, K., Jr., and Selenkow, H. A.: Serum placental lactogen (HPL) levels as an index of placental function, N. Engl. J. Med. 281:225, 1969.
15. Saxena, B. N., Refetoff, S., Emerson, K., Jr., and Selenkow, H. A.: A rapid radioimmunoassay for human placental lactogen; application to normal and pathologic pregnancies, Am. J. Obstet. Gynecol. 101:874, 1969.
16. Stafford, J. E. H., and Watson, D.: Total and unconjugated oestriol levels as a test of fetoplacental function. In International Atomic Energy Agency: Radio-

immunoassay and related procedures in medicine, vol. 2, Vienna, 1974, I.A.E.A., p. 57.

17. Taylor, E. S., Hagernac, D. P., Betz, G., Williams, K. L., and Grey, P. A.: Estriol concentrations in blood during pregnancy, Am. J. Obstet. Gynecol. **108:**868, 1970.

18. Tulchinsky, D., Hobel, C. J., and Korenman, S. G.: A radioligand assay for plasma unconjugated estriol in normal and abnormal pregnancies, Am. J. Obstet. Gynecol. **111:**311, 1971.

19. Tyrey, L., Handwerger, S., and Sherwood, L. M.: Human chorionic gonadotropin (HCG). In Jaffe, B. M., and Behrman H. R., editors: Methods of hormone radioimmunoassay, New York, 1974, Academic Press, Inc., p. 427.

20. Vaitukaitis, J. L., Braunstein, G. D., and Ross, G. T.: A radioimmunoassay which serially measures human chorionic gonadotropin in the presence of human luteinizing hormone, Am. J. Obstet. Gynecol. **113:**751, 1972.

12 HUMAN GROWTH HORMONE

Chemistry

Growth hormone (somatotropin) is a single-chain polypeptide of about 190 amino acids and has a molecular weight of about 21,500 daltons. The structure is highly species specific; thus only somatotropin of human extraction (human growth hormone, hGH) can be used in the assay. Two other hormones have similar structures: pituitary prolactin and human placental lactogen (hPL, or chorionic somatomammotropin). A "big" hGH, with a molecular weight of 40,000 to 45,000, also circulates in blood. "Big" hGH is transformed to hGH (molecular weight, 21,500) slowly in vitro.

Physiology

Somatotropin is an important regulator of intermediate metabolism. In addition to stimulating growth, somatotropin stimulates lipolysis, increases the glycogen stores in the liver, and acts as an insulin antagonist in skeletal muscles. Some of these effects are elicited via somatomedins, which are proteins produced in the liver and kidneys after stimulation by somatotropin.

Growth hormone is produced and secreted by the acidophilic cells of the anterior pituitary. The release is characterized by a low rate of basal secretion intermittently interrupted by episodes with a very high rate of release. These episodes will produce a peak in the secretion of hGH of approximately 30 to 120 minutes' duration. The release is influenced by hypothalamic releasing factors, which are transported to the anterior pituitary by the hypothalamic-hypophyseal portal vessels. A hypothalamic somatotropin release–inhibiting hormone, somatostatin, has been identified. Its structure is known, and it has also been synthesized and studied extensively during recent years. Somatostatin is probably produced in other endocrine cells as well and has been shown to inhibit not only the secretion of somatotropin but also the secretion of insulin and glucagon. A somatotropin-releasing hormone, analogous to other releasing hormones, has not yet been identified.

An increase in somatotropin release rate and a subsequent peak in plasma somatotropin concentration occur in response to a variety of stimuli, such as starvation, physical exercise, ingestion of proteins or amino acids, hypoglycemia, and nonspecific stress. During the first hours of sleep there is a marked increase in the secretion rate. Spontaneous peaks without obvious cause may also occur. Insulin hypoglycemia and amino acid function, especially that of arginine, the most active stimulator, will cause an increase in somatotropin secretion. Drugs with neuron-transmitting effects, such as L-dopa, also increase the secretion rate of somatotropin.

Conversely, secretion is inhibited by hyperglycemia and tranquilizing drugs, including barbiturates and chlorpromazine.

Somatotropin circulates freely in plasma and is not bound to any transporting protein. Its turnover rate in plasma is fairly rapid, with a half-life of approximately 30 minutes. Somatotropin is mainly degraded in the liver and is not secreted in the urine.

Method
Reagents

Human somatotropin of high purity is commercially available from several sources. An international standard has been established, and pure somatotropin is assumed to have a potency of about 2 units/mg. Human growth hormone serves as a reasonably good immunogen, and hGH antisera have been developed in guinea pigs, goats, and rabbits. Because of its homologous structure, hPL may cross-react in some somatotropin assays. The degree of cross-reactivity varies between individual antisera. Accordingly, some antisera may be used to measure hGH in the sera of pregnant women, whereas others may not.

In routine clinical work or other situations where plasma from pregnant women is assayed, the influence of hPL may be tested. The occurrence in plasma of hGH with a higher molecular weight, "big" hGH, has been reported. "Big" somatotropin cross-reacts with some somatotropin antisera. Its chemical structure has not been established. However, it constitutes only a small fraction of the circulating somatotropin, and its significance is not known. A somatotropin with altered biologic properties has been reported in acromegaly; but since this substance cross-reacts with somatotropin antibody, the use of the somatotropin assays for the clinical evaluation of cases with acromegaly is still valid.

Human somatotropin and somatotropin from higher primates can be assayed using antisera produced against human material. For assay of somatotropin of certain species, specific somatotropin and corresponding antisera are available from the National Pituitary Agency of the National Institutes of Health.

The chloramine-T and lactoperoxidase methods work well for iodination of somatotropin with ^{125}I.

Performance

Assays reported require from 1 to 6 days to complete. Most methods employ serum as a diluent for standards; in some assays serum from hypophysectomized patients is used. This is done to minimize the effects of nonspecific serum interference in the assay. Other methods have not been sensitive to these effects; for example, the method shown in Box 12-1.

A variety of techniques have been utilized for separating bound and free activity, including double antibody, chromatoelectrophoresis, ethanol, and dextran-coated charcoal.

Assay properties

Assay sensitivity ranges from 0.1 to 1 ng/ml. Many modifications of somatotropin assays have been reported; no single one seems to have absolute advantages. Most methods meet the requirements of being able to assay basal levels and are performed within 1 or 2 days.

Clinical applications
Pathophysiology

HYPOFUNCTION. Hyposecretion of somatotropin may occur either as an isolated deficiency of somatotropin or as a part of panhypopituitarism. The isolated deficiency is generally an inborn condition, without any familial history. The effect of the hypofunction usually is not recognized until the age of 3 to 4 years, although it may be traced earlier. It causes severe growth retardation—pituitary dwarfism. Pituitary dwarfism can be treated successfully by injections of human somatotropin as long as the epiphyseal growth zones in the skeleton are open. More generalized forms of hypopituitarism occur in association with pituitary tumors that are not hormone producing, such as craniopharyngioma and chromophobe adenoma. Other expanding processes in the sella region, such as histiocytosis, may cause pituitary insufficiency. Surgical ablation of the pituitary and Sheehan's syndrome (pituitary necrosis following severe postpartum hemorrhage) are two other causes of panhypopituitarism. Secondary hGH deficiency may occur in longstanding steroid therapy or in severe emotional disturbances, such as maternal deprivation. A relative decrease of the hGH secretion rate may occur secondary to abnormalities in other endocrine glands, such as hyper- or hypothyroidism. Accordingly, such abnormalities should be corrected before hGH secretion is tested, because a blunted response may otherwise be erroneously interpreted as primary pituitary insufficiency.

The hGH response to stimulation is greater in females than in males. This augmented response is related to higher estrogen levels.

hGH METHOD

Principle

Double antibody

$$R + [L + L^*] = [RL + RL^*] + [L + L^*]$$

Protocol

		Reagent	Volume
DAY 1	R	Guinea pig antiserum to hGH	200 μl
	L*	^{125}I-labeled hGH	200 μl
	L	Standard 3.1, 6.25, 12.5, 25, 50, 100 ng/ml Sample EDTA-plasma	100 μl

──────────── 24-48 hours, 4° C ────────────

DAY 3		Normal guinea pig serum (1:500)	50 μl
		Rabbit antiserum to guinea pig IgG (1:10)	50 μl

──────────── 18 hours, 4° C ────────────

DAY 4		Add diluent	500 μl
		Centrifugation, 2,500g, 15 minutes, 4° C	
		Decant supernatant	
		Count precipitate for 1 minute	

Reagents

R	Antiserum to hGH; no cross-reaction with hPL Avidity: $K_a \approx 2 \times 10^{10}$	
L*	hGH labeled with ^{125}I by lactoperoxidase (Appendix 17) Specific activity: 120-160 μCi/μg; separation on Sephadex G-50; T = 20,000 cpm ≈ 0.1 ng	
L	EDTA-plasma	
Diluent	Barbital-BSA (Appendix 34)	
	Appendix 28	

Box 12-1

hGH METHOD, cont'd
Alternatives

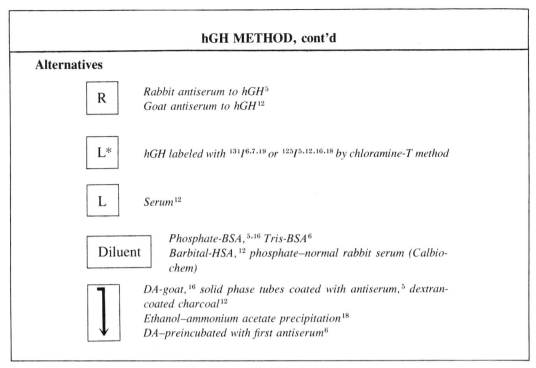

R   *Rabbit antiserum to hGH[5]*
      Goat antiserum to hGH[12]

L*   *hGH labeled with [131]I[6,7,19] or [125]I[5,12,16,18] by chloramine-T method*

L   *Serum[12]*

Diluent   *Phosphate-BSA,[5,16] Tris-BSA[6]*
      Barbital-HSA,[12] phosphate–normal rabbit serum (Calbiochem)

    DA-goat,[16] solid phase tubes coated with antiserum,[5] dextran-coated charcoal[12]
    Ethanol–ammonium acetate precipitation[18]
    DA–preincubated with first antiserum[6]

Box 12-1

Estrogen treatments of males increase their somatotropin secretion.

HYPERFUNCTION. Hypersecretion of somatotropin is usually caused by an acidophilic adenoma of the anterior pituitary. Clinically, it causes acromegaly in adults, and in the rare cases reported in childhood it causes gigantism. The secretion of somatotropin from such an adenoma is autonomous and does not respond to factors that normally change the secretion of hGH. In addition, the basal rate of secretion is elevated.

High levels of hGH have been reported in diabetic ketosis, malnutrition, and protein depletion. African pygmies have high levels in association with an end-organ failure to respond to hGH. Some patients with anorexia nervosa may have highly elevated levels, whereas others have low levels. Rare instances of elevated levels in which the effect of hGH is reduced occur in the so-called Laron type of dwarfism and in patients with hypothalamic tumors or malformations. Ectopic production of somato-tropin has been reported in pulmonary tumors as a possible cause of some cases of pulmonary osteoarthropathy.

Sampling

Because marked fluctuations in hGH concentration occur in normal individuals, random sampling does not give useful information. Accordingly, sampling should be performed when secretion is either stimulated or inhibited.

STIMULATION TEST. Stimulation tests are useful when there is clinical suspicion of hypofunction; samples should be collected when the secretion rate normally would be stimulated. Stimuli include infusion of insulin, arginine, L-dopa, and apomorphine. Sampling after exercise or after the first hours of sleep has been useful. The great variety of stimulation tests used reflects the fact that in a normal population none of these stimulation tests induces a response in all persons tested. Patients with insulin-induced hypoglycemia give the highest frequency of positive responses, and stimulation is achieved in 80% to 90% of normal individuals. The various stimulation tests used are outlined in Table 12-1, and the responses in normal individuals and in certain abnormal conditions are illustrated in Fig. 12-1. As a precaution, when the insulin hypoglycemia test is performed, an indwelling venous catheter should be maintained to permit infusion if prolonged or severe hypoglycemia occurs. This precaution is particularly important in patients with pituitary insufficiency who are occasionally prone to develop profound hypoglycemia when insulin is given. Blood glucose levels should be monitored during the test to ascertain that an adequate stimulation has been achieved, since there is significant individual variation in the sensitivity to insulin. A 50% decrease from fasting blood glucose level is generally regarded as adequate insulin response. The oral administration of L-dopa should be via tablets without a delayed-release effect, since the slow release and relatively low

Table 12-1. Tests of hGH secretion

Agent	Dose	Method of administration	Sample collection	
			Interval	Duration
Stimulation tests				
Insulin	0.1 IU/kg	Intravenous injection	30 minutes	90 minutes
L-Dopa	0.5 g	Oral administration	30 minutes	2 hours
Arginine	0.5 g/kg	Intravenous infusion	30 minutes	90 minutes
Glucagon	1 mg	Intravenous injection	30 minutes	2-3 hours
Apomorphine	0.75 mg	Subcutaneous injection	30 minutes	90 minutes
Inhibition test				
Glucose	50 g	Oral administration	30 minutes	2 hours

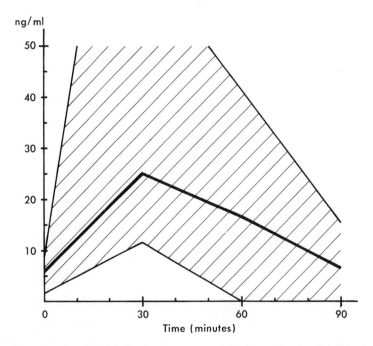

Fig. 12-1. Plasma levels of hGH following intravenous injection of insulin, 0.1 U/kg body weight (mean and 95% range).

serum concentration achieved may not cause the immediate stimulation of somatotropin desired. To increase the diagnostic accuracy of the stimulation test, combined tests (for example, the insulin hypoglycemia test immediately followed by an arginine infusion) have been proposed.

INHIBITION TEST. When hypersecretion of somatotropin is suspected, samples should be collected at a time when physiologic peaks in secretion do not normally occur. Sampling under conditions at which somatotropin is normally suppressed (inhibition testing) is the method of choice in this situation. It is known that hyperglycemia inhibits the release of somatotropin. A steady state of hyperglycemia produced by administration of a 50-g glucose load administered orally will inhibit the release of somatotropin. A glucose load administered intravenously should not be used, because the short-term injection of glucose and resulting peak in concentration are followed by a steadily falling level of blood glucose that will actually stimulate hGH secretion, even if this occurs at a hyperglycemic level. Accordingly, the hGH level will normally tend to increase during the latter phase of the orally administered glucose tolerance test. It is probably the same mechanism that is effective when glucagon is used as a stimulation test.

BLOOD SAMPLES. Venous blood is collected, and the assay is performed on either serum or plasma. Somatotropin is stable at room temperature in serum for a couple of days, but extended storage should be at $-20°$ C.

Reference values

Normal basal serum level: 4 ng/ml (< 5 ng/ml)

Normal stimulation response: 6-8 ng/ml above basal level

Interpretation of results

Decreased hGH response is best evaluated during a stimulation test. Peak values should reach at least 6 to 8 ng/ml above the basal level. If the test happens to be started when a spontaneous peak has occurred, the normal response to the stimulation may be inhibited; but a pretest value that is elevated significantly above the basal level indicates a normal secretory ability. Since the somatotropin response is slightly higher in females than in males, estrogen pretreatment of boys with suspected somatotropin deficiency has been used for more certain identification of the deficiency state. If the first test indicates somatotropin deficiency, a second test is usually performed to establish the diagnosis, since a blunted response sometimes occurs in normal individuals.

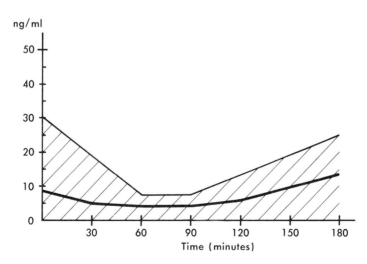

Fig. 12-2. Plasma levels of hGH after an oral glucose load (mean and 95% range).

Increased hGH response is best evaluated by an inhibition test. The basal level of secretion should be measured during the period of maximal hyperglycemia following a glucose load administered orally. In normal individuals this is less than 5 ng/ml. Abnormal secretion by an eosinophilic pituitary adenoma causes the average serum level to be elevated, although fluctuations in concentration may occur. In this situation an inhibition test may even cause a reverse reaction with an increased secretion. Such a reverse reaction is normally found in newborn babies. There is fairly good correlation between the levels of plasma somatotropin and the clinical activity of acromegaly. Somatotropin estimation is probably the most accurate method for evaluating the effect of surgery or radiation in acromegaly.

REFERENCES

1. Berson, S. A., and Yalow, R. S.: State of human growth hormone in plasma and changes in stored solutions of pituitary growth hormone, J. Biol. Chem. **241:** 5745, 1966.
2. Best, J. B., Catt, K. J., and Burger, H. G.: Arginine infusion and growth-hormone secretion, Lancet **2:** 1349, 1968.
3. Boden, G., and Soeldner, J. S.: A sensitive double antibody radioimmunoassay for human growth hormone (HGH); levels of serum HGH following rapid tolbutamide infusion, Diabetologia **4:**413, 1967.
4. Catt, K. J., Moffat, B., and Niall, H. D.: Human growth hormone and placental lactogen; structural similarity, Science **157:**321, 1967.
5. Catt, K. J., Tregear, G. W., Burger, H. G., and Skermer, C.: Antibody-coated tube method for radioimmunoassay of human growth hormone, Clin. Chim. Acta **27:**267, 1970.
6. Cerasi, E., Della Casa, L., Luft, R., and Roovete, A.: Determination of human growth hormone (HGH) in plasma by a double antibody radioimmunoassay, Acta Endocrinol. (Khb.) **53:**101, 1966.
7. Glick, S. M., Roth, J., Yalow, R. S., and Berson, S. A.: Immunoassay of human growth hormone in plasma, Nature **199:**784, 1963.
8. Goodman, A. D., Tanenbaum, R., and Rabinowitz, D.: Existence of two forms of immunoreactive growth hormone in human plasma, J. Clin. Endocrinol. Metab. **35:**868, 1972.
9. Hunter, W. M.: Radioimmunoassay of growth hormone (HGH, somatotrophin, STH) in plasma. In Brener, H., Hamel, D., and Knüskemper, H. L., editors: Methods of hormone analysis, New York, 1976, John Wiley & Sons, Inc., p. 1.
10. Hunter, W. M., and Greenwood, F. C.: A radioimmunoelectrophoretic assay for human growth hormone, Biochem. J. **91:**43, 1964.
11. Lazarus, L., and Young, J. D.: Radioimmunoassay of human growth hormone using ion exchange resin, J. Clin. Endocrinol. Metab. **26:**213, 1966.
12. Meek, J. C., Stoskopf, M. M., and Bolinger, R. E.: Optimization of radioimmunoassay for human growth hormone by the charcoal dextran technique, Clin. Chem. **16:**845, 1970.
13. Miles, L. E., and Hales, C. N.: Immunoradiometric assay of human growth hormone, Lancet **2:**492, 1968.
14. Mitchell, M. L., Collins, S., and Byron, J.: Radioimmunoassay of growth hormone by enzyme partition, J. Clin. Endocrinol. Metab. **29:**257, 1969.
15. Morgan, C. R.: Immunoassay of human insulin and growth hormone simultaneously using I^{125} and I^{131} tracers. Proc. Soc. Exp. Biol. Med. **173:**230, 1966.
16. Peake, G. T.: Growth hormone. In Jaffe, B. M., and Behrman, H. R., editors: Methods of hormone radioimmunoassay, New York, 1974, Academic Press, Inc., pp. 103-123.
17. Roth, J., Glick, S. M., Yalow, R. S., and Berson, S. A.: Hypoglycemia; a potent new stimulator to secretion of growth hormone, Science **140:**981, 1963.
18. Saito, T., and Saxena, B. B.: A sensitive, rapid, and economic radioimmunoassay of human growth hormone using ethanol-ammonium acetate, J. Lab. Clin. Med. **85:**497, 1975.
19. Schalch, D. S., and Parker, M. L.: A sensitive double antibody immunoassay for human growth hormone in plasma, Nature **230:**1141, 1964.
20. Thompson, R. G., Rodriguez, A., Kowaiski, A., and Blizzard, R. M.: Growth hormone; metabolic clearance rates, integrated concentrations and production ratio of normal adults and the effects of prednisone, J. Clin. Invest. **51:**3193, 1972.
21. Utiger, R. D., Parker, M. L., and Daughaday, W. H.: Studies on human growth hormone. I. A radioimmunoassay for human growth hormone, J. Clin. Invest. **41:**254, 1962.

13 RENIN-ANGIOTENSIN AND ALDOSTERONE

Renin, angiotensin, and aldosterone are important components of a system that regulates sodium balance, fluid volume, and blood pressure. In response to reduced renal perfusion, as would accompany decreased blood volume or decreased blood pressure, renin is secreted by the kidney into the blood, where renin acts enzymatically on a plasma globulin to produce angiotensin I. Angiotensin I is rapidly converted to angiotensin II by converting enzymes in the lung and plasma. Angiotensin II has a direct pressor effect on peripheral blood vessels and also stimulates aldosterone secretion by the adrenal. Aldosterone blocks excretion of sodium at the distal tubule. In this manner, angiotensin and aldosterone act to increase retention of sodium and thus raise blood pressure.

In this chapter methods of measurement of renin by means of radioimmunoassay (RIA) of angiotension I, as well as methods for measurement of aldosterone, are discussed.

RENIN-ANGIOTENSIN
Chemistry

The proteolytic enzyme renin cleaves the 57,000–molecular weight α_2-globulin, renin substrate, to form angiotension I, a decapeptide. Converting enzyme, which is found in the lung in high concentration, splits off the two carboxyl terminal amino acids to produce the octapeptide, angiotensin II. Angiotensin II has the following structure beginning from the amino end: Asp-Arg-Val-Tyr-Ileu-His-Pro-Phe. With different animal species, variability occurs only in the fifth amino acid from the aspartic end. The carboxyl end of the molecule appears to be of particular importance to the function of angiotensin II (Fig. 13-1).

Physiology

The enzyme renin is produced in the juxtaglomerular apparatus of the kidney. Renin is released into the circulation in response to a variety of circumstances that result in lowered blood pressure and reduced plasma volume. Both epinephrine and norepinephrine stimulate the renin release. In general, anything that induces decreased renal perfusion will cause an increase in renin secretion. This mechanism is apparently the cause for increased renin secretion in the upright posture and following arterial obstruction to renal blood flow. Similarly, dehydration, sodium depletion, and reduced concentration of serum proteins also increase renin secretion. These factors apparently lower the perfusion pressure in the kidney, which is the primary stimulus to renin release. The baroreceptors of the juxtaglomerular apparatus and sodium flux near the macula densa work together to control the amount of renin released into the circulation.

Renin secretion is decreased by angiotensin II by direct inhibition. Adrenergic blocking agents also suppress renin secretion.

Renin has a circulating half-time of 10 minutes in man. The half-time of angiotensin II is about 1 minute. Angiotensin II is the most potent pressor substance known. In addition, angiotensin II acts on the zona glomerulosa of the adrenal cortex to stimulate the production of aldosterone. Angiotensin II is rapidly broken down by angiotensinases in tissue and plasma. The concentration of renin is usually the rate

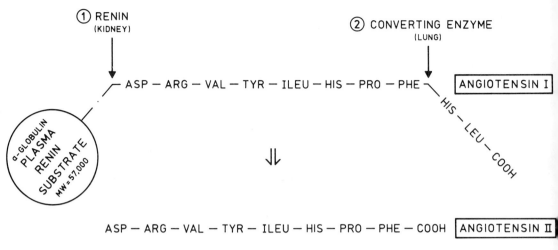

Fig. 13-1. Principles of formation of angiotensin II from renin substrate via angiotensin I.

limiting step in the reaction sequence shown in Fig. 13-1.

Method

Renin assay depended for many years on bioassay systems that were based on the pressor response of an intact animal or the response of an in vitro system such as the rat uterus, guinea pig ileum, or rabbit aorta. At present, renin assay is based on the enzymatic breakdown of plasma renin substrate by renin. Current methodology employs RIA to measure angiotensin I generated by this process. Two basic techniques have been employed: measurement of plasma renin activity (PRA) and measurement of plasma renin concentration (PRC). In addition, the concentration of the dominant plasma renin substrate (PRS) may also be measured. During these assays, the conversion of angiotensin I to angiotensin II is blocked by various agents.

DETERMINING PLASMA RENIN ACTIVITY. Measurement of PRA is performed on plasma samples without addition of exogenous renin or PRS. Angiotensin I is measured by RIA after incubation of the patient's plasma under standard conditions. The concentration of angiotensin I is a measure of the activity of renin under conditions that occur in the patient.

DETERMINING PLASMA RENIN CONCENTRA-

TION. In plasma, the amount of angiotensin I that is produced by the action of renin on its substrate depends on both the concentration of renin and the concentration of substrate. Therefore, the PRA is not necessarily related to PRC. This is particularly true in clinical states in which PRS concentrations vary, such as during pregnancy and oral contraceptive therapy, which elevate PRS concentrations.

In order to obtain better estimates of PRC, addition of excess heterologous PRS from cow or sheep combined with inactivation of endogenous renin substrate has been employed. In the presence of excess amounts of renin substrate, the rate of angiotensin I production depends only on the concentration of renin in plasma. The results of PRC measurements are expressed in terms of the maximal velocity of angiotensin I production (usually nanograms per milliliter per hour). These units can be converted to concentration of renin in Goldblatt units by comparison with the appropriate standard curve of angiotensin I production per unit of a renin standard.

DETERMINING PLASMA RENIN SUBSTRATE CONCENTRATION. The concentration of PRS may be determined by the addition of excess homologous renin to the plasma samples. Incubation is allowed to proceed for long enough to permit conversion of all renin substrate into angiotensin I. The amount of PRS is determined by reference to a standard curve of PRS concentration.

Reagents

The earliest antiangiotensin antibodies were developed by Deodhar, and the initial RIAs for angiotensin I were developed by Goodfriend and associates.

Angiotensin I has been made antigenic by coupling it to large molecules including albumin and succinylated polylysine. Adsorption to microparticles of carbon black has also been employed. Antisera have been produced primarily in rabbits.

Standards and material for preparations of immunogens may be obtained from the Medical Research Council, Division of Biological Standards, National Institute for Medical Research, Hampstead Laboratories, Holly Hill, London, England. Human renin (Research Standard A68/356) and angiotensin I standards are available. Commercially available monoiodinated angiotensin I and II can be obtained from New England Nuclear Corp., Boston, Mass. ^{125}I-labeled angiotensin I has been prepared by chloramine-T iodination with subsequent purification of the radiolabeled products on DEAE-Sephadex. An attempt is made to use only the monoiodinated angiotensins because these have much greater immunoreactivity than diiodinated forms.

Performance

One problem in the utilization of renin assay has been that conditions for assay have varied from laboratory to laboratory. There is still no widespread agreement on the ideal conditions of assay; however, a number of variables need to be considered, whether the assay is PRA, PRC, or PRS:

1. *Incubation pH*. Renin assay has been performed either at physiologic pH 7.4 or at the pH optimum (about 6.0) for the renin-catalyzed production of angiotensin I in plasma. Typically, incubation is employed at 37° C; under these circumstances, it is important to add additional buffers so that the pH does not rise during incubation.

2. *Effect of dilution*. In the assay of PRA, the reaction rate is dependent on the concentra-

tion of PRS present. Any dilution, therefore, will alter the rate at which the enzymatic reaction proceeds. Dilution of plasma is to be avoided as much as possible.

3. *Addition of enzymatic inhibitors*. Enzymatic inhibitors have been used to prevent degradation of angiotensin I produced from the action of renin on renin substrate. These enzyme inhibitors block the action of converting enzyme and angiotensinase activity. Converting enzyme is blocked by ethylenediamenetetraacetic acid (EDTA). For this reason, EDTA is used as an anticoagulant for blood samples to be assayed for renin activity. EDTA also blocks angiotensinase activity. In addition, other inhibitors have been employed during the incubation, including diisopropyl fluorophosphate (DFP) and dimercaprol (BAL). DFP is usually employed for incubations that proceed at pH 6.0. BAL and 8-hydroxyquinoline are usually employed at physiologic pH. As an alternative, phenylmethylsulfonyl fluoride (PMSF) has been used during incubation at pH 6.0.

4. *Incubation time*. For determining PRA, various incubation times ranging from 2 to 3 hours have been proposed. It is an important requirement that the generation of angiotensin I be linearly related to the time of incubation. Many investigators employ a standard incubation period of 3 hours and, if necessary, prolong the incubation for samples containing low renin concentrations or shorten it for those containing high renin concentrations.

Dextran-coated charcoal is the most common separation method employed. Refer to Box 13-1 for specific assay methods for PRA and PRC by means of measurement of angiotensin I by RIA. For further details on methodology see the work by Catt and Douglas (1974).

Assay properties

Most of the problems encountered occur at the enzymatic step. The RIA of angiotensin I is relatively straightforward.

PRA is by far the most widely used test.

Clinical applications
Pathophysiology

See section on physiology under Aldosterone. Rising renin levels result in increasing angio-

RENIN–ANGIOTENSIN I METHOD

Principle

Renin substrate $\xrightarrow[\text{Renin}]{}$ Angiotensin I (=L)

$$R + [L + L^*] = [RL + RL^*] + [L + L^*]$$

Charcoal adsorption

Protocol

	Reagent	Volume
DAY 1	*Plasma renin concentration*	
	EDTA-plasma	*500 μl*
	Renin substrate (sheep ≈ 4,000 ng/ml)[57]	*100 μl*
	First diluent	*500 μl*
	or	
	Plasma renin activity	
	EDTA-plasma	*1,000 μl*
	Second diluent	*50 μl*

3 hours, 37° C (generated plasma)
3 hours, 4° C (control plasma)

R	*Rabbit antiserum to angiotensin I*		*400 μl*
L*	*125I-labeled angiotensin I*		*50 μl*
L	Standard	*0, 62.5, 125, 250, 500, 1,000, 2,000, 4,000 pg/ml*	*200 μl*
	Sample	*Generated plasma sample*	

18-24 hours, 2-8° C

DAY 2 ↓ *Dextran-coated charcoal*   *400 μl*
Mix thoroughly and centrifuge 1,500g, 10 minutes
Immediately decant supernatant into another tube
Count tubes for 2 minutes

Reagents

R	*Rabbit antiserum to angiotensin I*
L*	*Angiotensin I labeled with 125I by lactoperoxidase (Appendixes 17 and 23)*
	Specific activity: 300 μCi/μg
L	*Generated and control plasma samples; the generation is stopped by adding 1.0 ml ice-cold first diluent*

Box 13-1

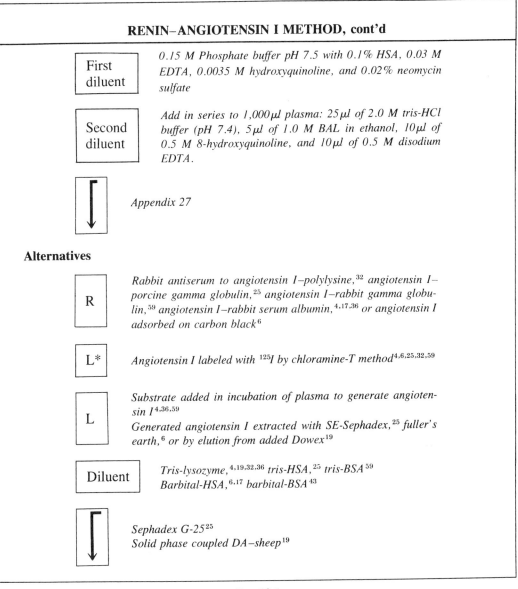

RENIN–ANGIOTENSIN I METHOD, cont'd

First diluent	*0.15 M Phosphate buffer pH 7.5 with 0.1% HSA, 0.03 M EDTA, 0.0035 M hydroxyquinoline, and 0.02% neomycin sulfate*
Second diluent	*Add in series to 1,000 µl plasma: 25 µl of 2.0 M tris-HCl buffer (pH 7.4), 5 µl of 1.0 M BAL in ethanol, 10 µl of 0.5 M 8-hydroxyquinoline, and 10 µl of 0.5 M disodium EDTA.*

Appendix 27

Alternatives

R	*Rabbit antiserum to angiotensin I–polylysine,[32] angiotensin I–porcine gamma globulin,[25] angiotensin I–rabbit gamma globulin,[59] angiotensin I–rabbit serum albumin,[4,17,36] or angiotensin I adsorbed on carbon black[6]*
L*	*Angiotensin I labeled with ^{125}I by chloramine-T method[4,6,25,32,59]*
L	*Substrate added in incubation of plasma to generate angiotensin I[4,36,59]* *Generated angiotensin I extracted with SE-Sephadex,[25] fuller's earth,[6] or by elution from added Dowex[19]*
Diluent	*Tris-lysozyme,[4,19,32,36] tris-HSA,[25] tris-BSA[59]* *Barbital-HSA,[6,17] barbital-BSA[43]*

Sephadex G-25[25]
Solid phase coupled DA–sheep[19]

Box 13-1

---

tensin II, which stimulates the production of aldosterone. Aldosterone directly inhibits the secretion of renin by the kidney (Fig. 13-2).

High renin output clinical states are usually associated with some readily identified abnormality in the feedback loop that controls renin and aldosterone secretion. In most instances of renin excess, aldosterone secretion is concomitantly stimulated, resulting in sodium retention and potassium loss. For example, in high renin output states associated with congestive heart failure, cirrhosis, and nephrotic syndrome, there is a reduction in renal perfusion pressure even though the total blood volume is expanded. In this situation, renin secretion increases. In another type of disorder associated with high renin output, such as primary renal disease, high renin output results from reduced renal perfusion and reduced sodium absorption. Although still controversial, this reduced renal

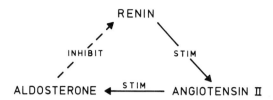

Fig. 13-2. Relationship between the formation of renin, angiotensin II, and aldosterone.

perfusion is thought to be the explanation for the rapidly increasing hypertension associated with malignant hypertension. Also, in some patients with essential hypertension, elevated PRA is present. These patients tend to respond to beta adrenergic blocking drugs, such as propranolol, with a lowering of their blood pressure.

Renin measurements have been used in the management of patients with renal vascular hypertension. The assay is performed as an adjunct to renal arteriography. Renin values are determined at the time of catheterization in both the ischemic and normal kidneys.

Low renin output clinical states occur when adrenal secretion of aldosterone becomes autonomous, as in aldosterone-secreting adenoma or bilateral adrenocortical hyperplasia. In this situation, secretion of renin by the kidneys is markedly inhibited. In addition, in about 30% of patients with essential hypertension, low renin output is observed along with low or normal aldosterone concentrations. Diuretics are the most effective therapeutic agents for the control of these patients' blood pressure.

Sampling

Since there is a significant diurnal variation in renin output, random sampling is not recommended. Usually, renin samples are obtained after a fasting patient has been in an upright position for 2 to 3 hours in the late morning. EDTA is the anticoagulant of choice, since heparin has been shown to inhibit the action of renin on its substrate. Samples should be stored in ice as quickly as possible in order to prevent the action of renin on its substrate until the appropriate inhibitors of angiotensin I degradation can be added to the system. Assays

should be performed as soon as possible, since there is some significant conversion of renin substrate to angiotensin I even at low temperatures.

Because a variety of factors influence PRA, in patients with low or elevated values it is usually desirable to repeat PRA or PRC under standardized conditions.

To substantiate low values, the patient may be placed on a low-sodium diet (10 mEq/day) for 5 days before testing. As an alternative, acute diuresis may be induced by giving the patient 120 mg furosemide orally on the morning of testing. The patient is then encouraged to ambulate for 3 to 4 hours, and a sample is drawn.

High renin values are confirmed by a protocol of high salt intake and recumbency. The patient is placed on a 150 to 200-mEq sodium diet for 5 days. After the patient has been recumbent overnight, a blood sample is drawn for plasma renin determinations.

Reference values

Normal values (mean ±SD) for PRA, PRC, and PRS are shown below (according to Catt and Douglas, 1974).

	Ambulatory patients
PRA (ng/ml/hr)	2.86 ± 2.1
PRC (microunits/ml)	44.0 ± 31.9
PRS (μg/ml)	1.56 ± 0.35

Interpretation of results

Renin secretion in normal individuals varies with posture; secretion is greater when the patient is in the upright position. Renin secretion is also increased by states that are associated with sodium retention in body fluids. During pregnancy and oral contraceptive therapy, all the parameters of renin activity are increased, including PRC, PRA, and PRS. In addition, there is a diurnal variation superimposed upon these changes, with the high point in the late morning and the low point in the evening.

Elevated plasma renin levels are found in a variety of hypertensive states, including unilateral renal disease, especially when associated with severe hypertension. Direct sampling of the renal vein of the affected kidney, with comparison to the contralateral side, is the most effective way to make the diagnosis of renovascular hypertension. A renal vein concentration ratio greater than 1.5:1 (ischemic to nonischemic kidney) when the patient is supine is evidence of significant renin production by the ischemic kidney. In addition, renin activity may be increased in other hypertensive disorders. Typically, renin levels are elevated in malignant hypertension, some forms of essential hypertension, and oral contraceptive–induced hypertension. Severe bilateral renal parenchymal disease may also cause elevated renin levels.

Decreased plasma renin levels are found in primary aldosteronism, in which an aldosterone-producing tumor in the adrenal gland has assumed autonomous function, which is not responsive to the suppressive effects of the renin–angiotensin system. In this case renin production is suppressed. Certain varieties of essential hypertension are also associated with low renin values. Hyperaldosteronism due to bilateral adrenal hyperplasia, exogenous mineralocorticoids including excessive ingestion of licorice, beta adrenergic blocking drugs, and certain varieties of essential hypertension all result in suppressed values.

Primary indications for testing include, first, the need to differentiate between adrenal and nonadrenal causes for hyperaldosteronism. If the adrenal is the cause, renin values are low; in nonadrenal causes, renin values are high. Second, testing may indicate which patients with renal artery stenosis require corrective surgery. Finally in patients with essential hypertension, renin determinations may be helpful in guiding selection of therapy.

ALDOSTERONE
Chemistry

The chemical structure of the mineralocorticoid aldosterone is shown in Fig. 13-3. The 21 carbons in the pregnane ring form the basic structure, which is common to all corticoids. The molecule contains a double bond at the fourth position, two keto groups at the 3 and 20 positions, and an aldehyde at position 18. The

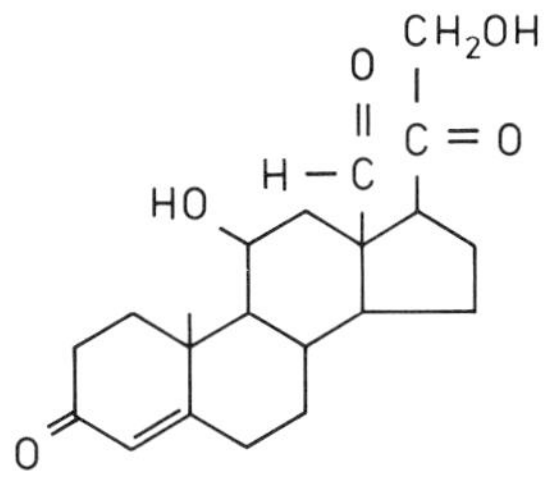

Fig. 13-3. Structure of aldosterone.

structure of aldosterone is identical in man and other mammals.

Physiology

Aldosterone is produced in the zona glomerulosa of the adrenal cortex. Like other steroids, cholesterol is the major precursor, and aldosterone is produced through a number of enzymatic steps of which progesterone and corticosterone are among the intermediate compounds produced. Normally, the enzymatic production of aldosterone from its precursors is very rapid, and the aldosterone is rapidly secreted into the blood. Little aldosterone is stored in the adrenal.

In man, aldosterone secretion is controlled as follows:

1. Angiotensin II stimulates the conversion of cholesterol to basic aldosterone precursors, resulting in accelerated production of aldosterone. The onset of action of angiotensin II is rapid, and the effect is abruptly stopped when angiotensin blood concentration in contact with the adrenal cells is reduced.
2. Serum potassium concentration has a direct effect on aldosterone secretion. Increasing potassium concentration causes increased aldosterone secretion, whereas decreased serum potassium concentration results in suppression of aldosterone.
3. Adrenocorticotropic hormone (ACTH) directly stimulates aldosterone production.
4. Reduced serum sodium concentration increases aldosterone secretion.

There is a diurnal rhythm to aldosterone secretion; greater secretion rates occur in the forenoon than the late afternoon. In this way aldosterone secretion parallels renin secretion.

Aldosterone secreted into the blood is rapidly

ALDOSTERONE METHOD

Principle Plasma aldosterone extracted with methylene chloride

Charcoal adsorption

$$R + [L + L^*] = [RL + RL^*] + [L + L^*]$$

Protocol

		Reagent	Volume
DAY 1	R	Rabbit antiserum to aldosterone-3-BSA	100 μl
	L*	(1,2-³H) Aldosterone	100 μl

		Standard	0, 20, 40, 80, 160, 320, 640, 1,280, 2,560, 5,120 pg/ml	100 μl
	L	Sample	Extracted sample	400 μl

Diluent	To standards	300 μl

――――――――― *2 hours, 4° C* ―――――――――

Dextran-coated charcoal 500 μl
10 minutes, 0° C
Centrifuge 2,500g, 15 minutes, 4° C
Decant supernatant into scintillation vial
with 10 ml Riafluor and count for 10 minutes

Reagents

R	Rabbit antiserum to aldosterone-3-carboxymethyloxime–BSA
L*	(1,2-³H) Aldosterone
L	EDTA-plasma; 1 ml is extracted with 10 ml methylene chloride. Evaporate at 37° C under N₂; dissolve residue in 1.5 ml diluent
Diluent	Phosphate-BSA (Appendix 34)

Alternatives

R *Rabbit antiserum to aldosterone-21–human gamma globulin,[50] aldosterone-3–human gamma globulin,[62] or aldosterone-3–rabbit serum albumin[49]; sheep antiserum to aldosterone-18,21-dihemisuccinate-BSA,[55,63] or aldosterone-γ-lactone[22]; guinea pig antiserum to aldosterone-γ-lactone[54]*

Box 13-2

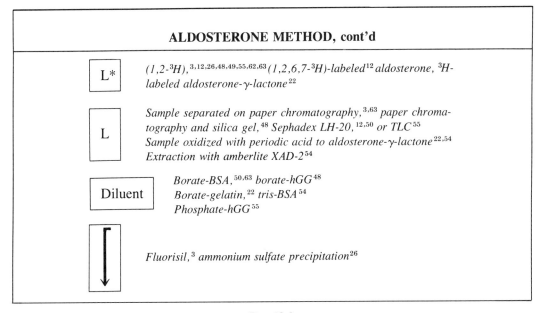

ALDOSTERONE METHOD, cont'd

L* — *(1,2-³H),*[3,12,26,48,49,55,62,63] *(1,2,6,7-³H)-labeled*[12] *aldosterone, ³H-labeled aldosterone-γ-lactone*[22]

L — *Sample separated on paper chromatography,*[3,63] *paper chromatography and silica gel,*[48] *Sephadex LH-20,*[12,50] *or TLC*[55] *Sample oxidized with periodic acid to aldosterone-γ-lactone*[22,54] *Extraction with amberlite XAD-2*[54]

Diluent — *Borate-BSA,*[50,63] *borate-hGG*[48] *Borate-gelatin,*[22] *tris-BSA*[54] *Phosphate-hGG*[55]

Fluorisil,[3] *ammonium sulfate precipitation*[26]

Box 13-2

cleared from the plasma; the half-life is 20 to 30 minutes. Although aldosterone has some affinity for transcortin, most of the aldosterone in plasma appears to be unbound. About 50μg to 150μg of aldosterone are produced per day under normal circumstances.

Aldosterone is metabolized predominantly within the liver and kidney. Predominant breakdown products are the tetrahydroaldosterone and the 18-glucuronide of aldosterone. These metabolites are excreted via the urine.

Aldosterone is the major mineralocorticoid in man and acts directly on the distal tubules of the kidney, causing increased resorption of sodium and increased secretion of potassium. Aldosterone is thought to share the mechanism of action of other steroids, whereby the lipid-soluble steroid easily passes through the plasma membrane of the cell and interacts with specific cytoplasmic receptors. This receptor-steroid complex migrates to the nucleus where it derepresses genes, resulting in formation of ribonucleic acid and new proteins.

Method

Measurement of aldosterone is much more technically challenging than measurement of other steroids because the normal blood con-

centrations are extremely low (about 10 pg/ml).

Bioassays provided the first tests of mineralocorticoid activity. These methods depend on changes in the concentration of sodium or potassium excreted by adrenalectomized animals. Although modifications that employed radioactive sodium-24 and potassium-22 gave improved sensitivity, these methods were cumbersome, and assay results were influenced by a host of extraneous factors. Simpson and associates isolated and determined the chemical structure of aldosterone; subsequently, a number of assays were developed based on the physical and chemical properties of the steroid. These chemical methods suffered from lack of specificity and required several preparatory chemical steps. Initial application of radioisotopes for in vitro assay employed double isotope derivative methods to measure aldosterone in urine and plasma. Although the double isotope derivative methods were very sensitive, they required considerable skill to perform and lacked specificity.

Since steroids are intrinsically nonimmunogenic, a major breakthrough in the development of RIAs for steroids was the discovery of methods for production of antibodies against steroids by first coupling the steroid to a carrier protein. The first application of aldosterone in plasma to RIA was developed by Mayes and associates. Since that time, a number of investigators have reported successful aldosterone RIAs.

Reagents

Aldosterone immunogens were first formed by conjugation of aldosterone-18,21-dihemisuccinate with bovine serum albumin. These antisera have too low a specificity to permit assay without previous chromatography. A number of animals have been utilized to raise antisera to aldosterone; however, rabbits and sheep are among those giving highest titers. Antisera conjugated to the 3 position on the steroid ring have also been employed, with highly improved specificity. An antiserum that was developed using aldosterone-18,21-dihemisuccinate is available from the Hormone Distribution Committee of the National Institutes of Health, Bethesda, Md.

Antisera specific enough to assay aldosterone in plasma extracts have been reported by several groups.

Tritiated aldosterone of high specific activity is usually added to the plasma sample before it is subjected to extraction in order to correct for losses during extraction. Many separation methods typically recover only 60% or less of the added aldosterone tracer.

Performance

Because of problems with antisera specificity, plasma samples are usually extracted and further purified before assay of plasma aldosterone. Various techniques have been utilized for this purpose: Sephadex LH-20, chromatography, thin-layer chromatography, paper chromatography, alkaline extraction after oxidation of aldosterone to aldosterone-γ-lactone, and extraction by aldosterone antibody and adsorption to fuller's earth.

Assay properties

Assay sensitivities of 2 to 3 pg per assay tube have been regularly reported. The coefficient of variation for most assays is about 10%. Some assay problems have been noted, particularly a relatively high nonspecific binding. This is probably due to impurities in the plasma extraction reagents.

Clinical applications

Pathophysiology

Hypersecretion of aldosterone occurs in two basic forms: (1) primary aldosteronism, in which autonomous function of the adrenal is observed; and (2) secondary aldosteronism, in which an extra-adrenal stimulation of the adrenals is the cause of the hyperaldosteronism observed.

There are three basic varieties of primary aldosteronism: (1) aldosterone-producing adenomas of the adrenal, which are usually unilateral; (2) idiopathic hyperaldosteronism, which is most commonly associated with bilateral adrenal hyperplasia (however, the adrenals may have a normal appearance); and (3) hyperaldosternism in which aldosterone levels are suppressible by exogenous administration of mineralocorticoids or glucocorticoids. The elevated aldosterone secretion that is seen in these syndromes is characterized by marked inhibition of plasma renin levels and associated aldosterone effect, including elevated total body sodium concentrations and hypokalemia with inappropriate potassium excretion. It is difficult to distinguish among the groups of primary aldosteronism, in particular between bilateral nodular adrenal hyperplasia and aldosterone-producing adenoma. One differential point is that in patients with adrenal adenomas, the usual increase of aldosterone with upright posture is not observed.

The most common forms of secondary hyperaldosteronism are edematous states associated with cirrhosis, nephrosis, and heart failure. In this situation, aldosterone is produced inappropriately since there is an excess of sodium and in most instances an associated hypokalemia.

Bartter's syndrome (hyperplasia of the juxtaglomerular apparatus) and malignant hypertension are also associated with hyperaldosteronism. All of the various forms of secondary hyperaldosteronism are in some way related to hypersecretion of renin with resultant overproduction of angiotensin II.

Hyposecretion of aldosterone occurs in Addison's disease. The lack of aldosterone results in impaired ability to excrete potassium and to conserve sodium. As long as the patient can take in adequate sodium, he may do relatively well. However, when the patient has vomiting, diarrhea, excessive sweating, or otherwise accelerated sodium loss, contraction of the blood volume with resulting reduced cardiac output and blood pressure will occur. If the condition is not treated with mineralocorticoids, shock and death may supervene. Renin secretion is concomitantly increased in this disorder.

Sampling

There is a diurnal variation of aldosterone secretion, and aldosterone secretion is stimulated by the upright posture. Accordingly, the time of sampling is controlled. For example, relatively low values of aldosterone serum concentration are noted in the morning (8 AM, with the patient still recumbent after sleeping all night). Higher values are seen when patient has been up and around for 2 to 3 hours, with a serum sample being drawn in the late morning. Thus, when hypersecretion of aldosterone is suspected, an early morning sample from the recumbent patient should be obtained. When low levels are suspected, a sample after ambulation is advised.

Both low and high values should be confirmed by measurement of serum levels under appropriate conditions of stimulation or inhibition of aldosterone secretion. For example, in order to evaluate low values, serum for aldosterone is drawn after a *stimulation test* is performed. The patient is placed on a salt-restricted (10 mEq NaCl) diet, along with potassium intake of 80 to 100 mEq/day, for 5 days. High values are evaluated by obtaining serum for aldosterone after an *inhibition test* performed 5 days after the patient has been placed on a high salt diet (150-200 mEq Na^+, 80 mEq K^+). *Mineralocorticoid suppression tests* may also be employed to evaluate high values. In this situation, 200μg of fludrocortisone acetate (Florinef) is given three times a day for 3 days before sampling. As an alternative, 11-desoxycorticosterone (DOC), 10 mg given intramuscularly twice a day for 3 days before testing, may also be used.

Reference values

Normal
  8 AM, patient supine, 40-102 pg/ml
  2-hour ambulation, 100-305 pg/ml

Interpretation of results

Elevated aldosterone levels are observed in both primary and secondary hyperaldosteronism (see Pathophysiology). In secondary hyperaldosteronism, increased renin levels are also observed; whereas in the primary forms, renin is suppressed. The distinction between the various forms of primary hyperaldosteronism is important, since adenomas overproducing aldosterone are the only group that is surgically responsive. Aldosterone secretion in the primary forms of hyperaldosteronism is not suppressed in response to the inhibition tests of salt loading. However, aldosterone secretion in some forms of the primary variety is suppressed after mineralocorticoid or glucocorticoid administration. Suppression does not occur in either the variety associated with aldosterone-producing adenoma or that associated with bilateral adrenal hyperplasia. Patients with adenomas have the most marked renin suppression, and plasma aldosterone levels actually decrease or stay about the same after the upright position is assumed. However, patients with bilateral adrenal hyperplasia have a normal response after 3 to 4 hours in the upright position, with a further increase of 2 to 4 times the baseline levels.

Decreased aldosterone levels that are resistant to stimulation are found in patients with excess of other mineralocorticoids in the circulation. This situation can occur in congenital adrenal hyperplasia, in which DOC is produced. Licorice ingestion will also cause aldosterone suppression. Certain adrenal tumors that produce nonaldosterone mineralocorticoids will also suppress aldosterone. In certain forms of essential hypertension, aldosterone secretion may also be decreased. In most of these states, renin is also reduced. However, in hypoaldosteronism due to primary adrenal failure, renin secretion is increased.

REFERENCES

1. Africa, B., and Haber, E.: The production and characterization of specific antibodies to aldosterone, Immunochemistry **8**:479, 1971.
2. Arnold, M. L., and James, V. H. T.: Determination of deoxycorticosterone in plasma; double isotope and immunoassay methods, Steroids **18**:789, 1971.
3. Bayard, F., Beitins, I. Z., Kowarski, A., and Migeon, C. J.: Measurement of plasma aldosterone by radioimmunoassay, J. Clin. Endocrinol. Metab. **31**:1, 1970.
4. Beckerhoff, R., Wilkinson, R., Lectscher, J. H., Netter, W., and Siegenthaler, W.: Bestimmung der Plasma-Renin-Konzeutration mittels Radioimmunoassays für Angiotensin, Klin. Wochenschr. **50**:702, 1972.
5. Biglieri, E. G., and others: Adrenal mineralocorticoids causing hypertension, Am. J. Med. **52**:623, 1972.
6. Boyd, G. W., Fitz, A. E., Adamson, A. R., and others: Radioimmunoassay determination of plasma-renin activity, Lancet **1**:213, 1969.
7. Boyd, G. W., Landon, J., and Peart, W. S.: Radioimmunoassay for determining plasma levels of angiotensin II in man, Lancet **2**:1002, 1967.
8. Boyd, G. W., and Peart, W. S.: The production of high titre antibody against free angiotensin II, Lancet **2**:129, 1968.
9. Brodie, A. H., and others: A method for the measurement of aldosterone in peripheral plasma using ^{3}H-acetic anhydride, J. Clin. Endocrinol. Metab. **27**:997, 1967.
10. Catt, K. J., Baukal, A. J., and Ashburn, M. J.: Radioimmunoassay determination of plasma renin parameters and circulating angiotensin II. In Fregly, M. J., and Fregly, M. S., editors: Oral contraceptives and hypertension, Gainesville, 1974, Dolphin Press, pp. 184-210.
11. Catt, K. J., and Cain, M. C.: Measurement of angiotensin II in blood, Lancet **2**:1005, 1967.
12. Catt, K. J., and Douglas, J.: The renin-angiotensin system and aldosterone. In Rothfeld, B., editor: Nuclear medicine in vitro, Philadelphia, 1974, J. B. Lippincott Co., pp. 306-314.
13. Coghlan, J. P., and Scoggins, B. A.: Measurement of aldosterone in peripheral blood of man and sheep, J. Clin. Endocrinol. Metab. **27**:1470, 1967.
14. Cohen, E. L., Conn, J. W., Lucas, C. P., and others: Radioimmunoassay for angiotensin I; measurement of plasma-renin activity, plasma renin concentration, renin substrate concentration and angiotensin I in normal and hypertensive people. In Genest, J., and Koiw, E., editors: Hypertension, New York, 1972, Springer-Verlag New York, Inc., pp. 569-582.
15. Conn, J. W., Cohen, E. L., and Roover, D. R.: Suppression of plasma renin activity in primary aldosteronism; distinguishing primary from secondary aldosteronism in hypertensive disease, J.A.M.A. **190**:213, 1964.
16. Deodhar, S.: Production and detection of anti-angiotensin, J. Exp. Med. **111**:429, 1960.
17. Dillon, M. J.: Measurement of plasma renin activity by semi–micro radioimmunoassay of generated angiotensin, J. Clin. Pathol. **28**:625, 1975.
18. Douglas, J. G., Hollifield, J. W., and Liddle, G. W.: Treatment of low-renin essential hypertension, J.A.M.A. **227**:518, 1974.
19. Drayer, J. I., and Benraad, T. J.: The reliability of the measurement of plasma renin activity by radioimmunoassay, Clin. Chim. Acta **61**:309, 1975.
20. Düsterdieck, G., and McElwee, G.: Estimation of angiotensin II concentration in human plasma by radioimmunoassay; some application to clinical and physiological states, Eur. J. Clin. Invest. **2**:32, 1971.
21. Ernst, C. B., Boakstein, J. J., Montie, J., and others: Renal vein renin ratios and collateral vessels in renovascular hypertension, Arch. Surg. **104**:496, 1972.
22. Farmer, R. W., Brown, D. N., and Howard, P. Y.: A radioimmunoassay for plasma aldosterone without chromatography, J. Clin. Endocrinol. Metab. **36**:460, 1973.
23. Freedlender, A. E., Fyhrquist, F., Hollemans, H. J. G.: Renin and the angiotensins. In Jaffe, B. M., and Behrman, H. R., editors: Methods of hormone radioimmunoassay, New York, 1974, Academic Press, Inc., pp. 455-469.
24. Ganguly, A., and others: Control of plasma aldosterone in primary aldosteronism; distinction between adenoma and hyperplasia, J. Clin. Endocrinol. Metab. **37**:765, 1973.
25. Giese, J., Jörgensen, M., Nielsen, M. D., Lund, J. O., and Munck, O.: Plasma renin concentration measured by use of a radioimmunoassay for angiotensin I, Scand. J. Clin. Lab. Invest. **26**:355, 1970.
26. Gomez-Sanchez, C., Kem, D. C., and Kaplan, N. M.: A radioimmunoassay for plasma aldosterone by immunologic purification, J. Clin. Endocrinol. Metab. **36**:795, 1973.
27. Goodfriend, T. L., and Ball, D.: Radioimmunoassay of angiotensin and measurement of renin activity, J. Lab. Clin. Med. **70**:884, 1967.
28. Goodfriend, T. L., Ball, D., and Farley, D.: Radioimmunoassay of angiotensin, J. Lab. Clin. Med. **72**:648, 1968.
29. Goodfriend, T. L., Levine, L., and Fasman, G. D.: Antibodies to bradykinin and angiotensin; a use of carbodiimides in immunology, Science **144**:1344, 1964.
30. Goodfriend, T. L., and Sehon, A. H.: Preparation of an estione-protein conjugate, Can. J. Biochem. Physiol. **36**:1177, 1958.
31. Gowenlock, A., and Wrong, O.: Hyperaldosteronism secondary to renal ischemia, Q. J. Med. **31**:323, 1962.
32. Haber, E., Koerner, T., Page, L. B., Climan, B., and Purnode, A.: Application of a radioimmunoassay for angiotensin I to the physiologic measurements of plasma renin activity in normal human subjects, J. Clin. Endocrinol. Metab. **29**:1349, 1969.
33. Haring, R., and others: The evaluation of titer and specificity of aldosterone binding antibodies in hyperimmunized sheep, Steroids **20**:73, 1972.
34. Harrop, G. A., and others: Studies on suprarenal cor-

tex; influence of corticol hormone upon excretion of water and electrolytes in suprarenalectomized dog, J. Exp. Med. **64:**233, 1936.

35. Hartman, F. A., and Spour, H. J.: Cortin and Na factor of the adrenal, Endocrinology **26:**871, 1940.

36. Hummerich, W., and Krause, D. K.: Improvement of renin determination in human plasma using a commonly available renin standard in a radioimmunological methods, Klin. Wochenschr. **53:**559, 1975.

37. Ito, T., and others: A radioimmunoassay for aldosterone in human peripheral plasma including a comparison of alternate techniques, J. Clin. Endocrinol. Metab. **34:**106, 1972.

38. Kliman, B., and Peterson, R. E.: Double isotope derivative assay of aldosterone in biological extracts, J. Biol. Chem. **235:**1639, 1960.

39. Laragh, J. H.: The role of aldosterone in man; evidence for regulation of electrolyte balance and arterial pressure by a renal-adrenal system which may be involved in malignant hypertension, J.A.M.A. **174:**293, 1960.

40. Laragh, J. H.: Interrelations between angiotensin, norepinephrine, aldosterone secretion and electrolyte metabolism in man, Circulation **25:**203, 1962.

41. Laragh, J. H.: The renin-aldosterone axis and blood pressure and electrolyte homeostasis. In Williams, R. H., editor: Textbook of endocrinology, Philadelphia, 1974, W. B. Saunders Co., p. 952.

42. Laragh, J. H., Baer, L., and others: Renin, angiotensin and aldosterone system in pathogenesis and management of hypertensive vascular disease, Am. J. Med. **52:**633, 1972.

43. Lash, B., and Fleisher, N.: Radioimmunoassay of angiotensin I for estimation of plasma renin activity, Clin. Chem. **20:**620, 1974.

44. Lee, M. R.: Renin and hypertension; a modern synthesis, Baltimore, 1969, The Williams & Wilkins Co.

45. Lieberman, S., and others: Steroid-protein conjugates their chemical, immunochemical and endocrinological properties, Recent Prog. Horm. Res. **15:**165, 1959.

46. Mader, W. J., and Buck, R. R.: Colorimetric determination of cortisone and related ketol steroids, Anal. Chem. **24:**666, 1952.

47. Martin, B. T., and Nugent, C. A.: A non-chromatographic radioimmunoassay for plasma aldosterone, Steroids **21:**169, 1973.

48. Mayes, D., Furnyama, S., Kim, D. C., and Nugent, C. A.: A radioimmunoassay for plasma aldosterone, J. Clin. Endocrinol. Metab. **30:**682, 1970.

49. McKenzie, J. K., and Clements, J. A.: Specific antibody for serum aldosterone utilizing increased antibody specificity, J. Clin. Endocrinol. Metab. **38:**622, 1974.

50. Newsome, H. H., Clements, A. S., and Hume, D. M.: Specificity of antisera to aldosterone and deoxycorticosterone (DOC). In International Atomic Energy Agency: Radioimmunoassay and related procedures in medicine, Vienna, 1974, I.A.E.A., pp. 79-85.

51. Nielsen, M. D., Jorgensen, M., and Giese, J.: ^{125}I-labelling of angiotensin I and II, Acta Endocrinol. (Kbh.) **67:**104, 1971.

52. Nowaczynski, W. J., and others: Microdetermination of corticosteroids with tetrazolium derivatives, J. Lab. Clin. Med. **45:**818, 1955.

53. Page, I. H., and McCubbin, J. W.: Renal hypertension, Chicago, 1968, Year Book Medical Publishers, Inc.

54. Roginsky, M. S., Panetz, A. I., and Gordon, R. D.: The use of amberlite XAD-Z columns for the determination of plasma aldosterone by radioimmunoassay, Clin. Chim. Acta **63:**303, 1975.

55. St. Cyr, M. J., and others: Quantitation of plasma aldosterone by radioimmunoassay, Clin. Chem. **18:**1395, 1972.

56. Simpson, S. A., and others: Adrenal cortex compounds and related substances. XCI. The isolation and properties of aldosterone, Helv. Chim. Acta **37:**1163, 1954.

57. Skinner, S. L.: Improved assay methods for renin concentration and renin activity in human plasma, Circ. Res. **20:**391, 1967.

58. Stason, W. B., Vallotton, M., and Haber, E.: Synthesis of an antigenic copolymer of angiotensin and succinylated poly-L-lysine, Biochim. Biophys. Acta **133:**582, 1967.

59. Stockigt, T., Collins, R. D., and Biblieri, E. G.: Determination of plasma renin concentration by angiotensin I immunoassay; diagnostic import of precise measurement of subnormal renin in hyperaldosteronism, Circ. Res. **28**(Suppl. 2):175, 1971.

60. Underwood, R. H., and Williams, G. H.: The simultaneous measurement of aldosterone, cortisol and corticosterone in human plasma by displacement analysis, J. Lab. Clin. Med. **79:**848, 1972.

61. Vallotton, M. B., Page, L. B., and Haber, E.: Radioimmunoassay of angiotensin in human plasma, Nature **215:**714, 1967.

62. Vetter, H., Vetter, W., and Siegenthaler, W.: Preparation of an antiserum specific to aldosterone and its application in radioimmunoassay. In International Atomic Energy Agency: Radioimmunoassay and related procedures in medicine, Vienna, 1974, I.A.E.A., pp. 87-96.

63. Williams, G. H., and Underwood, R. H.: Mineralocorticoids; aldosterone and deoxycorticosterone. In Jaffe, B. M., and Behrman, H. R., editors: Methods of hormone radioimmunoassay, New York, 1974, Academic Press, Inc., pp. 371-392.

14 PARATHORMONE AND CALCITONIN

Calcium ion is essential for a variety of important cellular functions, including muscular contraction, secretion, energy metabolism, and the action of neurotransmitters. The concentration of calcium in body fluids must be maintained within a rather narrow range for optimal body function.

CALCIUM HOMEOSTASIS

Calcium homeostasis is accomplished by the interaction of three hormones: parathyroid hormone (PTH), calcitonin, and 1,25-dihydroxycholecalciferol (vitamin D).

Change in the concentration of the free or ionized calcium in extracellular fluid is the trigger for the more active phases of calcium homeostasis. In response to a reduced free-calcium concentration, PTH is secreted. PTH exerts its action at intestinal, renal, and skeleton sites to mobilize calcium from the bone, decrease renal excretion, and increase calcium absorption. However, if the calcium concentration in biologic fluids increases, calcitonin is produced. This hormone lowers the serum calcium concentration primarily by inhibiting absorption of calcium from the hydroxyapatite in the skeleton. Vitamin D is essential for the skeletal actions of PTH and, in particular, for the mobilization of Ca^{++} from bone.

In this chapter parathormone and calcitonin radioimmunoassay (RIA) is discussed. The radioassay of vitamin D has not been widely applied clinically.

PARATHORMONE
Chemistry

Parathormone is an 84-amino acid polypeptide hormone with a molecular weight of 9,500.

Basically, there appears to be at least four naturally occurring forms of PTH: (1) an 11,500-molecular weight prohormone, primarily existing in the parathyroid gland; (2) a 9,500-molecular weight species, which is the most abundant storage form and primary secretagogue under normal conditions; (3) a 7,000-molecular weight form, primarily the carboxyl end of PTH (biologically inactive); and (4) a 4,500-molecular weight form, thought to be the amino end of the PTH molecule (biologically active).

Physiology

Parathormone is produced by the dark chief cells of the parathyroid gland. As mentioned above, the predominant hormone is an 84-amino acid polypeptide. The N-terminal end of of the molecule, consisting of 33 or 34 amino acids, is apparently where the biologic action of the hormone resides. The 11,500-molecular weight (about 100 amino acid chain length) constituent is now thought to be a prohormone, which under normal circumstances is converted to the 9,500-molecular weight hormone for storage within the parathyroid and subsequent secretion into the blood.

Serum calcium concentration correlates best with the 7,000- and 4,500-molecular weight constituents of parathormone. This has led some to believe that the 9,500-molecular weight product, which is the primary constituent in the parathyroid gland, is not an active form of the hormone.

Under normal circumstances, the predominant form of PTH that are circulating are the 9,500-(50% of total PTH), 7,000-, and 4,500-molecular weight forms. These last two types of PTH arise from peripheral enzymatic conversion of the 9,500–molecular weight species. The 7,000–molecular weight substance has a half-life of 2 to 4 hours in blood. The 9,500–molecular weight species has a half-life of about 30 minutes.

PTH is secreted (principally as the 9,500–molecular weight form) in response to a decrease in serum Ca^{++} concentration. This change occurs within 10 minutes of an abrupt Ca^{++} concentration decrement. PTH promotes an increase in Ca^{++} concentration in blood by (1) increasing the rate of osteocytic osteolysis in bone and the net rate of Ca^{++} resorption from bone, (2) increasing the absorption of Ca^{++} from the duodenum and jejunum, and (3) increasing the urinary excretion of phosphate and decreasing the urinary excretion of Ca^{++}. Phosphate metabolism is also important to calcium homeostasis. Free calcium and phosphate exist in equilibrium within the bloodstream, and the solubility product of calcium phosphate basically determines the relative concentration of both free calcium and phosphate in biologic tissues. Thus when PO_4 concentration decreases, Ca^{++} concentration increases. Similarly, when the concentration of Ca^{++} increases, parathormone secretion by the parathyroid is suppressed.

Method
Reagents

The first RIA for parathormone was developed by Berson and associates in 1963. This assay used bovine PTH for standard and iodination because of the lack of a suitable human PTH preparation. This deficiency has continued to be a problem for PTH RIAs, and today RIA methods are still based on heterologous antisera. Both bovine and porcine PTH has been used. Antisera have been raised in guinea pigs, rabbits, and chickens.

The production of antiserum that is sensitive enough to detect PTH in human serum has been difficult. This is in part related to the fact that, with heterologous antisera, the immunologic reactivity of human PTH is only 20% to 50% of the bovine or porcine PTH against which the antisera were raised. Also, the immunoheterogeneity of PTH in plasma must be kept in mind when antiserum and its reactivity are evaluated. Antisera produced against bovine PTH react particularly strongly against the 9,500–molecular weight component in plasma, whereas porcine PTH tends to react more with the 4,500–molecular weight form. Chloramine-T has been used primarily to iodinate the PTH ligand used.

Performance

Separation has been accomplished most frequently by the use of dextran-coated charcoal, although electrophoresis on cellulose acetate has also been used. Currently available methods require prolonged incubation of several days in order to achieve sufficient sensitivity for assay of human PTH.

Assay properties

PTH is very reactive in terms of adsorption to glass surfaces, and a relatively high proportion of serum must be utilized to block this tendency. In addition, PTH may be broken down in vitro by enzymes. Trasylol or rapid freezing of serum samples has been employed to prevent this breakdown. In most laboratories there have been considerable problems with overlap in the values of normal patients and of those who have hyperthyroidism.

An example of a PTH RIA is shown in Box 14-1.

Clinical applications
Pathophysiology

Parathormone immunoassay has been used primarily in the differential diagnosis of hypercalcemia. The causes of hypercalcemia are shown in the outline below.

HYPERCALCEMIA*

A. Neoplastic
1. Primary hyperparathyroidism
   a. Parathyroid adenoma
   b. Parathyroid hyperplasia
   c. Parathyroid carcinoma
2. Nonendocrine malignancies
   a. Bronchogenic carcinoma

*Adapted from Hamilton, C. R.: Radioimmunoassay of the calcium-regulative hormones. In Rothfeld, B., editor: Nuclear medicine in-vitro, Philadelphia, 1975, J. B. Lippincott Co.

PTH METHOD

Charcoal adsorption

Principle $R + [L + L^*] = [RL + RL^*] + [L + L^*]$

Protocol

		Reagent	Volume
DAY 1	R	Guinea pig antiserum to bovine PTH	100 μl
	L*	^{125}I-labeled PTH	100 μl
	L	Standard — 0, 40, 80, 160, 330, 660, 1,320, 2,630 pmol/liter in 10% normal pool serum	100 μl / 200 μl
		Sample — Serum	200 μl

──────── 96 hours, 4° C ────────

DAY 4	↓	Dextran-coated charcoal	1,000 μl

10 minutes, 4° C
Centrifugation 15 minutes, 2,500g, 4° C
Aspirate supernatant and count tubes for 5 minutes

Reagents

R — Guinea pig antiserum to bovine PTH; Trasylol added (1:1)

L* — Bovine PTH labeled with ^{125}I by lactoperoxidase separated on BioGel P-10 (Appendix 17)
Specific activity: 120-160 μCi/μg

L — Standards in diluent with 10% normal pool serum; serum samples

Diluent — Phosphate-buffer (Appendix 36)

↓ — Appendix 27

Alternatives

R — Guinea pig antiserum to porcine PTH[4]
Rabbit[15] or chicken[22] antiserum to bovine PTH

Box 14-1

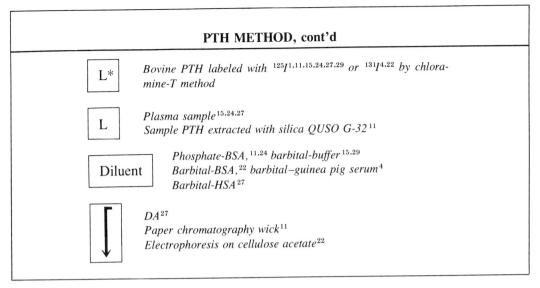

PTH METHOD, cont'd

L* — Bovine PTH labeled with ^{125}I[1,11,15,24,27,29] or ^{131}I[4,22] by chloramine-T method

L — Plasma sample[15,24,27]
Sample PTH extracted with silica QUSO G-32[11]

Diluent — Phosphate-BSA,[11,24] barbital-buffer[15,29]
Barbital-BSA,[22] barbital–guinea pig serum[4]
Barbital-HSA[27]

↓ — DA[27]
Paper chromatography wick[11]
Electrophoresis on cellulose acetate[22]

Box 14-1

  b. Breast carcinoma
  c. Lymphoma
  d. Multiple myeloma
  e. Leukemia
  3. Direct malignant bony involvement
B. Nonneoplastic
  1. Sarcoidosis
  2. Vitamin D intoxication
  3. Milk-alkali syndrome
  4. Addison's disease
  5. Thiazide diuretics

Good discrimination has been achieved in differentiating primary hyperparathyroidism from other states by antiserum that is directed toward the 7,000–molecular weight (C-terminal) component. Even in normocalcemic patients, PTH may be inappropriately high for the level of calcium in the blood in hyperparathyroidism.

Patients with hypercalcemia due to causes other than hyperparathyroidism have undetectable serum levels of PTH. These observations have been made primarily by Arnaud, who obtained two relatively monospecific antisera to the 9,500–molecular weight component, which he termed "glandular hormone," and the 7,000–molecular weight "circulating hormone." The two antisera showed markedly different results in patients with chronic renal failure. The 7,000–molecular weight fraction was elevated in virtually all patients with chronic renal failure, whereas the 9,500–molecular weight fraction was elevated in only a small minority of such patients. Similarly, the 7,000–molecular weight–directed antisera showed a high fraction of positive reactions in patients with primary hyperparathyroidism. Arnaud concluded that concentrations of the 9,500–molecular weight parathormone fraction reflect acute changes in secretory status of the gland, whereas the parathormone homeostasis in respect to calcium balance is most accurately reflected by the antiserum measuring the 7,000–molecular weight component. Since the 7,000–molecular weight fragment has a longer half-life in serum, this measurement is the better indicator of a state of chronic oversecretion by the parathyroid, as would occur in hyperparathyroidism. In chronic renal failure, for example, where oversecretion of PTH is common, particularly if patients are not being dialyzed frequently enough or if phosphate intake is too great, the antisera directed against the 7,000–molecular weight fraction show the oversecretion well. However, amino terminal–specific assays have been of use in localizing parathyroid adenomas. Because these

CALCITONIN METHOD

Principle

Double antibody

$$R + [L + L^*] = [RL + RL^*] + [L + L]$$

Protocol

		Reagent	Volume
DAY 1	R	*Antiserum to synthetic human calcitonin*	*200 μl*
	L*	*^{125}I-labeled calcitonin*	*200 μl*
	L	Standard: *0.156, 0.313, 0.625, 1.25, 2.50, 5.00 ng/ml in EDTA-plasma*	*100 μl*
		Sample: *EDTA-plasma*	

———————————— *72 hours, 4° C* ————————————

DAY 4	↓	*Normal rabbit serum (1:250)*	*50 μl*
		Goat antiserum to rabbit IgG (1:10)	*50 μl*

———————————— *18 hours, 4° C* ————————————

DAY 5	*Add diluent*	*500 μl*
	Centrifugation 2,500g, 15 minutes, 4° C	
	Decant supernatant	
	Count precipitate for 5 minutes	

Reagents

R — *Rabbit antiserum to synthetic human calcitonin coupled to BSA*
Avidity: $K_a \approx 6 \times 10^{10}$

L* — *Synthetic human calcitonin labeled with ^{125}I by lactoperoxidase (Appendix 17); separation on Sephadex G-25 (Appendix 19)*
Specific activity: 160-200 μCi/μg
T = 10,000 cpm ≈ 0.04 ng

L — *Standards: synthetic human calcitonin in hormone-free EDTA-plasma (from thyroidectomized patients)*
Sample: EDTA-plasma

Diluent — *Barbital-BSA (Appendix 34)*

Alternatives

R — *Guinea pig antiserum to calcitonin[28]*

Box 14-2

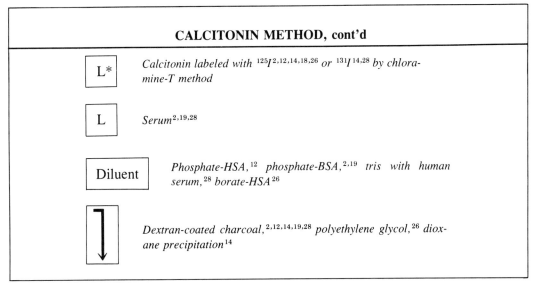

CALCITONIN METHOD, cont'd

L* — Calcitonin labeled with [125]I[2,12,14,18,26] or [131]I[14,28] by chloramine-T method

L — Serum[2,19,28]

Diluent — Phosphate-HSA,[12] phosphate-BSA,[2,19] tris with human serum,[28] borate-HSA[26]

Dextran-coated charcoal,[2,12,14,19,28] polyethylene glycol,[26] dioxane precipitation[14]

Box 14-2

antisera more accurately reflect acute secretion in the region of parathyroid adenomas, they have been used at the time of surgery to localize parathyroid adenomas. Certain malignancies also can produce PTH that is immunologically indistinguishable from that produced by the parathyroid gland (see outline on p. 197 and Chapter 19). There is an additional group of patients in whom hypercalcemia is also related to a tumor product, but this tumor product is apparently different from parathormone.

Sampling

PTH serum samples are usually obtained in the early morning, since there is a diurnal variation of PTH, with a peak in the evening and lowest values in the morning. In addition, sampling of thyroid veins at the time of surgery has been of great value in preoperative localization of abnormal parathyroid tissue.

Reference values

Normal range: 120-260 pmol-equivalents/liter = 1.1-2.5 ng/ml

Interpretation of results

Elevated values of PTH are found in hyperparathyroidism. The test has been useful, particularly when compared with the serum Ca^{++} value; at high serum Ca^{++} values, PTH levels in plasma should be low. Some antisera reported can separate completely patients with parathyroid adenomas from normal patients. That which we have available to us shows elevated values in only about 80% of patients with primary hyperparathyroidism. In secondary hyperparathyroidism, the values are much higher. Thus, when the PTH concentration is inappropriately elevated for a given Ca^{++} value, overproduction of PTH is likely. The source of PTH overproduction may be more elusive, however, since both a parathyroid adenoma and a nonendocrine neoplasm can produce PTH. Selective venous sampling from the thyroid veins may be the best way to localize PTH overproduction to a particular parathyroid. Renal failure is associated with elevated PTH values, and the degree of renal osteodystrophy is thought to correlate with PTH concentration.

Decreased values of PTH are found in forms of hypercalcemia that are not dependent on PTH overproduction. For example, some malignant tumors, such as those of the breast, produce hypercalcemia without detectable PTH activity. Other common causes of hypercalcemia that have been associated with low PTH values are shown in the outline on p. 197.

CALCITONIN
Chemistry

Calcitonin is a 32-amino acid polypeptide hormone having a disulfide bridge at the amino terminal end of the molecule and also has proline as a C-terminal amino acid. The molecular weight of this hormone is 3,400. There are very wide differences in structure between calcitonin of various species. The entire molecule appears to be necessary for biologic activity.

It has recently been shown that there is a larger molecular weight compound circulating in plasma with similar immunoreactivity to calcitonin. The exact nature of this compound is not known.

Physiology

Calcitonin is produced by thyroid parafollicular cells in mammals and by the ultimobranchial organ in fish. Calcitonin lowers the concentration of calcium and phosphate in the blood by directly inhibiting the rate of bone resorption. In humans, calcitonin is produced in the C cells, which are small groups of interstitial and parafollicular cells in the thyroid. Some of these cells may also be scattered throughout the parathyroid gland and even in the thymus tissue.

Calcitonin is normally present in human urine. The usual concentration is less than 1 ng/ml; very high values up to 3μg/ml have been observed in patients with medullary carcinoma. The finding of biologically active calcitonin levels in human urine suggests that low levels are present in serum even though the relative insensitivity of most current assay methods does not permit routine detection.

With increasing concentration of serum Ca^{++} above 9 mg/100 ml, the rate of secretion of calcitonin is directly stimulated. Calcitonin acts directly on bone to decrease the rate of bony remodeling. For this reason, calcitonin has been used therapeutically in Paget's disease and appears to be effective therapy in this disorder.

Method
Reagents

Heterologous assays for calcitonin are not possible because of the wide difference in structure between calcitonin of various species. With the availability of human calcitonin, specific assays were developed. Human calcitonin has been synthesized by Ciba-Geigy in Basel, Switzerland and by N. V. Organon, Oss, The Netherlands. As a standard for RIA, the MRC human synthetic calcitonin has been utilized. This is available from the National Institute for Medical Research, London. Human ligand must be used to measure human calcitonin. The ligand has also been prepared by 1 N HCl extracts of large tumor deposits of medullary carcinoma.

Human calcitonin antisera have been developed in both guinea pigs and rabbits. Since the amino acid sequence of human calcitonin is quite different from the calcitonin of these species, no conjugation is necessary.

Performance

A variety of methods have been employed for separation of antibody-bound and unbound calcitonin, including chromatoelectrophoresis, dextran-coated charcoal, and dioxane precipitation.

Assay properties

Most of the early techniques were not able to detect normal calcitonin levels in serum. Recently, assays have been developed with the capability of measuring these levels in man, and these methods are finding growing application.

A method for RIA of calcitonin is shown in Box 14-2.

Clinical applications
Pathophysiology

In patients with medullary carcinoma of the thyroid gland, calcitonin measurements are useful as an early indication of malignancy. Medullary carcinoma arises as a malignancy of the C cells of the thyroid. Calcitonin measurements are particularly valuable in screening family members of patients with a hereditary tendency to medullary carcinoma.

Calcitonin levels have also been detected in the serum of patients with pseudohypoparathyroidism and chronic hypocalcemia, as well as of patients with carcinoid tumors.

Sampling

Either serum or plasma can be used in radioassay; no differences between the two sampling methods are noted. Calcitonin is stable in plasma that is kept at $-20°$ C. Random serum samples are primarily taken.

Reference values

Normal range: 0.02-0.4 ng/ml (plasma)

Interpretation of results

Elevated calcitonin levels are found in patients with medullary carcinoma of the thyroid. Levels ranging from a few ng/ml to several μg/ml have been found in these patients. This is by far the most common situation in which increased levels exist. Rarely, malignant tumors will produce ectopic calcitonin. The assay is of value both in the primary diagnosis of medullary carcinoma and in the follow-up of these patients. Medullary carcinoma has been recognized with increasing frequency with the wider availability of RIA methods.

REFERENCES

1. Almqvist, S., Hjern, B., and Wåsthed, B.: The diagnostic value of a radioimmunoassay for parathyroid hormone in human serum, Acta Endocrinol. (Kbh.) **78**:493, 1975.
2. Almqvist, S., Telenius-Berg, M., and Wåsthed, B.: Serum calcitonin in medullary thyroid carcinoma, Acta Med. Scand. **196**:177, 1974.
3. Arnaud, C. D., Goldsmith, R. S., Sizenore, G. W., and others: Studies on the characterization of human parathyroid hormone in hyperparathyroid serum; practical considerations. In Frame, B., and others, editors: Clinical aspects of metabolic bone disease, Amsterdam, 1973, Excerpta Medica.
4. Arnaud, C. D., Tsao, H. S., and Littledike, T.: Radioimmunoassay of human parathyroid hormone in serum, J. Clin. Invest. **50**:21, 1971.
5. Arnaud, C. D., Tsao, H. S., and Oldham, S. B.: Native human parathyroid hormones; an immunochemical investigation, Proc. Natl. Acad. Sci. USA **67**:415, 1970.
6. Berson, S. A., and Yalow, R. S.: Parathyroid hormone in plasma in adenomatous hyperplasia, uremia and bronchogenic carcinoma, Science **154**:907, 1966.
7. Berson, S. A., and Yalow, R. S.: Immunochemical heterogeneity of parathyroid hormone in plasma, J. Clin. Endocrinol. Metab. **28**:1037, 1968.
8. Berson, S. A., Yalow, R. S., Aurbach, G. D., and Potts, J. T., Jr.: Immunoassay of bovine and human parathyroid hormone, Proc. Natl. Acad. Sci. USA **49**:613, 1963.
9. Bileziklan, J. P., Doppman, J. L., Shimkin, P. M., and others: Preoperative localization of abnormal parathyroid tissue; cumulative experience with venous sampling and arteriography, Am. J. Med. **55**:505, 1973.
10. Canterbury, J. M., Levey, G. S., and Reiss, E.: Activation of renal cortical adenylate cyclase by circulating immunoreactive parathyroid hormone fragments, J. Clin. Invest. **52**:524, 1973.
11. Christensen, M. S.: Sensitive radioimmunoassay of parathyroid hormone in human serum using a specific extraction technique, Scand. J. Clin. Lab. Invest. **36**:313, 1976.
12. Clark, M. B., Byfield, P. H. G., Boyd, O., W., and Foster, V. U.: A radioimmunoassay for human calcitonin, Lancet **2**:74, 1969.
13. Copp, D. H., Cameron, E. C., Cheney, B. A., and others: Evidence for calcitonin; a new hormone from the parathyroid that lowers blood calcium, Endocrinology **70**:638, 1962.
14. Deftos, L. J.: Immunoassay for human calcitonin. I. Method, Metabolism **20**:1122, 1971.
15. Deftos, L. J.: Parathyroid hormone. In Jaffe, B. M., and Behrman, H. R., editors: Methods of hormone radioimmunoassay, New York, 1974, Academic Press, Inc., pp. 231-247.
16. Doppman, J. L., and Hammond, W. G.: The anatomic basis of parathyroid venous sampling, Radiology **95**:603, 1970.
17. Habener, J. F., Powell, D., Murray, T. M., and others: Parathyroid hormone; secretion and metabolism in vivo, Proc. Natl. Acad. Sci. USA **68**:2986, 1971.
18. Hamilton, C. R.: Radioimmunoassay of the calcium–regulative hormones. In Rothfeld, B., editor: Nuclear medicine in-vitro, Philadelphia, 1975, J. B. Lippincott Co.
19. Heynen, G., and Franchimont, P.: Human calcitonin radioimmunoassay in normal and pathological conditions, Eur. J. Clin. Invest. **4**:213, 1974.
20. Kaufmann, H. T., Aurbach, G. D., Dawson, B. F., Niall, H. D., Deftos, L. J., and Potts, J. T., Jr.: Isolation and characterization of bovine parathyroid isohormones, Biochemistry **10**:2779, 1971.
21. Melvin, K. E. W., Miller, H. H., and Tashjian, A. H.: Early diagnosis of medullary carcinoma of the thyroid gland by means of calcitonin assay, N. Engl. J. Med. **285**:1115, 1971.
22. Reiss, E., and Canterbury, J. M.: Experience with radioimmunoassay of parathyroid hormone in human sera, Proc. Soc. Exp. Biol. Med. **128**:501, 1968.
23. Saaman, N. A., Hill, C. S., and Schultz, P. N.: Immunoreactive calcitonin in medullary carcinoma of the

thyroid and in maternal and cord serum, J. Lab. Clin. Med. **81:**671, 1973.

24. Schopman, W., Hackeng, H. L., and Leguin, R. M.: A radioimmunoassay for parathyroid hormone in man. I. Development of a radioimmunoassay for bovine PTH, Acta Endocrinol. (Kbh.) **63:**643, 1970.

25. Segre, G. V., Habener, J. F., Powell, D., and others: Parathyroid hormone in human plasma; immunochemical characterizations and biological implications, J. Clin. Invest. **51:**3163, 1972.

26. Silva, O. L., Snider, R. H., and Becker, K. L.: A radioimmunoassay of calcitonin in human plasma, Clin. Chem. **20:**337, 1974.

27. Tanaka, M., Abe, K., Adachi, I., Yamaguchi, K., Miyakawa, S., Hirakawa, H., and Kumasaka, S.: Radioimmunoassay specific for amino (N) and carboxyl (C) terminal portion of parathyroid hormone, Endocrinol. Jpn. **22:**471, 1975.

28. Tashjian, A. H., Jr., and Voelkel, E. F.: Human calcitonin; application of affinity chromatography. In Jaffe, B. M., and Behrman, H. R., editors: Methods of hormone radioimmunoassay, New York, 1974, Academic Press, Inc., pp. 199-214.

29. Woo, J., and Singer, F. R.: Radioimmunoassay for human parathyroid hormone, Clin. Chim. Acta **54:** 166, 1974.

15 INSULIN

Chemistry

Insulin is a two-chain (A and B chains) polypeptide with a molecular weight of about 6,000 daltons. The A chain has 21 amino acids and the B chain 30. The two chains are joined by two disulfide bridges. In addition, the A chain contains one disulfide bridge. Insulin varies very little between mammalian species. Only one amino acid residue is different in human and porcine insulin, and three amino acids in bovine insulin. For this reason most assays for human insulin work with ligand and radioligand based on insulin from either of these species, whereas the standards are human insulin. Insulin is synthesized via the prohormone proinsulin, which differs from insulin by the so-called connecting peptide (C-peptide). This is a single-chain, 31–amino acid polypeptide that connects the N-terminal of the A chain with the C-terminal of the B chain via three arginine residues. This piece is split off by a trypsinlike enzyme, and the insulin is stored in the cytoplasmic granules characteristic of the beta cell. Equimolar amounts of the C-peptide are released together with insulin upon secretion.

Physiology

Insulin is an important regulator of carbohydrate and lipid metabolism. It is believed to have its main influence in modifying the transport of glucose into the cell and then secondarily inhibiting lipolysis and gluconeogenesis and promoting lipogenesis and the synthesis of glycogen.

Insulin is produced and secreted by the beta cells of the pancreatic islets. A small amount of proinsulin is released at the same time. Normally, proinsulin constitutes less than 20% of the insulin secreted. The release of insulin is stimulated and inhibited by a wide variety of agents, the major physiologic stimulator being the blood glucose level. Changes in release rate occur very rapidly; an intravenous load of glucose causes a rapid increase in the release rate within a couple of minutes, producing a peak in plasma insulin level 5 to 25 times above the baseline level. The plasma level of insulin will therefore closely follow that of glucose, but it is modified by a variety of other stimuli or inhibitors. Examples of stimulators are glucagon and gastrointestinal hormones such as secretin and gastric inhibitory peptide, vagal stimulation, and increased plasma levels of amino acids. Inhibitors are catecholamines and somatostatin. The secretion of insulin in response to most stimuli occurs in two phases (early and late response), which are particularly apparent after an acute stimulus such as an intravenous injection of glucose or tolbutamide. The early response to such a stimulus reaches its peak value 4 to 8 minutes after the beginning of the injection, whereas the peak of the late response occurs much later in relationship to the duration of the stimulus. The action of insulin is also modified by other hormones; in particular, epinephrine, glucagon, and growth hormones have anti-insulin effects.

Insulin is not bound to any transporting protein in plasma. Its turnover rate is rapid, with a half-life of less than 4 minutes. Since insulin is secreted into the portal circulation, all insulin appearing in the peripheral circulation has passed through the liver. The liver takes up about half of the insulin coming through the portal vein. The hepatic insulin extraction is not constant but varies with insulin and glucose

---

INSULIN METHOD

Principle

Ethanol precipitation

$$R + [L + L^*] = [RL + RL^*] + [L + L^*]$$

Protocol

		Reagent	Volume
DAY 1	R	Guinea pig antiserum to insulin	$200\,\mu l$
	L*	^{125}I-labeled insulin	$200\,\mu l$
	L	Standard — h-insulin 6.25, 12.5, 25, 50, 100, 200 $\mu U/ml$	$100\,\mu l$
		Sample — Plasma	

──────────── *18 hours, 4° C* ────────────

DAY 2	↓	Plasma to standards	$100\,\mu l$
		Barbital-BSA to samples	$100\,\mu l$
		99.5% ethanol	$1,800\,\mu l$

Centrifugation 2,500g, 15 minutes, 25° C
Decant supernatant
Count precipitate for 1 minute

Reagents

R	Antiserum to porcine insulin Avidity: $K_a = 4 \times 10^{10}$
L*	Labeled with ^{125}I by lactoperoxidase (Appendix 17) Specific activity: 150-200 $\mu Ci/\mu g$; separation on cellulose (Appendix 20) $T = 20,000\ cpm \approx 0.1\ ng$
L	EDTA-plasma
Diluent	Barbital-BSA (Appendix 34)
↓	Appendix 24

Box 15-1

INSULIN METHOD, cont'd		
Alternatives		
R	*Guinea pig antiserum to bovine insulin*[3,29]	
L*	*Insulin labeled with* ^{125}I[3,14] *or* ^{131}I[13] *by chloramine-T method*	
L	*Serum*[2,13,18,24]	
Diluent	*Barbital-HSA,*[14,29] *phosphate-BSA*[2,3,10] *Phosphate-HSA,*[11,28] *borate-BSA*[18,24]	
↓	*DA-rabbit,*[10,24] *DASP-rabbit (BioRIA, Montreal) DA added with first antiserum (Wellcome) Dextran-coated charcoal,*[2,13] *polyethylene glycol*[18] *Zirconyl-phosphate + ammonium acetate*[3] *Talc tablet,*[14] *solid phase antiserum coupled to Sephadex*[28]	

Box 15-1

concentration. The C-peptide circulates in plasma with a considerably longer half-life than insulin because C-peptide is extracted much less efficiently by the liver.

Insulin secretion shows large variation between individuals. This normal variation is related to the amount and type of food intake, particularly in terms of carbohydrate content. Insulin secretion is influenced by the amount of body fat, since obesity is associated with markedly elevated insulin secretion, in terms of both basal secretion and the response to stimuli.

Methods

Reagents

Insulin of high purity from various species is readily available commercially. Insulin antisera are also available. There are a great number of insulin radioimmunoassay (RIA) kits on the market. Radioligand may be produced by chloramine-T methods or lactoperoxidase. Most antisera are produced in guinea pigs, since rabbits usually give poor insulin antisera. This is probably due to the close similarity of rabbit

insulin to human, bovine, and porcine insulin. Guinea pig insulin exhibits marked structural differences from insulin of other species.

Performance

The available methods differ essentially in the method chosen for separation of bound and free activity, including double antibody and ethanol precipitation, buffer flow chromatography, solid phase coupled antibodies, and active charcoal adsorption. For most assays, a 0.5 M phosphate buffer, around pH 7.4, has been used. In some cases, 0.1 M borate or barbital buffers of pH 8.6 have been employed. The choice of buffer system has had little effect on sensitivity or precision.

Assay properties

Proinsulin cross-reacts to a certain degree in insulin RIAs, but it is normally of minor importance, since proinsulin usually constitutes less than 20% of the plasma insulin and the immunologic reactivity of proinsulin is less than insulin in most assay systems. Assay sensitivity is typically in the range of 1 to 2 μU/ml. Since the insulin assay was the first RIA developed, it is not surprising that it is one of the best characterized and most reproducible of all assays. This is also true, in general, of the many kit modifications.

A routine RIA for insulin is described in detail in Box 15-1.

Despite the small difference in the structure of insulin between different species, insulin of bovine or porcine origin, which is used for therapeutic purposes in human diabetic patients, usually induces antibodies against insulin in treated patients. This is probably due to the presence of degraded or modified insulin molecules in the insulin preparations, since antibodies are less likely to be developed during treatment with recently developed insulin preparations of higher purity. However, such endogenous antibodies will interfere in the assay; thus a regular insulin assay on plasma from such individuals will not give adequate results. For this reason, it is important that the assayist be aware of this source of error, because if not revealed by adequate control tubes, endogenous antibody will give erroneous results, which will cause misinterpretation of the clinical picture. The influence of such exogenous binders is discussed at length on pp. 68-69.

Insulin antibodies may be assayed by a slight modification of the insulin RIA.

Clinical applications
Pathophysiology

HYPOFUNCTION (DIABETES AND PREDIABETES). Classic insulin-requiring juvenile diabetes is characterized by a much reduced secretion of insulin and nonresponsiveness of the beta cell to all known stimuli. Milder forms of diabetes are associated with a decreased secretion of insulin in response to most stimuli. However, it has been suggested that increased insulin secretion may occur in certain phases of the milder forms of the disease. These findings have not been completely verified and are probably explained by the difficulties in establishing the range of normality for the individual. Usually it is not possible to demonstrate abnormal insulin secretion until glucose tolerance tests or fasting blood glucose show pathologic values. Therefore, insulin assay has not proved to be of much value for the clinical workup or management of the patient with suspected or established diabetes mellitus.

Recent interest has focused on the possibility of identifying various types of *prediabetes*. It has been shown that relatives of diabetic patients have decreased insulin secretion, particularly with regard to the early phase of insulin release. However, this view has been challenged by others, and it is still an open question whether a low insulin response in the presence of completely normal blood glucose levels and glucose tolerance tests has any bearing on the risk of developing an overt diabetic state later on. Long-term prospective studies are obviously needed to settle this question.

HYPERFUNCTION. Hypersecretion of insulin may cause hypoglycemia. Hypersecretion may be due to insulin-producing adenomas of the beta cells of the pancreatic islets. These are usually benign, but malignant metastasizing varieties have been described. The majority of patients with hypoglycemia, however, do not have islet tumors or hyperinsulinemia. This is particularly true in newborns, the age group in which hypoglycemia is most prevalent. Rarely, hyperinsulinism occurs because of production of insulin or insulinlike material by a non–beta cell tumor. This has been described particularly in association with retroperitoneal sarcomas but also with other tumors, such as cancer of the lung. Because of the intermittent nature of insulin secretion and the rapid turnover of insulin, it is sometimes difficult to establish the hyperinsulinemic state. However, like many tumors of endocrine organs, insulin-producing tumors are often characterized by autonomous secretion, which is not responsive to agents that normally inhibit insulin secretion. Also, insulin-secreting tumors frequently show exaggerated responses to normal stimuli of insulin secretion.

Sampling

Insulin is usually measured in plasma or serum. Methods have been described for assay on urine, but these do not have general application because of interference of urine constituents other than insulin in the assay. For this reason, it is usually necessary to extract insulin from the urine.

Plasma insulin must be measured under specified standard conditions, either while the patient is fasting or during a particular test situation, usually a stimulation test. There is a correlation between basal insulin levels and the insulin response to stimuli, but the response pattern after stimulation gives more information than measurement of the basal level alone. Common *stimulation tests* used are as follows.

1. *Oral glucose tolerance test.* Various dose schedules have been used, such as 100 g, 1.75 g/kg body weight, or 40 g/m² body surface area. Samples are collected every 10 minutes for the first 30 minutes and then every 15 or 30 minutes up to 3 hours.

2. *Intravenous glucose tolerance test.* A total dose of 25 g has frequently been employed, but this standard dose causes a proportionally high stimulation in small individuals such as children and understimulation in obese individuals. For this reason a dose of 0.5 g/kg body weight or 50 g/1.73 m² body surface area will give a more standardized stimulation. It is important that the first samples be collected

early in this test, since the peak value of the early insulin response occurs within 3 to 6 minutes after glucose injection has begun. Therefore, timing of the samples should be set at the beginning (0 minutes) of the glucose injection. An example of the schedule for collection in this test is 0, 4, 6, 10, 20, 30, 45, and 60 minutes.

3. *Intravenous administration of tolbutamide (1 g, or in children 20 mg/kg body weight) or glucagon (1 mg).* These stimuli may also be used to test insulin secretion. Because the response is as rapid as that induced by intravenous administration of glucose, the same sampling schedule may be used here.

The *inhibition tests* clinically involve prolonged fasting, from 24 to 72 hours, with several samples collected every day.

BLOOD SAMPLES. Venous blood is collected and the assay performed either on serum or plasma. Heparin may influence the results in double-antibody assays. Samples not assayed the same day should be stored at −20° C. Autonomous insulin secretion by an adenoma may be established by means of inhibition tests, in which the autonomous secretion does not show the normal decrease of a fasting level.

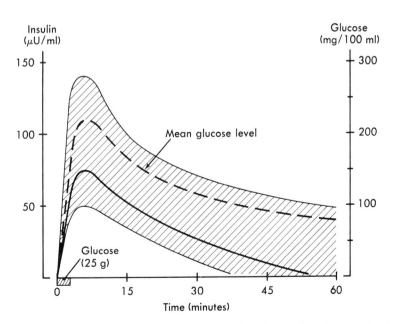

Fig. 15-1. Plasma insulin (continuous lines = mean and 95% range) and mean blood glucose (interrupted line) levels following an intravenous glucose load.

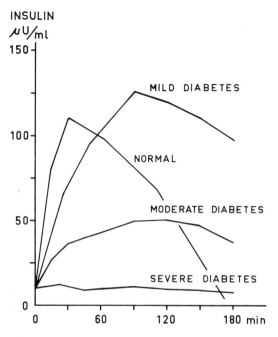

Fig. 15-2. Typical insulin responses to an oral glucose load (50 g) in normal individuals and various stages of diabetes.

Reference values

Different types of assays or different laboratories produce different results. The absolute figures given here should be regarded only as a guide. The normal basal insulin level is 5 to 25 mU/liter. The normal response to any of the above-mentioned stimuli shows wide variation. The early response to the intravenous tests reaches a peak value of 50 to 200 mU/liter (Fig. 15-1) at 3 to 6 minutes, after which it decreases, often quite parallel to the fall in blood glucose levels. The response to an oral glucose load is also highly variable (Fig. 15-2).

Interpretation of results

ELEVATED LEVELS. The most common cause of hyperinsulinemia is obesity. Obesity may be associated with both high fasting insulin levels and very high responses to all stimuli. Obesity is therefore a potential difficulty when one is attempting to diagnose insulin-producing tumors. Hyperinsulinemia due to insulin-secreting adenomas may be demonstrated by different approaches. Adenomas frequently show exaggerated responses to any stimuli. Peak values above 250 mU/liter following intravenous ad-

ministration of glucose, tolbutamide, or glucagon have been reported as highly suggestive (in the absence of obesity) of organic hyperinsulinemia. During an inhibition test, such as prolonged fasting, the autonomous secretion from an adenoma will not show the normal decrease to basal secretion; and peaks in the secretion, without any exogenous stimulation, may be observed.

In the workup of the patients with hypoglycemic conditions, single samples collected during hypoglycemic attacks may be quite valuable in establishing the diagnosis of an insulin-producing tumor. A high insulin plasma concentration in the absence of obesity, when blood glucose values are low, is highly suggestive of autonomous insulin secretion. However, it is important to realize that the finding of normal basal insulin levels during a hypoglycemic phase does not rule out the possibility of an insulin-producing tumor; because of the short half-life of insulin in plasma (less than 4 minutes), the insulin causing the hypoglycemia may have disappeared from plasma when the sample was collected.

It has been reported that insulin-producing

tumors secrete proinsulin in a higher proportion than does the normal beta cell; thus assay of this prohormone has been suggested as a more specific test.

DECREASED LEVELS. Low fasting insulin levels or responses cannot in themselves be taken as an indicator of a diabetic disorder or predisposition. However, in combination with decreased glucose tolerance, such abnormal insulin responses suggest the likelihood of this diagnosis. Maturity-onset diabetes is associated with a ranging degree of decreased response and is correlated with the progress of the disease (Fig. 15-2). An absent response to oral administration of glucose is an indication of threatened absolute insulin deficiency, which will require insulin therapy sooner or later.

REFERENCES

1. Adams, P. W., and Oakley, N. W.: Oral contraceptives and carbohydrate metabolism. In Pyke, D. A., editor: Clinics in endocrinology and metabolism, vol. 1, Philadelphia, 1972, W. B. Saunders Co.
2. Albano, J. D., Ekins, R. P., Maritz, G., and others: A sensitive, precise radioimmunoassay of serum insulin relying on charcoal separation of bound and free hormone moieties, Acta Endocrinol. (Kbh.) **70:**487, 1972.
3. Coffey, I. W., Nagy, C. F., Lenusky, R., and Hansen, H. I.: A radioimmunoassay for plasma insulin using zirconyl phosphate gel, Biochem. Med. **9:**54, 1974.
4. Duckworth, W. C., Kitabchi, A. E., and others: Direct measurement of plasma proinsulin in normal and diabetic subjects, Am. J. Med. **53:**418, 1972.
5. Ellenberg, M., and Rifkin, H., editors: Diabetes mellitus; theory and practice, New York, 1970, McGraw-Hill Book Co.
6. Fajans, S. S.: What is diabetes; definition, diagnosis, and course, Med. Clin. North Am. **55:**793, 1971.
7. Fajans, S. S., and Sussman, K. E., editors: Diabetes mellitus; diagnosis and treatment, vol. 3, New York, 1971, American Diabetes Association.
8. Freinkel, N.: The effect of pregnancy on insulin homeostasis, Diabetes **13:**260, 1964.
9. Gorden, P., and Roth, J.: Plasma insulin; fluctuations in the "big" insulin component in man after glucose and other stimuli, J. Clin. Invest. **48:**2225, 1969.
10. Hales, C. N., and Randle, P. J.: Immunoassay of insulin with insulin-antibody precipitate, Biochem. J. **88:**137, 1963.
11. Heding, L. G.: Determination of total serum insulin (IRI) in insulin-treated diabetic patients, Diabetologia **8:**260, 1972.
12. Heding, L. G.: Radioimmunological determination of human C-peptide in serum, Diabetologia **11:**541, 1975.
13. Herbert, V., Lau, K., Gottlieb, C. W., and Bleicher, C. J.: Coated charcoal immunoassay of insulin, J. Clin. Endocrinol. Metab. **25:**1375, 1965.
14. Kagan, A.: Radioimmunoassay of insulin, Semin. Nucl. Med. **5:**183, 1975.
15. Kitabchi, A. E., Duckworth, W. C., Brusch, J. C., and Heinemann, M.: Direct measurement of proinsulin in human plasma by the use of an insulin-degrading enzyme, J. Clin. Invest. **50:**1792, 1971.
16. Lefebvre, P., and Unger, R. H., editors: Glucagon: molecular physiology, clinical and therapeutic implications, Oxford, 1972, Pergamon Press Ltd.
17. Melani, F., Rubenstein, A. H., Oyer, P. E., and Steiner, D. F.: Identification of proinsulin and C-peptide in human serum by a specific immunoassay, Proc. Natl. Acad. Sci. USA **67:**148, 1970.
18. Nakagawa, S., Nakayama, H., Sasaki, T., and others: A simple method for the determination of serum free insulin levels in insulin-treated patients, Diabetes **22:**590, 1973.
19. Porte, D., Jr., and Robertson, R. P.: Control of insulin secretion by catecholamines, stress, and the sympathetic nervous system, Fed. Proc. **32:**1792, 1973.
20. Pyke, D. A., editor: Clinics in endocrinology and metabolism. I. Diabetes and related disorders, Philadelphia, 1972, W. B. Saunders Co.
21. Rimoin, D. L.: Inheritance in diabetes mellitus, Med. Clin. North Am. **55:**807, 1971.
22. Rubenstein, A. H., and Steiner, D. F.: Proinsulin, Ann. Rev. Med. **22:**1, 1971.
23. Rull, J. A., Conn, J. W., and others: Levels of plasma insulin during cortisone glucose tolerance tests in "nondiabetic" relatives of diabetic patients, Diabetes **19:**1, 1970.
24. Soeldner, J. S., and Slone, D.: Critical variables in the radioimmunoassay of serum insulin using the double antibody technique, Diabetes **14:**771, 1965.
25. Steiner, D. F., and Freinkel, N., editors: Handbook of physiology. I. Endocrinology, Washington, D.C., 1972, American Physiological Society.
26. Steiner, D. F., Oyer, P., Cho, S., and others: Structural and immunological studies on human proinsulin. In Rodriguez, R. R., and Vallance-Owen, J., editors: Diabetes (Proceedings of the Seventh Congress of the International Diabetes Federation), Amsterdam, 1971, Excerpta Medica Foundation, pp. 281-291.
27. Swerdloff, R. S., Pozefsky, T., and others: Influence of age on the intravenous tolbutamide response test, Diabetes **16:**161, 1967.
28. Velasco, C. A., Cole, H. S., and Camerini-Davalos, P. A.: Radioimmunoassay of insulin, Clin. Chem. **20:**700, 1974.
29. Yalow, R. S., and Berson, S. A.: Immunoassay of endogenous plasma insulin in man, J. Clin. Invest. **39:**1157, 1960.

16 GASTRIN

The gastrointestinal hormones are produced in the gut and have their principal action on digestive organs. To date seven hormones have been identified: secretin, gastrin, cholecystokinin-pancreozymin, vasoactive intestinal peptide, gastric inhibitory peptide, motilin, and enteroglucagon.

Radioimmunoassays (RIAs) have been developed for secretin, cholecystokinin-pancreozymin, vasoactive intestinal peptide, and gastrin. The main problem in the development of these tests was the isolation of sufficiently pure hormone preparations to serve as immunogen, since the cells producing the gastrointestinal hormones are scattered throughout a large area of gut mucosa. A secondary problem in RIA development has been that the immunologic response to the hormone is inconsistent. Conjugation of the hormones to a larger molecule, such as albumin, results in more consistently good RIA antisera.

Gastrin RIA is the only one of these methods in widespread clinical use.

Chemistry

The substance that was originally isolated from the stomach as "gastrin" is a heptadecapeptide (17 amino acids). This substance (human) has been synthesized and is available in pure form.

A variety of congeners of gastrin have been isolated from biologic systems. These differ chiefly by variation in the number of amino acids in the polypeptide chain. Gastrin congeners of 34, 17, and 13 amino acid residues have been isolated. An additional gastrin has been termed "big-big" gastrin by Yalow and Berson. The exact chain length of this sub-

stance is not known. An additional gastrin congener has been reported that is also incompletely characterized. The substance is called component I of Rehfeld. Each of these substances can exist in sulfated or nonsulfated forms with respect to the carboxyl-terminal tyrosine residue.

In shorthand notation these substances are referred to by the designation for gastrin, followed by the chain length of the polypeptide residues. Thus the 34 amino acid gastrin material becomes G-34. In addition, if this material contains a sulfate residue, it is called G-34-II. The more common nonsulfated form is called G-34-I, or simply G-34. G-34 is also used as a generic term to refer to both the sulfated and nonsulfated forms. Thus, according to this nomenclature, there are G-34, G-17, and G-13 forms. Big-big gastrin and component I of Rehfeld are gastrins for which there is no shorthand notation.

A parallel notation has been employed, principally by Yalow and Berson. From largest to smallest, there is "big-big" gastrin, "big" gastrin (G-34), "little" gastrin (G-17), and "mini" gastrin (G-13). The physiologically active portion of the gastrin molecule is the carboxyl-terminal tetrapeptide region with the following structure: Tyr-Met-Asp-Phe-NH$_2$. Pentagastrin, a commercially available synthetic pentapeptide, consists of the biologically active C-terminal tetrapeptide amide plus beta alanine in a terminal group (tertiary butyloxycarbonyl).

Physiology

Gastrin (G-17) is by weight the most powerful known stimulator of gastric acid secretion.

Gastrin also stimulates the stomach to secrete pepsin and intrinsic factor, the pancreas to secrete pancreatic juices, and the small intestine to secrete secretin. In addition to its effect on secretion, gastrin increases the muscular tone of the lower esophageal sphincter, stomach, small intestine, large intestine, gallbladder, and uterus. Gastrin relaxes the sphincter of Oddi. Other gastrin effects include promoting growth of stomach mucosa and increasing blood flow through gastric, pancreatic, and small intestinal capillary beds. The gastrin-producing cells are distributed throughout the upper small intestine and stomach, with the major concentration in the stomach. The principal site of gastrin production is the mucosa of the gastric antrum and proximal duodenum. Most gastrin in the antrum is G-17; however, the more distally one goes in the gut, the greater the proportion of G-34 that is found. In the proximal jejunum, only G-34 or big-big gastrin is found.

The cells that produce gastrin are called G cells. G cells have a flasklike shape with a broad base and narrow neck extending to the mucosal surface.

Release of gastrin from the intestinal mucosa may be provoked by vagal stimulation, insulin-induced hypoglycemia, ingestion of protein, and increases in serum calcium. Acid within the lumen of the stomach effectively inhibits gastrin secretion and blocks the effect of stimulatory influences.

Serum gastrin shows considerable structural heterogeneity. Big-big gastrin accounts for the majority of serum gastrin in normal individuals during the fasting state. G-34 gastrin is the predominant serum form in nonfasting states. Once gastrin is within the blood, disappearance half-times are as follows: G-17, 3.0 minutes; G-34, 9 minutes; big-big gastrin, 90 minutes. There is no demonstrable difference between the sulfated and nonsulfated forms with respect to clearance half-times.

Distribution space is approximately 11% of body weight, or two times plasma volume.

Big-big gastrin has no biologic activity; G-34 gastrin has about one half of the biologic activity of the G-17 form.

Gastrin is degraded principally by the kidney. Very little gastrin is excreted into the urine.

Method

Bioassay techniques for assessment of gastrin activity are not sufficiently sensitive to measure the picogram quantities of gastrin circulating in serum. The initial RIAs capable of measuring normal fasting serum gastrin levels were described by Hansky and Cain and by McGuigan and Trudeau; these assays utilized the G-17 material for preparation of radioligand and for standard.

Reagents

Gastrin antibodies can be produced by use of either pure or semipurified preparations of gastrin as immunogen. Hansky and Cain, and McGuigan and Trudeau used synthetic gastrin I conjugated to serum albumin as immunogen. Yalow and Berson utilized pork gastrin as immunogen in partially purified preparations. Antibodies have been developed in guinea pigs and rabbits by use of standard immunization schedules and techniques. Conjugated human gastrin provokes a consistent antibody response.

Synthetic human gastrin is available in purified form from Imperial Chemical Industries (ICI) of Britain. Standards are available from the Medical Research Council of England for pork gastrin II and synthetic human gastrin I. Gastrin is stable and, if frozen, may be stored for prolonged periods without loss of immunoreactivity. Since gastrin is insoluble at acidic pH, standards should be prepared in slightly alkaline buffers.

Heptadecapeptide gastrin has been successfully iodinated by the chloramine-T and lactoperoxidase techniques. Specific activities of 500 mCi/mg can be obtained.

Performance

The time of incubation for these assays varies from 3 to 4 hours up to several days. Several separation techniques have been utilized, including charcoal, ethanol precipitation, anion exchange resins, and double-antibody precipitation.

Assay properties

The typical sensitivity for most assays is on the order of 5 to 10 pg/ml. Big-big gastrin, G-

GASTRIN METHOD

Principle

Anion exchange resin

$$R + [L + L^*] = [RL + RL^*] + [L + L^*]$$

Protocol

		Reagent	Volume
DAY 1	R	*Rabbit antiserum to synthetic human gastrin I*	*1,000 µl*
	L*	*^{125}I-labeled gastrin*	*250 µl*
	L	Standard *15.6, 31.3, 62.5, 125, 250, 500, 1,000 ng/liter* Sample *Serum*	*250 µl*

———————————— *72 hours, 4° C* ————————————

DAY 4	↓	*30 mg Amberlite CG 4B 200 mesh in barbital-BSA* *Mix by rotation of assay tubes for 5 minutes*	*300 µl*

Centrifugation 2,500g, 15 minutes
Decant supernatant into plastic tubes
Count supernatant for 10 minutes

Reagents

R — *Rabbit antiserum to synthetic human gastrin I, covalently bound to BSA*
Avidity: $K_a = 2 \times 10^{12}$ liter/mol

L* — *Synthetic human gastrin I labeled with ^{125}I by lactoperoxidase (Appendix 17)*
Specific activity: 320-400 µCi/µg
Separation on Sephadex G-10 (Appendix 19)
T = 2,000 cpm ≈ 4 pg

L — *Serum*

Diluent — *0.02 M barbital-HSA (Appendix 34)*

Alternatives

R — *Guinea pig antiserum to porcine gastrin A[28]*
Chicken antiserum to porcine gastrin[10]

Box 16-1

	GASTRIN METHOD, cont'd
L*	*Gastrin labeled with $^{131}I^{15}$ or $^{125}I^{6,8,10,12,23,24,28}$ by chloramine-T method*
L	*Plasma*[6]
Diluent	*Phosphate-ovalbumin,*[15] *phosphate-HSA*[10] *Phosphate-BSA,*[24] *barbital–egg albumin*[12]

DA-goat,[15] *ethanol precipitation*[10]
Dextran-coated charcoal[8,24]
Solid phase antiserum coupled to cellulose[23]

Box 16-1

34, and G-17 are all measured as "gastrin" activity by RIA. Although this may complicate interpretation of results, the assay itself has usually been relatively straightforward and reliable.

A specific method for gastrin RIA is shown in Box 16-1.

Clinical applications

Pathophysiology

The Zollinger-Ellison syndrome (ulcerogenic islet cell tumor) consists of severe ulcer disease associated with markedly increased gastric acid secretion in the presence of a nonbeta islet cell tumor. This disorder, by some estimates, accounts for about 1% of the patient population with peptic ulcer disease. The gastrin-secreting tumors are usually located in the pancreas and contain large amounts of gastrin. Patients with Zollinger-Ellison syndrome have markedly elevated fasting serum gastrin concentrations. In addition, these serum levels of gastrin are not affected by the normal stimuli that increase gastrin concentrations, such as a protein-rich meal or histamine provocation. However, with intravenous calcium infusion, patients with Zollinger-Ellison tumors show remarkable increases in serum gastrin concentration. These patients also exhibit an abnormal response to secretin administration. In patients with Zollinger-

Ellison syndrome, secretin may cause an increase rather than the usual decrease in serum gastrin levels.

In patients with pernicious anemia and other causes of atrophic gastritis, significant increases in serum gastrin concentrations are observed. In addition, in patients with gastric ulcer disease, serum gastrin levels may be elevated. These elevations both in pernicious anemia and in gastric ulcer tend to correlate with a relative decrease in acid production in these two conditions. The increase in serum gastrin is viewed as a compensatory accompaniment of these disorders.

Gastrin serum levels in patients with duodenal ulcer disease are not increased when compared with the levels in the normal patient population. These levels may be relatively increased, however, since there is relatively more acid production than would be expected from the serum gastrin level. It may be related to the fact that in patients with duodenal ulcers, the normal inhibition of gastrin secretion by acid is somewhat blunted.

Sampling

Morning fasting gastrin samples are usually obtained, since serum gastrin concentrations both in normal individuals and patients with peptic ulcer disease are lowest during the early morning hours (3:00 AM to 7:00 AM), rise during the day, and begin to fall at about 10:00 PM. Gastrin is relatively stable in serum and, particularly if frozen, may be stored for prolonged periods.

PROVOCATIVE TESTS. To evaluate the rate of secretion, a variety of stimulation and inhibition tests have been developed. Stimulation of gastrin secretion has been achieved by feeding the patient a 180-gm protein meal and then taking blood samples at 15-minute intervals for the next 2 hours. The normal subject increases baseline values from 50% to 150%. Patients with Zollinger-Ellison syndrome do not respond to a test meal. In the special situation where Zollinger-Ellison syndrome is suspected, a calcium infusion test may be performed, in which Ca^{++} is infused intravenously (Ca^{++} gluconate at 5 mg/kg/hr over a 3-hour period), and blood samples are taken every 15 minutes. A secretin stimulation test is also used. Secretin, 1 to 2 units/kg, is rapidly infused, and samples are taken at 5-minute intervals for the first 30 minutes, then every 10 minutes for 1 hour. In Zollinger-Ellison syndrome both Ca^{++} and secretin increase the level of gastrin by more than 50%, or 200 pg/ml. However, a minority of patients with Zollinger-Ellison syndrome do not respond to these two tests. Normal subjects show no change, or a slight decrease in serum gastrin values, in response to both a secretin challenge and Ca^{++} infusion.

The stimulation test that we have found most useful is the glucagon infusion test. In this situation 1 mg glucagon is given by intravenous push. Samples are obtained over the next 1 hour at 5-minute intervals. Normal subjects respond with a slight decrease of basal gastrin values. Patients with Zollinger-Ellison syndrome have a marked increase in gastrin levels, with a peak 5 to 15 minutes after glucagon infusion.

Reference values

Normal basal secretion: 20-160 pg/ml
Normal stimulation response
  180-gm protein meal: 50-150% increase in basal secretion, peak at 15-30 minutes after eating
  Secretin, glucagon: no change, or decrease in serum gastrin levels after administration
  Ca^{++} infusion: rise of less than 500 pg/ml over 4-hour infusion duration

Interpretation of results

The major indication for gastrin RIA is the patient who is suspected of having Zollinger-Ellison syndrome. Other indications for gastrin measurement are patients who have severe ulcer disease with diarrhea, or who require surgery; those who have recurrent ulcers after gastrointestinal surgery; and those whose basal rate of acid excretion exceeds 10 mEq HCl per hour, with associated symptoms of peptic ulcer disease.

Elevated values of serum gastrin are found in patients with Zollinger-Ellison syndrome. Basal values that range from 300 up to 350,000 pg/ml have been observed. Patients with Zollinger-Ellison syndrome do not respond normally to the usual stimuli of gastrin secretion. A test meal causes no change in serum concentration. However, the majority of patients with Zollinger-Ellison syndrome will show a paradoxically increased secretion of gastrin in response to secretin or glucagon infusion. Ca^{++} infusion causes an increase of greater than 500 pg/ml in most instances. Elevated serum values are also observed in patients with pernicious anemia or other diseases associated with gastric achlorhydria. Levels of several thousand picograms per milliliter have been observed. However, these patients show a normal response to secretin and glucagon. Patients with renal failure may also have elevated values because of delayed excretion and delayed metabolic degradation of gastrin. Similarly, patients with major resection of the intestine may have increased levels for unknown reasons. After vagotomy, basal and postprandial gastrin levels are elevated because of reduced acid production. Minimal degrees of gastrin elevation may be found in patients with duodenal ulcer disease. These patients typically have a greater response to a protein-rich meal and Ca^{++} infusion than do normal subjects.

Decreased values of serum gastrin are found in patients following gastrectomy. The gastrin level is a useful way to follow patients with

Zollinger-Ellison syndrome after resection surgery.

REFERENCES

1. Berson, S. A., and Yalow, R. S.: Radioimmunoassay in gastroenterology, Gastroenterology **62:**1061, 1972.
2. Bloom, S. R., Polak, J. M., and Pearse, A. G.: Vasoactive intestinal peptide and watery-diarrhoea syndrome, Lancet **2:**14, 1973.
3. Boden, G., and Chey, W. Y.: Preparation and specificity of antiserum to synthetic secretin and its use in radioimmunoassay (RIA), Endocrinology **92:**1617, 1973.
4. Colin-Jones, D. G., and Lennard-Jones, J. E.: The detection and measurement of circulating gastrin-like activity by bioassay, Gut **13:**88, 1972.
5. Englert, E.: Radioimmunoassay (RIA) of cholecystokinin (CCK), Clin. Res. **21:**207, 1973.
6. Ganguli, P. C., and Hunter, W. M.: Radioimmunoassay of gastrin in human plasma, J. Physiol. (Lond.) **220:**499, 1972.
7. Go, V. L., Ryan, R. J., and Summerskill, W. H.: Radioimmunoassay of porcine cholecystokinin-pancreozymin, J. Lab. Clin. Med. **77:**684, 1971.
8. Hansky, J., and Cain, M. D.: Radioimmunoassay of gastrin in human serum, Lancet **2:**1388, 1969.
9. Hansky, J., Soveny, C., and Korman, M. G.: The effect of glucagon on serum gastrin. I. Studies in normal subjects, Gut **14:**457, 1973.
10. Jeffcoate, S. L.: Radioimmunoassay of gastrin; specificity of gastrin antisera, Scand. J. Gastroenterol. **4:** 457, 1969.
11. Korman, M. G., Soveny, C., and Hansky, J.: The effect of glucagon on serum gastrin. II. Studies in pernicious anemia and Zollinger-Ellison syndrome, Gut **14:**459, 1973.
12. Kumar, M. S., and Deodhar, S. D.: An improved radioimmunoassay of serum gastrin using a commercial kit, Clin. Chim. Acta **61:**191, 1975.
13. McGuigan, J. E.: Antibodies to the carboxyl-terminal tetrapeptide amide of gastrin in guinea pigs, J. Lab. Clin. Med. **71:**964, 1968.
14. McGuigan, J. E.: The radioimmunoassay of gastrin; clinical considerations, J.A.M.A. **235:**405, 1976.
15. McGuigan, J. E., and Trudeau, W. L.: Studies with antibodies to gastrin; radioimmunoassay in human serum and physiological studies, Gastroenterology **58:** 139, 1970.
16. McGuigan, J. E., and Trudeau, W. L.: Differences in rates of gastrin release in normal persons and patients with duodenal ulcer disease, N. Engl. J. Med. **288:**64, 1973.
17. Newton, W. T., McGuigan, J. E., and Jaffe, B. M.: Radioimmunoassay of peptides lacking tyrosine, J. Lab. Clin. Med. **75:**886, 1970.
18. Reeder, D. D., Becker, H. D., Smith, N. J., Rayford, P. L., and Thompson, J. C.: Radioimmunoassay of cholecystokinin, Surg. Forum **23:**361, 1972.
19. Reeder, D. D., Becker, H. D., Smith, N. J., Rayford, P. L., and Thompson, J. C.: Measurement of endogenous release of cholecystokinin by radioimmunoassay, Ann. Surg. **178:**304, 1973.
20. Rehfeld, J. F.: Three compounds of gastrin in human serum; gel filtration studies on the molecular size of immunoreactive serum gastrin, Biochim. Biophys. Acta **285:**364, 1972.
21. Rehfeld, J. F., and Stadil, F.: Production and evaluation of antibodies for the radioimmunoassay of gastrin, Scand. J. Clin. Lab. Invest. **30:**221, 1972.
22. Rehfeld, J. F. and Stadil, F.: Gel filtration studies on immunoreactive gastrin in serum from Zollinger-Ellison patients, Gut **14:**369, 1973.
23. Rehfeld, J. F., and Stadil, F.: Radioimmunoassay for gastrin employing immunoabsorbent, Scand. J. Clin. Lab. Invest. **31:**459, 1973.
24. Schrumpf, E., and Sand, T.: Radioimmunoassay of gastrin with activated charcoal, Scand. J. Gastroenterol. **7:**683, 1972.
25. Straus, E., and Yalow, R. S.: Studies on the distribution and degradation of heptadecapeptide, big, and big big gastrin, Gastroenterology **66:**936, 1974.
26. Walsh, J. H.: Clinical significance of gastrin radioimmunoassay, Semin. Nucl. Med. **5:**247, 1975.
27. Walsh, J. H., and Grossman, M. I.: Gastrin (parts I and II), N. Engl. J. Med. **292:**1324, 1377, 1975.
28. Yalow, R. S., and Berson, S. A.: Radioimmunoassay of gastrin, Gastroenterology **58:**1, 1970.
29. Yalow, R. S., and Berson, S. A.: Size and charge distinction between endogenous human plasma gastrin in peripheral blood and heptadecapeptide gastrins, Gastroenterology **58:**609, 1970.
30. Yalow, R. S., and Berson, S. A.: And now, "big, big" gastrin, Biochem. Biophys. Res. Comm. **48:**391, 1972.
31. Young, J. D., Lazarus, L., Chisholm, D. T., and Atkinson, F. F. U.: Radioimmunoassay of secretin in human serum, J. Nucl. Med. **9:**641, 1968.
32. Young, J. D., Lazarus, L., Chisholm, D. J., and Atkinson, F. F. U.: Radioimmunoassay of pancreozymin in human serum, J. Nucl. Med. **12:**743, 1969.

17 HEMATOPOIETIC SYSTEM

Cyanocobalamin
Folate

Radioligand assays have been principally employed on a research basis for the evaluation of a wide variety of substances related to red blood cell production and, to a lesser extent, to coagulation. A list of those developed is shown in Table 17-1. Vitamin B_{12} and folate assays are the tests most broadly applied clinically.

CYANOCOBALAMIN
Chemistry

Cyanocobalamin (vitamin B_{12}) is a glycoprotein complex with a molecular weight of 1,200. The molecule contains cobalt as an integral part of the molecular structure.

The term "cobalamin" is used to describe vitamin B_{12} minus the cyanide group, and "cyanocobalamin" is a term used to describe vitamin B_{12} itself. Other "cobalamins" of importance include hydroxycobalamin, in which the $-OH$ group replaces the $-CN$ of cyanocobalamin; aquocobalamin, in which $-H_2O$ replaces the $-CN$ of cyanocobalamin. The active form of vitamin B_{12} in vivo is called coenzyme B_{12}, in which the $-CN$ of cyanocobalamin is replaced by 5'-deoxyadenosine. Vitamin B_{12} coenzyme is quite unstable in the presence of light and is rapidly oxidized to aquocobalamin. In the presence of potassium cyanide, aquocobalamin is converted back to cyanocobalamin. This fact is employed in several assays to make sure that the vitamin B_{12} is in a form that is readily measured by the test system.

Physiology

Coenzyme B_{12} is essential to a variety of enzymatic reactions. The coenzyme serves as a methyl donor in the production of essential nucleic acids and nuclear protein. Coenzyme B_{12} is essential to normal maturation and division of cells. The cyanocobalamins are essential for normal growth, hematopoiesis, production of epithelial cells, and maintenance of myelin in a functional state within the central nervous system. Cyanocobalamin is present in animal proteins. In the normal individual, ingested cyanocobalamin forms a complex with intrinsic factor (IF) in the stomach. IF is a 55,000–molecular weight glycoprotein produced by the gastric parietal cells. Two molecules of cyanocobalamin complex with two molecules of IF. This tetramer then passes down the intestinal lumen to the terminal ileum, where absorption normally takes place by direct attachment of the complex to the ileal mucosa and then by transfer of vitamin B_{12} into the blood. Once absorbed into the blood, the vast majority of vitamin B_{12} circulates bound to plasma protein.

In man, there are two primary transporting plasma proteins: transcobalamin I and transcobalamin II. Transcobalamin I is an α-globulin and is primarily responsible for maintaining the level of vitamin B_{12} in serum. Transcobalamin II, a β-globulin, is involved in transfer of cyanocobalamin into cells. In addition, transcobalamin III, an inter-α-globulin, also participates in transport. The avidity of these proteins for vitamin B_{12} is high, with K_a's in the order of 10^{11} or 10^{12} liter/mole. Unbound cyanocobalamin in the blood is rapidly filtered by the renal glomerulus.

Cyanocobalamin is stored in the liver. Under normal circumstances, the human liver contains a year's supply of vitamin B_{12}. About $0.1 \mu g$ of vitamin B_{12} is the minimal daily requirement for this vitamin. The recommended intake of the vitamin is about $2 \mu g$/day for adults, $2.5 \mu g$/day

Table 17-1. Radioligand assays of the hematopoietic system

Assays	References
Competitive protein binding systems	
Vitamin B_{12} (cyanocobalamin)	Barakat and Ekins, 1961
	Rothenberg, 1961
	Lau and others, 1965
Folic acid	Rothenberg, 1965
Methyltetrahydrofolic acid	Waxman and others, 1971
Radioimmunoassays	
Fibrinogen, fibrin degradation products	Catt and others, 1968
Fibrinogen fragment D	Plow and Edgington, 1973
Fibrinopeptides A and B	Nossel and others, 1971
Plasminogen and plasmin	Rabiner and others, 1969
Antihemophilic factor	Hoyer, 1972
Prothrombin	Johnston and others, 1972
Ferritin	Reller, 1971
	Addison and others, 1972
Erythropoietin	Fisher and others, 1971
Anti-D immunoglobulin	Hughes-Jones, 1967
	Hughes-Jones and Stevenson, 1968
	Hughes-Jones and others, 1972

for pregnant and lactating women, and $0.3\mu g/$ day for children.

Method

The radioligand assay for vitamin B_{12} was one of the first developed. Two factors favored development of this method. First, vitamin B_{12} contains cobalt as part of its natural structure. A radioactive isotope of cobalt, such as ^{57}Co or ^{60}Co, may be relatively easily substituted for the native cobalt within the molecule. Thus the radioligand is easily produced. Second, naturally occurring binders for vitamin B_{12} are readily available. Transcobalamin I, a highly avid binding protein, circulates in plasma. This substance can be used as a highly specific receptor in a radioligand assay. IF is also an avid binder for vitamin B_{12} and may be used as a receptor.

A radioimmunoassay (RIA) for vitamin B_{12} has recently been developed, although it has not yet been fully evaluated clinically.

Reagents

Some methods utilize unique receptors, such as transcobalamin I of patients with chronic myelogenous leukemia, chicken serum, and fish serum. Most methods utilize IF as receptor. Although charcoal has become the most popular separation reagent, DEAE cellulose, dialysis, and absorbent columns have also been utilized to separate vitamin B_{12}. ^{57}Co is usually used to label the radioligand.

Performance

In methods so far developed, some technique for blocking the binding of vitamin B_{12} and naturally occurring binding proteins in serum is employed. Most commonly, samples are acidified and boiled to disrupt this binding.

Cyanide or albumin added to the serum samples after dissociation from serum proteins has been suggested to improve the stability of cyanocobalamin in serum.

Assay performance times are typically short, ranging from 30 minutes to a few hours.

Assay properties

The binding of cyanocobalamin to exogenous binders must be disrupted without destroying vitamin B_{12} reactivity. In the lower end of the normal range and below, biologically inactive

CYANOCOBALAMIN (VITAMIN B$_{12}$) METHOD†

Principle

DEAE cellulose

$$R + [L^* + L] = [RL + RL^*] + [L + L^*]$$

Protocol

		Reagent	Volume
DAY 1	R	*Pooled human serum*	*30-150 μl*
	L*	*^{57}Co-cyanocobalamin (100 pg)*	*100 μl*
	L {Standard / Sample}	*Cyanocobalamin 10, 25, 100, 200, 400, 600, 900, pg/ml*	*4.0 ml*
		Boiled acidified (acetate-cyanide) serum extracts	*4.0 ml*

——————— *90 minutes, room temperature* ———————

Diluent	*Tris buffer (pH 8.5)*	*10.0 ml*
↓	*DEAE cellulose*	*300 mg*

——————— *Mix (Kahn shaker) 15 minutes* ———————

Centrifuge
Decant
Count cellulose

Reagents

R — *Pooled human serum, 200-300 ml from one or several donors; a volume is chosen for assay that binds 100 pg of ^{57}Co-vitamin B$_{12}$ to 50-60%; this is usually in the order of 30-150 μl*

L* — *^{57}Co-cyanocobalamin (Amersham/Searle)*
Specific activity: 100 μCi/μg
Diluted to about 100 pg/100 μl (100 pg = 23-28,000 cpm)

L {Standard / Sample}
Standard — Cyanocobalamin crystalline from Schwarz-Mann
Sample — Boiled acidified acetate/CN serum extract

† Adapted from Frenkel, E. P., and others: Radioisotopic assay of serum vitamin B$_{12}$ with the use of DEAE cellulose, J. Lab. Clin. Med. **68:**510, 1966.

Box 17-1

CYANOCOBALAMIN (VITAMIN B₁₂) METHOD, cont'd

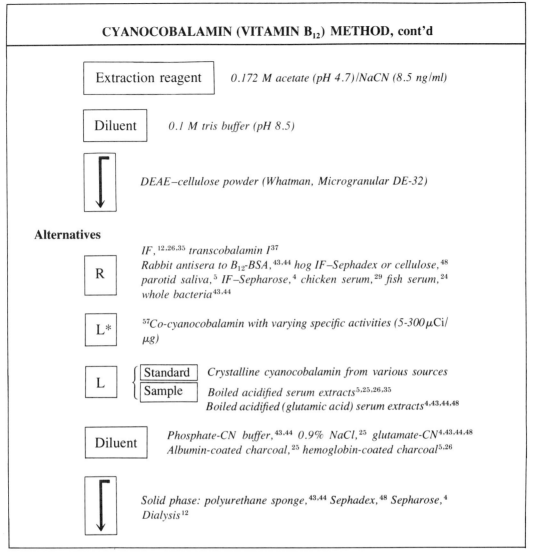

Extraction reagent	*0.172 M acetate (pH 4.7)/NaCN (8.5 ng/ml)*
Diluent	*0.1 M tris buffer (pH 8.5)*
↓	*DEAE–cellulose powder (Whatman, Microgranular DE-32)*

Alternatives

R — *IF,[12,26,35] transcobalamin I[37]*
Rabbit antisera to B₁₂-BSA,[43,44] hog IF–Sephadex or cellulose,[48] parotid saliva,[5] IF–Sepharose,[4] chicken serum,[29] fish serum,[24] whole bacteria[43,44]

L* — *[57]Co-cyanocobalamin with varying specific activities (5-300 μCi/μg)*

L —
Standard | *Crystalline cyanocobalamin from various sources*
Sample | *Boiled acidified serum extracts[5,25,26,35]*
Boiled acidified (glutamic acid) serum extracts[4,43,44,48]

Diluent — *Phosphate-CN buffer,[43,44] 0.9% NaCl,[25] glutamate-CN[4,43,44,48]*
Albumin-coated charcoal,[25] hemoglobin-coated charcoal[5,26]

↓ — *Solid phase: polyurethane sponge,[43,44] Sephadex,[48] Sepharose,[4] Dialysis[12]*

Box 17-1

substances may cross-react, giving falsely high levels of measured vitamin B₁₂. Most assays give sensitivities in the order of 10 to 30 pg/ml.

A radioassay for vitamin B₁₂ is shown in Box 17-1.

Clinical applications

Pathophysiology

VITAMIN B₁₂ DEFICIENCY STATES. When coenzyme B₁₂ is lacking, a characteristic defect develops in cells of many different tissues. The nucleus is unable to mature normally and does not divide appropriately. The nucleus takes on an unusual appearance, with the formation of nucleoli and enlargement. This produces a megaloblastic cell. In particular, those organ systems are affected which contain the most rapidly proliferating cells in the body, such as the hematopoietic cells and cells of the gut mucosa. In prolonged vitamin B₁₂ deficiency, the central nervous system is also affected.

Most deficiency states are due to malabsorption of the vitamin. Malabsorption of vitamin B_{12} may be caused by the inability of the gastric parietal cells to secrete IF, as in pernicious anemia or following gastric resection. Malabsorption of the IF–vitamin B_{12} complex is seen with inflammatory disease of the ileum or following surgical resection of the terminal ileum. In addition, malabsorption of vitamin B_{12} is sometimes associated with bacterial overgrowth within the gut. Malabsorption is sometimes associated with parasitic infestation, such as with *Diphyllobothrium latum,* or after surgery, particularly when a blind loop is created in the Billroth I operation for duodenal ulcer.

Dietary deficiency of vitamin B_{12} may occur in strict vegetarians and in their breast-fed infants. Pathologic manifestations of vitamin B_{12} deficiency usually do not appear before the serum levels fall to less than 100 pg/ml. At this stage the liver contains less than 0.1 μg (normal liver contains 1-10μg cyanocobalamin). The degree of involvement of the hematologic or nervous system may vary from case to case of vitamin B_{12} deficiency; in general, the two major manifestations do not necessarily correlate because of the varying amounts of folate ingested by such patients. Folate is partially effective in reversing the hematologic manifestations of the disease, but not the neurologic manifestations.

Sampling

Random serum samples may be employed.

Reference values

Regardless of the method employed, the normal range in serum is 200 to 900 pg/ml.

Interpretation of results

Radioassay of vitamin B_{12} gives values for serum concentrations that generally correspond well with values from microbiologic assay methods. However, with values below the normal range, radioassay methods generally give higher results than do the bioassay techniques. This is a problem in screening patients for vitamin B_{12} deficiency, since an occasional patient will have a measured serum concentration in the low normal range when the microbiologic assay shows no effective vitamin B_{12} in serum.

The reasons for this discrepancy between bioassay and radioassay are not clear at this time. If a patient is suspected of having pernicious anemia, with assay values measuring in the low normal range, a microbiologic assay should be performed to rule out vitamin B_{12} deficiency.

LOW VALUES. Values less than 100 pg/ml are almost always associated with vitamin B_{12} deficiency. However, falsely low levels of vitamin B_{12} have been reported in patients taking very large doses of ascorbic acid. Similarly, falsely low levels of vitamin B_{12} have also been associated with high concentrations of fluoride in serum.

ELEVATED VALUES. Values greater than 1,000 pg/ml are found in hepatic disorders (such as hepatitis) in which there is a release of cyanocobalamin into the blood and in myeloproliferative disorders in which there is abnormal elevation of specific binding proteins. This particularly occurs in chronic myelogenous leukemia, with changes in transcobalamins I and III.

FOLATE
Chemistry

"Folate" is a generic term used to describe folic acid and its biologically important derivatives. The parent compound, folic acid (pteroyltriglutamic acid [PGA]), is rapidly reduced in vivo to tetrahydrofolic acid (THFA). Methyl-THFA (MTHFA) is the principal coenzyme in vivo, and it is this form that is measured in most radioassay systems.

Physiology

MTHFA serves to transfer 1-carbon units in a variety of enzymatic reactions; in particular, in the production of purines and pyrimidine nucleotides, essential precursors to deoxyribonucleic acid synthesis.

Folate is not synthesized in vivo. The adult dietary requirement is about 50μg/day. Folate requirements are considerably greater during childhood (100μg/day), pregnancy (400μg/day), and lactation (300μg/day). Folate is found in nearly all foodstuffs, including liver, yeast, fresh green vegetables, and fruits. However, the folate content of these foods is greatly reduced by cooking, and the normal adult requirement of $50\mu g$/day may not be met if the diet does not contain fresh vegetables or fruit.

Folate in food is in the form of a polyglutamate. This is broken down within the gut, and folate in the monoglutamate form is rapidly absorbed primarily through the proximal small intestine. Folic acid is rapidly absorbed into the blood and, once within the blood, is rapidly converted to a variety of active folate forms, particularly THFA. The majority of folate circulates in plasma bound to plasma protein. Normal folate stores are about 5 to 10 mg distributed primarily within the liver. The main storage form is MTHFA. MTHFA is also the predominant form that circulates in human plasma.

Method

A microbiologic assay that employs *Lactobacillus casei* has been available for clinical studies. These organisms require *N*-MTHFA for growth. These tests are somewhat difficult to perform and usually require an overnight incubation. A variety of substances, including antibiotics and folate antagonists, interfere with interpretation of the test results.

Radioligand assays for folate compounds were initially developed by Rothenberg and by DaCosta and Rothenberg. These methods utilized an enzyme, dihydrofolate reductase, and antibody to bovine albumin conjugate of PGA as binders. PGA, although not the biologically important form, was measured in these assay systems. With the discovery of specific folate-binding proteins in milk, radioligand assays that were capable of measuring MTHFA were developed.

Reagents

Most radioligand assays now utilize milk proteins or more purified β-lactoglobulin, the dominant folate binder in milk. The ^{3}H-labeled MTHFA has relatively low specific activity and is quite unstable. Hence its use as radioligand is not practical. ^{3}H-labeled PGA has been most widely used as radioligand, even though PGA is not the biologically active folate form in vivo. MTHFA is usually used as a standard; and, because MTHFA competes with PGA for the receptor, a satisfactory assay is possible in

most systems. Recently, iodinated tracers have been introduced, and their use is becoming widespread.

Performance

The assay is usually performed in a sequential manner, with the MTHFA in serum added first and the ^{3}H-labeled PGA added after an interval of incubation. The reaction between MTHFA and milk binder is favored by this incubation scheme, compensating for the higher affinity of PGA for the milk binder.

If the pH is relatively alkaline (pH 9.0), PGA and MTHFA are quite similar in their binding with milk proteins. The use of ^{3}H-labeled PGA in the assay limits sensitivity because of low count rate. The monoiodinated monotyramine of PGA has been used as radioligand in the assay of folate. The ^{125}I-labeled PGA gives higher count rates than does the tritiated form.

Assay properties

The use of alkaline pH for the reaction mixture (pH 9.3) and ^{125}I-labeled PGA makes possible the use of PGA as standard. This technique offers the advantage of a relatively short counting time and the more stable PGA as ligand. This method works because at pH 9.3, the milk binder binds PGA and MTHFA equally well.

Endogenous protein binders may interfere with the reaction of the receptor and MTHFA in serum. Various extraction procedures (see Box 17-2, Alternatives) and the use of raw milk as a binder have been employed to reduce this problem. MTHFA may also tend to be relatively unstable in serum.

An overview of a folate radioassay is shown in Box 17-2.

Clinical applications
Pathophysiology

Malabsorption of folate may occur in intestinal disorders such as sprue, but the most common cause of folate deficiency is dietary. In certain disease states, hyperutilization of folate may occur and result in deficiency. This can be found in pregnancy, hemolytic anemia, some malignancies, and during lactation.

A number of drugs that are folate antag-

FOLATE METHOD

Principle

Charcoal

$$R + [L + L^*] = [RL + RL^*] + [L + L^*]$$

Protocol

		Reagent	Volume
DAY 1	R	β-lactoglobulin, purified	0.1 ml
	L*	³H-PGA (250 pg)	0.1 ml
	L { Standard	MTHFA (Waxman)	0.5 ml
	Sample	Boiled acidified (phosphate ascorbate) serum extracts	
	Diluent	0.3 M Na₂HPO₄	0.5 ml

——————————— 35 minutes, room temperature ———————————

Hemoglobin-coated charcoal   1.0 ml

Centrifuge at 2,000 rpm, 20 minutes
Count supernatant in liquid scintillation counter

Reagents

R   *125 mg β-lactoglobulin (Sigma) dissolved in 0.1 M phosphate buffer (pH 7.4)*

L*   *³H-PGA (Amersham/Searle)*
Specific activity: 35-43 mCi/mg
Diluted to approximately 250 pg/0.1 ml (250 pg = 2,000 cpm)

L { Standard   *MTHFA (Waxman, Mt. Sinai)*
Sample   *Serum should be frozen if not immediately assayed; stored in 0.1 M phosphate buffer (pH 6.1) containing 200 mg/100 ml ascorbic acid*

Diluent   *0.3 M NaH₂PO₄ (pH 7.4)*

Norit A Charcoal in 0.5 gm/100 ml hemoglobin

Box 17-2

FOLATE METHOD, cont'd

Alternatives

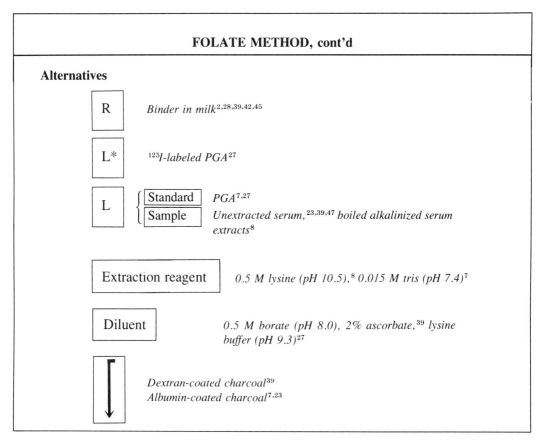

| R | *Binder in milk*[2,28,39,42,45] |

| L* | [125]*I-labeled PGA*[27] |

| L | Standard | *PGA*[7,27] |
| | Sample | *Unextracted serum,*[23,39,47] *boiled alkalinized serum extracts*[8] |

| Extraction reagent | *0.5 M lysine (pH 10.5),*[8] *0.015 M tris (pH 7.4)*[7] |

| Diluent | *0.5 M borate (pH 8.0), 2% ascorbate,*[39] *lysine buffer (pH 9.3)*[27] |

Dextran-coated charcoal[39]
Albumin-coated charcoal[7,23]

Box 17-2

---

onists, such as methotrexate and pentamidine, may induce a deficiency state. Some drugs, such as oral contraceptives, phenytoin, and ethanol, impair absorption of folate. Deficiency of folate can develop within 4 to 6 weeks of reduced absorption of the compound.

Like vitamin B_{12}, folic acid is essential to rapidly dividing cellular systems. In folate-deficient states, nuclear maturation is delayed, and megaloblastic changes occur in blood cells, small intestinal cells, and other rapidly proliferating tissues within 3 to 4 months.

Sampling

Fasting serum samples should be used, since serum folate levels may vary significantly after eating. The samples should be separated and frozen for storage as soon as possible after drawing because MTHFA is relatively unstable

when held at room temperature for prolonged periods. Ascorbic acid has also been used to stabilize MTHFA in serum.

Reference values

Serum levels
  Normal levels in serum: 3-20 ng/ml
  Folate deficiency states: <3 ng/ml
  Aqueous extracts of red blood cells: 210 ± 57 ng/ml

Interpretation of results

The fasting serum folate levels employed for the screening examination correlate well with microbiologic estimates. Elevations in the serum folate concentration are not uncommon in patients with vitamin B_{12} deficiency. Values below the normal range (3 ng/ml) are associated with folate deficiency. Clinically, folate deficiency is common in malabsorption states, pregnancy, alcoholism, and malignancy. Since serum values fluctuate significantly with dietary alterations, measurement of folate levels in aqueous extracts of red blood cells has been widely employed to give an estimate of tissue folate stores.

REFERENCES

1. Addison, G. M., Beamish, M. R., Hales, C. N., Hodgkins, M., Jacobs, A., and Llewellin, P.: An immunoradiometric assay for ferritin in the serum of normal subjects and patients with iron deficiency and iron overload, J. Clin. Pathol. **25:**326, 1972.
2. Archibald, E. L., Mincey, E. K., and Morrison, R. T.: Estimation of serum proteins by competitive protein binding assay, Clin. Biochem. **5:**232, 1972.
3. Barakat, R. M., and Ekins, R. P.: Assay of vitamin B_{12} in blood; a simple method, Lancet **2:**25, 1961.
4. Boguslaski, R. C., and Rathjen, C. P.: A column radioassay for the quantification of vitamin B_{12}, Clin. Chim. Acta **62:**349, 1975.
5. Carmel, R., and Coltman, C. A., Jr.: Radioassay for serum vitamin B_{12} with the use of saliva as the vitamin B_{12} binder, J. Lab. Clin. Med. **74:**967, 1969.
6. Catt, K. J., Hirsch, J., Castelan, D. J., Niall, H. D., and Tregear, G. W.: Radioimmunoassay of fibrinogen and its proteolysis products, Thromb. Diath. Haemorrh. **20:**1, 1968.
7. DaCosta, M., and Rothenberg, S. P.: Identification of an immunoreactive folate in serum extracts by radioimmunoassay, Br. J. Haematol. **21:**121, 1971.
8. Dunn, R. T., and Foster, L. B.: Radioassay of serum folate, Clin. Chem. **19:**1101, 1973.
9. Fisher, J. W., Thompson, J. F., and Espada, J.: A radioimmunoassay for human urinary erythropoietin, Isr. J. Med. Sci. **7:**873, 1971.
10. Frenkel, E. P., Keller, S., and McCall, M. S.: Radioisotopic assay of serum vitamin B_{12} with the use of DEAE cellulose, J. Lab. Clin. Med. **68:**510, 1966.
11. Frenkel, E. P., McCall, M. S., and White, J. D.: Recognition and resolution of errors in the radioisotopic assay of serum vitamin B_{12}, Am. J. Clin. Pathol. **53:**891, 1970.
12. Friedner, S., Josephson, B., and Levin, K.: Vitamin B_{12} determination by means of radioisotope dilution and ultrafiltration, Clin. Chim. Acta **24:**171, 1969.
13. Ghitis, J.: The folate binding in milk, Am. J. Clin. Nutr. **20:**1, 1967.
14. Givas, J. K., and Gutcho, S.: pH dependence of the binding of folates to milk binder in radioassays of folates, Clin. Chem. **21:**427, 1975.
15. Herbert, V., Wasserman, L. R., Frank, O., Pasher, I., and Baker, H.: Values of fasting serum "folic acid" levels, Fed. Proc. **18:**246, 1959.
16. Hillman, R. S., Oakes, M., and Finkolt, C.: Hemoglobin-coated charcoal radioassay for serum vitamin B_{12}; a simple medication to improve intrinsic factor reliability, Blood **34:**385, 1969.
17. Hoyer, L. W.: Immunologic studies of antihemophilic factor (AHF, factor VIII). IV. Radioimmunoassay of AHF antigen, J. Lab. Clin. Med. **80:**822, 1972.
18. Hughes-Jones, N. C.: The estimation of the concentration and equilibrium constant of anti-D, Immunology **12:**565, 1967.
19. Hughes-Jones, N. C., Norley, I., and Hunt, V.: Automatic red cell washing machine for quantitative assay of anti-D concentration, Vox Sang. **22:**268, 1972.
20. Hughes-Jones, N. C., and Stevenson, M.: The anti-D content of IgG preparations for use in the prevention of Rh hemolytic disease, Vox Sang. **14:**401, 1968.
21. Jacob, E., and O'Brien, H. A.: A simple assay of intrinsic factor–vitamin B_{12} complex employing the binding intrinsic factor antibody, J. Clin. Pathol. **25:**320, 1972.
22. Johnston, M. F., Kipfer, R. K., and Olson, R. E.: Studies of prothrombin biosynthesis in cell-free systems. I. Comparison of coagulation and immunochemical assays, J. Biol. Chem. **247:**3987, 1972.
23. Kamen, B. A., and Caston, J. D.: Direct radiochemical assay for serum folate; competition between 3H-folic acid and 5 methyltetrahydrofolic acid for a folate binder, J. Lab. Clin. Med. **83:**164, 1974.
24. Kim, H. R., Buchanan, J. W., D'Antonio, R., Larson, S. M., Morgan, R. P., Thorell, J. I., McIntyre, P. A., and Wagner, H. N., Jr.: Toadfish serum as a binder for in-vitro assay of vitamin B_{12}, J. Nucl. Med. **17:**737, 1976.
25. Lau, K. S., Gottlieb, C., Wassemar, L. P., and Herbert, V.: Measurement of serum vitamin B_{12} level using radioisotope dilution and coated charcoal, Blood **26:**202, 1965.
26. Lin, Y. K., and Sullivan, L. W.: An improved radioisotope dilution assay for serum vitamin B_{12} using hemoglobin-coated charcoal, Blood **39:**426, 1972.
27. Longo, D. L., and Herbert, V.: Radioassay for serum and red cell folate, J. Lab. Clin. Med. **87:**138, 1976.
28. Mincey, E. K., Wilcox, E., and Morrison, R. T.: Estimation of serum and red cell folate by simple radiometric technique, Clin. Biochem. **6:**274, 1973.
29. Newmark, P. A., Green, R., Musso, A. M., and Molbin, D. L.: A comparison of the properties of chicken serum with other vitamin B_{12} binding proteins used in radioisotope dilution methods for measuring serum vitamin B_{12} concentrations, Br. J. Haematol. **25:**339, 1973.
30. Nossel, H. L., Younger, L. R., Wilner, G. D., Procupez, T., Canfield, R. E., and Bulter, V. P., Jr.: Radioimmunoassay of human fibrinopeptide, Proc. Natl. Acad. Sci. USA **68:**2350, 1971.
31. Plow, E., and Edgington, T. S.: Discriminating neoantigenic differences between fibrinogen and fibrin derivatives, J. Clin. Invest. **52:**273, 282, 1973.
32. Rabiner, S. F., Goldfine, I. D., Hart, A., Summaria, L., and Robbins, K. C.: Radioimmunoassay of human plasminogen and plasmin, J. Lab. Clin. Med. **74:**265, 1969.
33. Raven, J. L., Robson, M. B., Morgan, J. O., and Hoffbrand, A. V.: Comparison of three methods for

measuring vitamin B_{12} in serum; radioisotopic, euglena gracilis and Lactobacillus leichmanii, Br. J. Haematol. **22**:21, 1972.

34. Reller, H.: Radioimmunologischer Nachweis von Ferrilin met aer "solid Phase" methode, Pathol. Microbiol. (Basel) **37**:201, 1971.

35. Rothenberg, S. P.: Assay of serum vitamin B_{12} concentration using Co^{57}, B_{12}, and intrinsic factor, Proc. Soc. Exp. Biol. **108**:45, 1961.

36. Rothenberg, S. P.: A radioenzymatic assay for folic acid, Nature **206**:1154, 1965.

37. Rothenberg, S. P.: A radioassay for serum B_{12} using unsaturated transcobalamin I as the B_{12} binding protein, Blood **31**:44, 1968.

38. Rothenberg, S. P., DaCosta, M., and Lawson, J.: The determination of erythrocyte folate concentration using a two-phase ligand-binding radioassay, Blood **43**:437, 1974.

39. Rothenberg, S. P., DaCosta, M., and Rosenberg, Z.: A radioassay for serum folate; use of a two-phase sequential-incubation, ligand-binding system, N. Engl. J. Med. **286**:1335, 1972.

40. Rudzki, Z.: The clinical value of the radioassay of serum folate, J. Lab. Clin. Med. **87**:859, 1976.

41. Scott, J. M., Bloomfield, F. J., Slebbins, R., and Herbert, V.: Studies on derivation of transcobalamin III from granulocytes; enhancement by lithium and elimination by fluoride of in-vitro increments in vitamin B_{12} binding capacity, J. Clin. Invest. **53**:228, 1974.

42. Tajuddin, M., and Gardyna, H. A.: Radioassay of serum folate, with use of a serum blank and nondialyzed milk as folate binder, Clin. Chem. **19**:125, 1973.

43. Van De Wiel, D. F., Goedemans, W. T., De Vries, J. A., and Woldring, M. G.: Radioimmunoassay of vitamin B_{12} using a polyurethane sponge and competitive protein binding assay using Lactobacillus leichmannii. In International Atomic Energy Agency: Radioimmunoassay and related procedures in medicine, vol. 2, Vienna, 1974, I.E.A.E., p. 185.

44. Van De Wiel, D. F., Goedemans, W. T., and Woldring, M. G.: Production and purification of antibody against protein–vitamin B_{12} conjugates for radioimmunoassay purposes, Clin. Chim. Acta **56**:143, 1974.

45. Waxman, S., and Schreiber, C.: Characteristics of folic acid-binding protein in folate deficient serum, Blood **42**:291, 1973.

46. Waxman, S., and Schreiber, C.: Measurement of serum folate levels and serum folic acid-binding protein by ^{3}H-PGA radioassay, Blood **42**:281, 1973.

47. Waxman, S., Schreiber, C., and Herbert, V.: Radioisotopic assay for measurement of serum folate levels, Blood **38**:219, 1971.

48. Wide, L., and Killander, A.: A radiosorbent technique for the assay of serum vitamin B_{12}, Scand. J. Clin. Lab. Invest. **27**:151, 1971.

18 IMMUNOGLOBULIN E

The concentration of most immunoglobulins in plasma is high enough to permit their measurement with chemical or conventional (nonradioactive) immunologic methods. However, the most recently discovered class of immunoglobulins, IgE, circulates in concentrations so low as to be undetectable with these methods. The reagins, which are a type of antibody involved in certain hypersensitivity reactions, belong to this class of immunoglobulins. It has been shown that quantitation of IgE, in terms of both the total concentration and the occurrence of specific IgE antibodies against certain allergens, is a valuable test for the evaluation of allergic conditions and other diseases of the immunologic system.

Chemistry

IgE has a molecular weight of about 200,000 daltons. Its structure corresponds to that of the other immunoglobulins, with two heavy chains and two light chains joined by disulfide bridges. Like other immunoglobulins, it can be fragmented by enzymes such as trypsin and papain into Fab and Fc fragments.

Physiology

The normal function of IgE in the nonallergic human is not known. In healthy persons, the average plasma IgE concentration is about $100\mu g$/liter, which is a very small fraction of the total immunoglobulin concentration of 10 g/liter. Elevated IgE levels are found in patients with atopic types of allergic diseases, in association with certain parasitic infections, and in a few rare diseases associated with immune defects.

Method

The total concentration of IgE in plasma may be assayed with any radioimmunoassay (RIA)

system that utilizes a specific method for separation of antibody-bound and free activity. Since the ligand and radioligand in this assay are immunoglobulins themselves, methods isolating all immunoglobulins cannot be utilized. A second antibody method with specific IgG antibodies not cross-reacting with human IgE could be used. The most commonly used methods utilize antibodies bound to a solid phase, either as a competitive method or as a noncompetitive (sandwich) test. Assay sensitivity on the order of 1 to 2 ng/ml is achieved by most tests.

An example of an RIA for IgE is shown in Box 18-1.

The concentration of specific IgE antibodies is assayed by an immunosorbent technique with the antigen (allergen) coupled to a nonsoluble matrix (immunosorbent). This insolubilized allergen is incubated with serum from a patient suspected of being sensitive against this allergen. After incubation, the immunosorbent is washed. If the serum contained antibodies against the allergen, they will bind to the immunosorbent. After washing, the solid phase allergen is incubated with an antiserum against IgE labeled with [125]I. If the serum sample contained any IgE antibodies against the allergen, the labeled antibodies will bind to the immunosorbent. The principles and performance of the method are given in Box 18-2. A list of available allergens for testing is shown in Table 18-1.

Clinical applications

Pathophysiology

Individuals with a disposition to develop atopic allergic reactions may produce reagins against one or more allergens (the material to which the allergic reaction occurs). The reactions occur when such individuals are exposed

TOTAL IgE ASSAY†

Principle   S-R + [L + L*] → [S-RL + S-RL*] $\overset{\text{Wash}}{+}$ [L + L*]

Protocol

		Reagent	Volume
DAY 1	S-R	Sephadex–anti-IgE	1,000 μl
	L*	^{125}I-labeled IgE	100 μl
	L	Standard 0, 1, 2, 5, 10, 15, 50, 100, 200, 400 units/ml Sample Serum diluted 10×	100 μl

———————— Incubate overnight at 25° C under vertical rotation ————————

DAY 2   Centrifuge 2,000g, 2 minutes, and aspirate supernatant down to 5 mm from bottom of tube; add 2 ml 0.9% saline, and centrifuge 2,000g, 2 minutes; aspirate supernatant; repeat washing 3 times
Count tubes for 2-5 minutes

Reagents

S-R   Rabbit antiserum coupled to Sephadex

L*   IgE labeled with ^{125}I

Alternatives

R   Sheep antiserum to IgE[2,14]

L*   Label antiserum to IgE with ^{125}I (sandwich technique)[4]
IgE labeled with ^{131}I[7] or ^{125}I[2,10,14] by chloramine-T method

Diluent   Phosphate-HSA,[2,10,14] phosphate-BSA,[7] borate–normal rabbit serum

Antiserum coupled to cellulose,[2,10] or plates[14]
Ammonium sulfate precipitation[3]
DA-goat[7]

†Phadebas IgE test, Pharmacia Diagnostics AB.

Box 18-1

SPECIFIC IgE ASSAY
(ANTIBODY AGAINST A SPECIFIC ALLERGEN)†

Principle

$$\text{S-L} + \text{R}_L \xrightarrow{\text{Wash}} \text{S-LR}_L + \text{R}^*_R \xrightarrow{\text{Wash}} \text{S-LR}_L\text{R}_R + \text{R}^*_R$$

Protocol

		Reagent	*Volume*
DAY 1	S-L	*Allergen coupled to paper disc*	
	R_L Standard / Sample	*Reference serum* / *Plasma or serum*	*50 μl*

——————————— *3 hours, 25° C* ———————————

Aspirate solution, add 2.5 ml 0.9% saline; let tubes stand 10 minutes, and aspirate solution
Repeat twice
Count disc for 2 minutes

R^*_R — *^{125}I-labeled antiserum to IgE*   *50 μl*

——————————— *18 hours, 25° C* ———————————

DAY 2

Aspirate solution, add 2.5 ml 0.9% saline; let tubes stand 10 minutes, and aspirate solution
Repeat twice
Count disc for 2 minutes

Reagents

R^*_R — *^{125}I-labeled antiserum to IgE (antibodies to IgE are purified by immunoadsorption)*

L — *Serum (IgE)*

S-L — *Allergen covalently coupled to paper disc*

Rabbit antiserum to IgE labeled with ^{125}I

† Phadebas RAST, Pharmacia Diagnostics AB

Box 18-2

SPECIFIC IgE ASSAY
(ANTIBODY AGAINST A SPECIFIC ALLERGEN), cont'd

Alternatives

| S-L | *Allergen-coated test tubes,*[9,12,15] *IgE-coated tubes*[17] |

| L* | [131]*I-labeled*[8] *or* [125]*I-labeled allergen,*[1,6] [125]*I-labeled IgE*[9,12,15] |

| R$_R$ | *Rabbit anti-IgE,*[9,12] *goat anti-IgE*[15] |

| R$_L$ | *Immunoabsorbent extraction of allergen-specific IgE; measure extracted IgE*[5,13] |

| 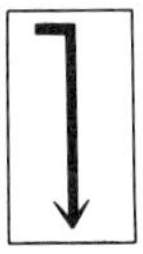 ↓ | *Ammonium sulfate precipitation,*[1] *solid phase coupled antiserum*[6] |

Box 18-2

---

to material to which they are hypersensitive. The reaction itself is believed to be elicited by the following mechanism. The heavy chain of the IgE molecule has a specific ability to bind to the surface of mast cells and basophilic granulocytes. When the allergen is brought into contact with cells having IgE on their surface, the allergen is bound to the IgE molecule. This binding elicits a chain of enzymatic reactions within these cells and causes the release of vasoactive substances, such as histamine, which provoke the allergic symptoms. The allergens are usually glycoproteins with molecular weights of 10,000 to 30,000 daltons. They occur frequently in materials known to cause allergy, such as pollen, animal epithelium, mold, certain foods, and pharmaceuticals.

Sampling

Random serum sampling is acceptable.

Reference values

Plasma levels are given in gravimetric units (micrograms per liter) or as units per milliliter of a standard established by the World Health Organization. One unit is approximately equal to 0.02μg. IgE levels in children are low, about 10μg/liter up to age 3 years, then increasing to 50μg to 100μg/liter from age 10 years and up. Values above 200μg/liter are indicative of an atopic genesis of the disease.

Interpretation of results

ELEVATED TOTAL CONCENTRATION OF IgE. Elevated plasma concentrations of IgE occur in a number of atopic allergic conditions. Mea-

Table 18-1. Allergens available for testing of reagins (specific IgE antibodies)

Type of allergen	Trivial name	Latin name
Grass pollen	Sweet vernal grass	Anthoxanthum odoratum
	Bermuda grass	Cynodon dactylon
	Cocksfoot	Dactylis glomerata
	Meadow fescue	Festuca elatior
	Ryegrass	Lolium perenne
	Timothy grass	Phleum pratense
	Common reed	Phragmites communis
	Meadow grass	Poa pratensis
	Redtop, Bent grass	Agrostis stolonifera
Weeds	Common ragweed	Ambrosia elatior (artemisiifolia)
	Western ragweed	Ambrosia psilostachya
	Giant ragweed	Ambrosia trifida
	False ragweed	Franseria acanthicarpa
	Wormwood	Artemisia absinthium
	Mugwort	Artemisia vulgaris
	Marguerite	Chrysanthemum leucanthemum
	Dandelion	Taraxacum vulgare
	Plantain (English), ribwort	Plantago lanceolata
	Goosefoot, lamb's-quarter	Chenopodium album
	Slatwort (prickly), Russian thistle	Salsola kali (pestifer)
	Goldenrod	Solidago virgaurea
Tree pollen	Box elder	Acer negundo
	Gray elder	Alnus incana
	Common silver birch	Betula verrucosa
	Hazel	Corylus avellana
	Beech	Fagus grandifolia
	Mountain cedar	Juniperus mexicana
	Oak	Quercus alba
	Elm	Ulmus americana
	Olive	Olea europaea
	Walnut	Juglans californica
	Maple leaf	Platanus acerifolia
	Willow	Salix caprea
Mites		Dermatophagoides pteronyssinus
		Dermatophagoides farinae
House dust	(Greer Labs)	
	(Hollister-Stier Labs)	
	(Bencard)	
Molds and yeasts		Penicillium notatum
		Cladosporium herbarum (Hormodendrum)
		Aspergillus fumigatus
		Mucor racemosus
		Alternaria tenuis
Epithelia	Cat epithelium	
	Dog epithelium	
	Horse dander	
	Cow dander	
Insects	Bee venom	Apis mellifera

Table 18-1. Allergens available for testing of reagins (specific IgE antibodies)—cont'd

Type of allergen	Trivial name	Latin name
Food	Egg white	
	Milk	
	Fish (cod)	
	Peanuts	
	Hazelnut	
	Almond	
	Crab	
	Shrimp	

surement of total IgE concentrations may therefore be of value for the evaluation of diseases that may be caused by reagins. This includes diseases of the respiratory tract, such as bronchial asthma or other types of obstructive bronchitis and chronic or relapsing rhinitis. Various skin disorders of dermatitis type, particularly in connection with rhinitis or bronchial asthma and relapsing urticaria, may occur in young persons. Furthermore, IgE concentrations may be high in parasitic infections and in immunedeficient diseases, such as Wiskott-Aldrich syndrome.

SPECIFIC IgE ANTIBODIES. Specific antibodies to various allergens may be present in cases of exogenously caused bronchial asthma, allergic rhinitis, atopic eczema, and so forth. Accordingly, the test may be performed for the same reasons as allergy provocation tests. There are many reports of a high correlation between the in vivo allergy tests and the IgE-specific antibody tests. The radioassay, however, is much easier to perform than are provocation tests and has the great advantage of not being associated with significant discomfort or risk to the patient. However, in most allergic conditions it is necessary to utilize combinations of both in vitro and in vivo tests to achieve a correct diagnosis.

The results of tests that measure the presence of specific IgE antibodies to certain allergens are semiquantitative, since the patient's serum is tested against reference sets of matched allergen preparations and reference sera. The correlation between provocation tests and the specific IgE antibody test improves with

increasing serum titers of the specific IgE antibody.

REFERENCES

1. Ahlstedt, S., Belin, L., Eriksson, N. E., and Hansson, L. Å.: Quantity and avidity of antibodies against birch pollen in atopic patients during hyposensitization, Int. Arch. Allergy Appl. Immunol. **48:**632, 1975.
2. Bazaral, M., Orgel, H. A., and Hamburger, R. N.: IgE levels in normal infants and mothers and an inheritance hypothesis, J. Immunol. **107:**794, 1969.
3. Carson, D., Metzger, H., and Bazin, H.: A simple radio-immunoassay for the measurement of human and rat IgE levels by ammonium sulphate precipitation, J. Immunol. **115:**561, 1975.
4. Ceska, M., and Lundkvist, U.: A new and simple radioimmunoassay method for the determination of IgE, Immunochemistry **9:**1021, 1972.
5. Dessaint, J. P., Bout, D., Fruit, J., and Capron, A.: Serum concentration of specific IgE antibody against Aspergillus fumigatus and identification of the fungal allergen, Clin. Immunol. Immunopathol. **5:**314, 1976.
6. Foucard, T., and Johansson, S. G. O.: Immunological studies in vitro and in vivo of children with pollenosis given immunotherapy with an aqueous and glutaraldehyde-treated tyrosine-adsorbed grass pollen extract, Clin. Allergy **6:**429, 1976.
7. Gleich, G. J., Averbeck, A. K., and Swedlund, H. A.: Measurement of IgE in normal and allergic serum by radioimmunoassay, J. Lab. Clin. Med. **77:**690, 1971.
8. Ishizaka, K., Ishizaka, T., and Hornbrook, M. M.: Allergen-binding activity of γE, γG and γA antibodies in sera from atopic patients; in vitro measurements of reaginic antibody, J. Immunol. **98:**490, 1967.
9. Kelly, J. F., and Patterson, R.: Allergy to snake venom; the use of radioimmunoassay for the detection of IgE antibodies against antigens not suitable for cutaneous tests, Clin. Allergy **3:**385, 1973.
10. McLaughlan, P., Stanworth, D. R., Kennedy, J. F., and Cho Tun, H.: Use of antibody-coupled cellulose as immunosorbent in the estimation of human immunoglobulin E (γE), Nature (New Biol.) **232:**245, 1971.

11. Özkaragöz, K., Smith, H. J., Gökcen, M., and Saraclar, I.: The radioallergosorbent test (RAST) in the diagnosis of atopic allergy, Acta Allergol. (Kbh.) **29:**96, 1974.

12. Patterson, R., Schatz, M., Fink, J. N., DeSwarte, R. S., Roberts, M., and Cugell, P.: Pigeon breeders' disease. I. Serum immunoglobulin concentrations; IgG, IgM, IgA, and IgE antibodies against pigeon serum, Am. J. Med. **60:**144, 1976.

13. Schellenberg, R. R., and Adkinson, N. F., Jr.: Measurement of absolute amounts of antigen-specific human IgE by a radioallergosorbent (RAST) elution technique, J. Immunol. **115:**1577, 1975.

14. Smith, H. J., Ozkaragöz, K., and Gokcen, M.: A simplified radioimmunoassay technique for measuring human IgE, J. Allergy Clin. Immunol. **50:**193, 1972.

15. Thompson, R. A.: Specific antibodies in allergic subjects, Int. Arch. Allergy Appl. Immunol. **45:**170, 1973.

16. Wide, L., Bennich, H., and Johansson, S. G. O.: Diagnosis of allergy by an in-vitro test for allergen antibodies, Lancet **2:**1105, 1967.

17. Zeiss, C. R., Pruzansky, J. J., Patterson, R., and Roberts, M.: A solid phase radioimmunoassay for the quantitation of human reaginic antibody against ragweed antigen E, J. Immunol. **110:**414, 1973.

19

TUMOR PRODUCTS

Carcinoembryonic antigen
Alpha-fetoprotein

Measurement of tumor-specific products in body fluids may in the future offer a selective way to detect human neoplasms at a curable stage in their natural history. This has been realized for some tumors, which produce hormones that call attention to their presence by inducing hormonal effects, such as gynecomastia and Cushing's syndrome, or which occur in specific situations (for example, post partum), when the tumors are still small enough to be amenable to specific therapy. The best example of this situation is certain trophoblastic tumors, which elaborate human chorionic gonadotropin (hCG). Since this hormone is normally not present in the nonpregnant individual, its presence in serum indicates a neoplastic state. Significant hCG may be detected by radioimmunoassay (RIA) methods when the tumor is about 1 mm³ in size. Subsequent measurements of hCG levels are, then, a very reliable guide to tumor responsiveness. Human chorionic gonadotropin is present in significant amounts in virtually all patients with choriocarcinoma and chorioadenomas.

Hormones may also be elaborated by non-endocrine tumors in amounts sufficient to cause specific hormone-related syndromes. Measurement of the specific hormones produced has been a reliable guide to both the presence of malignancy and the response of the tumor to antineoplastic therapy.

The ectopic production of hormone by non-endocrine neoplasms appears to be a manifestation of a general phenomenon of the neoplastic state in which genes that are normally repressed in adult life become derepressed and tumor-associated antigens are produced. These prod-

ucts may be polypeptide hormones, or parts of hormones, or substances that were normal constituents of the fetal stage of the cell's life cycle. Some other products produced by tumors are like those that are normally produced by the placenta. These products are called "oncofetal" and "oncoplacental" antigens, respectively, and may be elaborated into the serum in sufficient quantity to serve as "markers" for the neoplastic process. (See Table 19-1 for a list of the tumor products produced by nonendocrine neoplasms, for which RIAs are available.) Several reviews on this topic have appeared. Unfortunately, in the majority of instances the clinical utility of these neoplastic markers is limited. Essentially, none of the products listed is unique to tumors, but all are products that are inappropriate to normal adult tissues.

The hormonal products are produced by normal glandular tissue; thus it is usually overproduction or production that fails to respond to normal homeostatic mechanisms that allows the detection of ectopic hormone secretion.

The oncoplacental and oncofetal products are abnormal in the adult, but they too are not diagnostic of malignancy. Frequently, when tissue undergoes dysplastic changes that may precede neoplasia, the dysplastic tissue may be sufficiently altered to produce oncofetal or oncoplacental antigens. For example, heavy smokers with chronic bronchitis and bronchial epithelial dysplasia have mildly elevated carcinoembryonic antigen levels.

The ideal method for detecting tumor products would be extremely sensitive and specific for neoplasia. The levels of the tumor product in the blood should correlate with the total mass

Table 19-1. Tumor products (nonendocrine neoplasms) for which RIAs are available

Product	Reviews
Ectopic hormones*	Lipsett and others, 1964
Calcitonin, chorionic gonadotropin, corticotropin, erythropoietin, follicle-stimulating hormone, gastrin, glucagon, insulin, kinins, parathormone, prolactin, prostaglandins, renin, secretin, somatomammotropin, thyrotropin, vasopressin	Gordon and Roof, 1972 Odell, 1974
Oncofetal antigens	Dykes and King, 1972
Carcinoembryonic antigen	Kraft, 1972
Alpha-fetoprotein	Laurence and Neville, 1972
	Chayvialle and others, 1974
Oncoplacental antigens	Rosen and others, 1975
Placental lactogen	
Human chorionic gonadotropin	
Placental alkaline phosphatase	

*In alphabetical order only.

of tumor present. Such a method would be useful for:

1. Screening for cancer in high-risk patient populations
2. Assisting in establishing a specific diagnosis of cancer
3. Helping to localize tumors
4. Monitoring tumor response to therapy

At present only hCG RIA for the diagnosis of choriocarcinoma and chorioadenoma is widely used for screening for neoplasia. RIA for the oncofetal antigens, carcinoembryonic antigen (CEA) and alpha-fetoprotein (AFP), has also been widely useful clinically. RIA for hCG is discussed in Chapter 11. CEA and AFP are discussed in detail in the remainder of this chapter.

CARCINOEMBRYONIC ANTIGEN
Chemistry

CEA is a stable glycopeptide complex with a molecular weight of 150,000 to 200,000. This substance has β-globulin mobility on agar gel electrophoresis. CEA is soluble in perchloric acid and 50% ammonium sulfate solution. The sedimentation coefficient varies from 7S to 8S. Preparations of this antigen are heterogeneous with respect to size, charge, density, and isoelectric point behavior of various isomers. Six or more such isomers have been observed. Variations in sialic acid content may account for most of these differences. One isomer, CEA-S, with isoelectric point 4.5 and molec-

ular weight 181,000, is reported to be more specific for adenocarcinoma of the colon than are other isomers, although this point cannot be considered proven. CEA is often obtained from large tumors and may be purified to the order of 20 mg from 1 kg of tumor. Most methods for preparation of a ligand depend on perchloric acid extraction of tumor homogenates with ammonium sulfate precipitation of non-CEA protein material. Further purification may be obtained by absorption with various blood group antigens on Sepharose agar and treatment with varying concentrations of perchloric acid.

Physiology

CEA is a normal product of human development and occurs in the fetal colon. CEA may also be found as a normal constituent of adult tissues, such as the glycocalyx of the adult large intestine.

Method

Gold and Freedman found a tumor-specific antigen (CEA) that was present in perchloric acid extracts of cancer of the colon and fetal intestine, but not the adult intestine. These authors subsequently developed an RIA for CEA that showed great promise for selective diagnosis of gastrointestinal malignancy. Several subsequent RIAs have been developed. CEA RIA is currently in widespread use for evaluation of patients with a variety of neoplasms.

Reagents

Perchloric acid extraction of human tumors or fetal tissue is used to obtain CEA for use as immunogen. Rabbits and goats have been most extensively used to produce the antisera. The antisera produced may be made more specific by absorption with normal tissue antigens that are structurally similar to CEA. Perchloric acid extracts of spleen may serve as antigen for this purpose. CEA is readily iodinated by the chloramine-T or lactoperoxidase method.

Performance

The early methods utilized perchloric acid extraction of plasma with subsequent prolonged dialysis of the extract to remove the perchloric acid material. This dialysis required 36 to 48 hours, and in the Thomson technique the extract was subsequently lyophilized. This method works better in smaller volumes. Egan and associates have developed a double-antibody method that measures CEA in unextracted serum. Except for a higher upper limit of normal (12.5 ng/ml) with this method, results are comparable to those of other methods.

Heparin interferes with the zirconyl gel separation method. See Box 19-1 for a specific CEA method.

Clinical applications
Pathophysiology

CEA is located on the luminal surface of the mucosal cell. The antigen actually appears to be in the glycocalyx that coats the membrane of the cells and is thus external to the cell membrane itself. Two factors appear to be important as a cause for increased serum levels of CEA in malignancy. Tumor cells produce a greater quantity of this antigen. In addition, rapidly growing tissue results in disruption of blood-tissue barriers, so that what is produced in the tissues is more accessible to the blood. A variety of malignant tumors produce CEA in abundance (Table 19-2), and levels are higher in cases of metastatic tumor than in localized tumor. Antibodies to CEA are found in the blood of patients with tumors. Originally it was thought that CEA antibodies were present only in patients with localized disease, but this has been difficult to verify in later studies.

Table 19-2. Diseases associated with elevated plasma CEA levels*

Disease	Percent positive
Malignant	
Pancreas	92
Colon	75
Rectum	75
Lung	72
Other gastrointestinal malignancy	67
Breast	52
Benign	
Pancreatitis	50
Cirrhosis	42
Chronic lung disease	38
Inflammatory bowel disease	21
Benign breast tumor	4

*Data from Laurence, D.J. R., and Neville, A. M.: Fetal antigens and their role in the diagnosis and clinical management of human neoplasm; a review, Br. J. Cancer **26:**335, 1972.

Sampling

Random samples of plasma (usually with the use of EDTA as anticoagulant) are employed most commonly. CEA is stable in the frozen state for prolonged periods.

Reference values

Normal:
Extracted serum: <2.5 ng/ml (Thomson and others, 1969)
Unextracted serum: <12.5 ng/ml (Egan and others, 1972; Laurence and Neville, 1972); <3 ng/ml (Box 19-1)
"Malignant" range:
>40 ng/ml (Egan and others, 1972; Laurence and Neville, 1972)
Unextracted serum: 5-100 ng/ml (Box 19-1)

Interpretation of results

In the original evaluation by Thomson and associates of 36 patients with colon cancer, 35 were correctly identified as having CEA in their serum and thus being suspect for colon malignancies. Later workers, however, have shown a broader, less specific reactivity to the appearance of CEA in blood so that a variety of gastrointestinal tumors in the esophagus, stomach,

CEA METHOD

Principle

Double antibody

$$R + [L + L*] = [RL + RL*] + [L + L*]$$

Protocol

		Reagent	Volume
DAY 1	**R**	*Rabbit antiserum*	*250 µl*
	L	Standard: *0, 1.6, 3.12, 6.25, 12.5, 25.50, 100 ng/ml* Sample: *EDTA-plasma*	*500 µl*

———————— *72 hours, 4° C* ————————

DAY 4	**L***	*^{125}I-labeled CEA*	*250 µl*

———————— *72 hours, 4° C* ————————

DAY 7		*Normal rabbit serum 1:250*	*250 µl*
		Goat antirabbit serum 1:10	*250 µl*

———————— *24 hours, 4° C* ————————

DAY 8

Centrifuge 2,500g, 30 minutes; decant supernatant and centrifuge 2,500g, 15 minutes; count precipitate for 5 minutes

Reagents

R — *Rabbit antiserum to CEA*
Avidity: $K_a \approx 5.3 \times 10^{10}$
The extended incubation periods and sequential addition of radioligand were needed to achieve sufficient sensitivity to measure unextracted serum

L* — *CEA labeled with ^{125}I by lactoperoxidase; separated on Sephadex G-50 (Appendix 17)*
Specific activity: 6-8 µCi/µg

L — *Standards diluted in normal pooled EDTA-plasma*
Sample: EDTA-plasma

Diluent — *Barbital-BSA (Appendix 34)*

Appendix 28

Box 19-1

CEA METHOD, cont'd

Alternatives

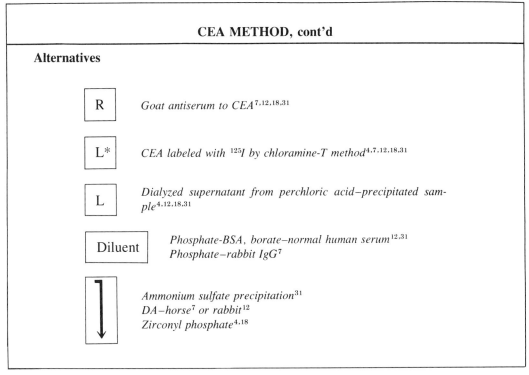

| R | *Goat antiserum to CEA*[7,12,18,31] |

| L* | *CEA labeled with* ^{125}I *by chloramine-T method*[4,7,12,18,31] |

| L | *Dialyzed supernatant from perchloric acid–precipitated sample*[4,12,18,31] |

| Diluent | *Phosphate-BSA, borate–normal human serum*[12,31] *Phosphate–rabbit IgG*[7] |

Ammonium sulfate precipitation[31]
DA–horse[7] *or rabbit*[12]
Zirconyl phosphate[4,18]

Box 19-1

---

pancreas, and colon result in significant elevation of CEA blood concentration. Furthermore, some patients with benign conditions, such as cirrhosis, pancreatitis, chronic bronchitis, and inflammatory bowel disease, may also have modest elevation of CEA levels. However, very high levels of CEA are most often found in disseminated malignancies. There is a "malignant range" of assay values (>40 ng/ml, >10 ng/ml, >5 ng/ml, depending on the methods used). Serum samples with values in this range are very likely to be due to malignant conditions.

The main utility of measuring CEA appears to be the evaluation of patients who have already been documented to have tumors. Response of patient tumor to a given modality of therapy appears to correlate well with the concentration of CEA in serum. CEA levels have in particular been used as indicators of recurrence of tumor after surgical treatment of colon carcinoma.

ALPHA-FETOPROTEIN

AFP has been known to be associated with liver malignancies ever since Tatarinov noted this substance in the sera of patients with hepatoma. RIA methods have shown this substance to be detectable in increased amounts in a significant number of patients with hepatoma, teratocarcinoma, and metastatic tumors to the liver.

Chemistry

AFP has the electrophoretic mobility of an α_1-globulin and a molecular weight of 60,000-70,000. The sedimentation coefficient of this substance is 4.5. Four percent of the molecule is carbohydrate.

Physiology

AFP is a normal constituent of the fetus of several species, including man. In human fetuses, the normal transition from AFP to serum albumin as the dominant serum protein begins at about the thirteenth week of gestation. The peak concentration of AFP in the fetus is 3 to 4 mg/ml, whereas in the normal adult levels as high as 25 ng/ml are distinctly uncommon. As exception to this is in pregnancy; levels of over 100 ng/ml are frequently seen in the third trimester. Increased levels (to 1,000 ng/ml) may occur in maternal plasma at the time of fetal death. AFP appears to play the same role in fetal life that serum albumin plays in adult life.

Method

Initial studies were dependent on rather insensitive methods to detect AFP in serum. Zone electrophoresis methods had a limit of sensitivity of greater than $300\mu g/ml$. Immunodiffusion methods improved the sensitivity to a level of 50 ng/ml. The major breakthrough, however, came when RIA techniques were developed. These methods can reliably detect AFP in the 1 to 3 ng/ml range.

Reagents

RIAs developed to date employ fetal serum or purified AFP as standard. The AFP may be readily iodinated by the chloramine-T method. Assay sensitivity is in the order of 1 ng/ml for most recent assays.

Clinical applications
Pathophysiology

AFP is found as a normal constituent of human serum; but in diseases of the liver, particularly in the malignant liver, massive elevations may be noted. Not all cells in a hepatoma or regenerating liver produce AFP. The properties of cells that contribute to production of AFP have been reviewed by Abelev.

Sampling

Random serum sampling is most commonly employed.

Reference values

Normal adults: 3-25 ng/ml
Pregnant women: up to 120 ng/ml

Interpretation of results

Elevated values of AFP are seen in both benign and malignant liver disease. Values above 1,000 ng/ml in an adult are almost always associated with primary liver malignancy, however. Hepatomas, metastatic liver involvement, and teratomas give markedly elevated values.

REFERENCES

1. Abelev, G. I.: Production of embryonal serum α-globulin by hepatomas; review of experimental and clinical data, Cancer Res. **28:**1344, 1968.
2. Bagshawe, K. D.: Tumor-associated antigens, Br. Med. Bull. **30:**68, 1974.
3. Chayvialle, J. A. P., Touillon, C., Crozier, C., and Lambert, R.: Radioimmunoassay of α-fetoprotein in human serum; clinical value in patients with liver disease, Digestive Dis. **19:**1102, 1974.
4. Chu, T. M., and Reynoso, G.: Evaluation of a new radioimmunoassay method for carcinoembryonic antigen in plasma, with use of zirconyl phosphate gel, Clin. Chem. **18:**918, 1972.
5. Dykes, P. W., and King, J.: Carcinoembryonic antigen (CEA), Gut **13:**1000, 1972.
6. Edgington, T. S., Astasita, R. W., and Plow, E. F.: Association of an isomeric species of carcinoembryonic antigen with neoplasia of the gastrointestinal tract, N. Engl. J. Med. **293:**103, 1975.
7. Egan, M. L., Lautenschleger, J. T., Coligan, J. E., and Todd, C. W.: Radioimmune assay of carcinoembryonic antigen, Immunochemistry **9:**289, 1972.
8. Gold, P., and Freedman, S. O.: Demonstration of tumor-specific antigens in human colonic carcinomata by immunological tolerance and absorption techniques, J. Exp. Med. **121:**439, 1965.
9. Gold, P., and Freedman, S. O.: Specific carcinoembryonic antigens of the human digestive system, J. Exp. Med. **122:**467, 1965.
10. Gold, P., and Freedman, S. O.: Cellular location of carcinoembryonic antigens of the human digestive system, Cancer Res. **28:**1331, 1968.
11. Gordon, G. S., and Roof, B. S.: "Humors from tumors"; diagnostic potential of peptides, Ann. Intern. Med. **76:**501, 1972.
12. Khoo, S. K., and MacKay, I. R.: CEA in serum in diseases of the liver and pancreas, J. Clin. Pathol. **26:**470, 1973.
13. Kraft, S. C.: "Humors from tumors"; carcinoembryonic antigen, alpha-fetoprotein, and digestive system cancer, Ann. Intern. Med. **76:**502, 1972.
14. Laurence, D. J. R., and Neville, A. M.: Fetal antigens and their role in the diagnosis and clinical management of human neoplasm; a review, Br. J. Cancer **26:**335, 1972.
15. Le Bel, J. S., Deodhar, S. D., and Brown, C. H.: Newer concepts of cancer of the colon and rectum; clinical evaluation of a radioimmunoassay for CEA, Dis. Colon Rectum **15:**111, 1972.
16. Li, M. C., Hertz, R., and Spencer, D. B.: Effect of methotrexate therapy upon choriocarcinoma and chorioadenoma, Proc. Soc. Exp. Biol. Med. **93:**361, 1956.
17. Lipsett, M. D., Odell, W. D., and others: Humoral

syndromes associated with non-endocrine tumors, Ann. Intern. Med. **61:**733, 1964.

18. Lo Gerfo, P., Krupey, J., and Hansen, H. J.: Demonstration of an antigen common to several varieties of neoplasia; assay using zirconyl phosphate gel, N. Engl. J. Med. **285:**138, 1971.

19. Martin, F., and Martin, M. S.: Demonstration of antigens related to colonic cancer in the human digestive system, Int. J. Cancer **6:**352, 1970.

20. Martin, F., and Martin, M. S.: Radioimmunoassay of carcinoembryonic antigen in extracts of human colon and stomach, Int. J. Cancer **9:**641, 1972.

21. Moore, T. L., Kupchik, H. Z., Marcon, N., and Zamchek, N.: Carcinoembryonic antigen assay in cancer of the colon and pancreas and other digestive tract disorders, Am. J. Dig. Dis. **16:**1, 1971.

22. Odell, W. D.: Humoral manifestations of non-endocrine neoplasms; ectopic hormone production. In Williams, R. H., editor: Textbook of endocrinology, ed. 5, Philadelphia, 1974, W. B. Saunders Co., pp. 1105-1116.

23. Rosen, S. W., Weintraub, B. D., Vaitukaitis, J. L., Sussman, H. H., Heishman, J. M., and Nuggia, F. M.: Placental proteins and their sub-units as tumor markers, Ann. Intern. Med. **82:**71, 1975.

24. Ross, G. T., Hammond, C. B., and others: Chemotherapy of metastatic and non-metastatic gestational trophoblastic neoplasms, Tex. Rep. Biol. Med. **24:** 326, 1966.

25. Rothfeld, B., and Larson, S. M.: Tumor antigens. In Rothfeld, B., editor: Nuclear Medicine in vitro, Philadelphia, 1974, J. B. Lippincott Co., pp. 315-322.

26. Ruoslahti, E., and Seppälä, M.: Studies of carcinofetal proteins. III. Development of a radioimmunoassay for α-fetoprotein; demonstration of α-fetoprotein in serum of healthy human adults, Int. J. Cancer **8:**374, 1971.

27. Ruoslahti, E., and Seppälä, M.: Normal and increased alpha-fetoprotein in neoplastic and non-neoplastic liver disease, Lancet **2:**278, 1972.

28. Ruoslahti, E., Seppälä, M., Vuopio, P., Sallsela, E., and Peltokallio, P.: Radioimmunoassay of alpha-fetoprotein in primary and secondary cancer of the liver, J. Natl. Cancer Inst. **49:**623, 1972.

29. Silver, H. K. B., Gold, P., Feder, S., Freedman, S. O., and Shuster, J.: Radioimmunoassay for human alpha-1 fetoprotein, Proc. Natl. Acad. Sci. USA **70:** 526, 1973.

30. Tatarinov, Y.: Presence of embryonal α-globulin in the serum of a patient with primary hepatocellular carcinoma, Vopr. Med. Khim. **10:**90, 1964.

31. Thomson, D. M. P., Krupey, J., Freedman, S. O., and Gold, P.: The radioimmunoassay of circulating carcinoembryonic antigen of the human digestive system, Proc. Natl. Acad. Sci. USA **64:**161, 1969.

32. Von Kleist, S., Chavenel, G., and Burtin, P.: Identification of an antigen from normal human tissue that cross reacts with carcinoembryonic antigen, Proc. Natl. Acad. Sci. USA **69:**2492, 1972.

20 PHARMACOLOGY

Digoxin

The application of radioimmunoassay (RIA) to the measurement of serum drug levels promises to be of increasing importance in the next decade. Basically, sensitive and specific methods that are easily automated are needed to monitor therapy for clinical uses of drugs as well as to provide a sound basis for evaluation of drug pharmacodynamics.

Despite the need for accurate measurement of drug levels in clinical practice, RIA for drugs has been relatively late in developing. This is primarily the result of two factors. Most drugs are too small to be immunogenic unless coupled to some larger molecule. Also, labeled derivatives, which could serve as radioligand in an assay system, have only recently been developed for many important drugs.

The problems of development of antisera and of labeled derivatives of drugs for use in assay were first solved for digitoxin by Oliver and associates in the late 1960s. Since that time, a number of RIAs for drugs have been developed (see list below). For a recent review of the topic of drug RIA, see the works by Landon and Moffat (1976) and Spector (1974).

RADIOASSAY MEASUREMENT OF DRUGS

Adriamycin[70]	Diazepam[12]
Amphetamine[44]	Digitoxin[49]
Barbitone (barbital)[63]	Digoxin[59]
Bleomycin[7]	Ethinyl estradiol[28]
Cannabis[39]	Fluoximesterone[13]
Chlordiazepoxide[16]	Gentamicin[37]
Chlorpromazine[62]	Isoniazid[56]
Codeine[65]	Medroxyprogesterone[15]
Corticosteroids[9]	Mestranol[28]
Daunomycin[11]	Methadone[35]
Dexamethasone[14]	Methotrexate[26]
Methylprednisolone[14]	Pentobarbital[64]
Morphine[65]	Phenobarbital[11,43,44]
Norethisterone[71]	Phenytoin[69]
Norgestrel[71]	Prednisone[12]
Ouabain[57]	Sulthiame[53]
Pentazocine[73]	Tubocurarine[25]

The application of RIA to measurements of digitalis is probably the most widely used of this new class of assays, although there is growing application for measurements of serum levels of antibiotics, drugs subject to abuse, and antineoplastic agents. RIA for urine screening for opiates, barbiturates, and other drugs of abuse has become widely accepted as a sensitive and specific test for use in monitoring compliance in drug abuse treatment programs. A number of methods are available, including screening for barbiturates, cannabis products, amphetamines, and opiates in serum and urine. Some of these techniques are also useful in quantitating blood and urine concentrations. Basically, RIAs employ drug derivatives conjugated to proteins such as bovine serum albumin and bovine γ-globulin to produce immunogen for preparation of antisera. Tritiated drug derivatives have so far been primarily used, and ammonium sulfate precipitation has been a particularly popular separation technique. Reported studies have been limited to scattered short reports endorsing the general concept, and published clinical experience with these methods is limited.

Gentamicin is an aminoglycoside antibiotic that is effective against a variety of gram-negative organisms. Use of this drug is associated with significant toxicity, particularly otic and renal damage. The toxicity is dose related,

242

however, and monitoring of serum drug levels has been suggested as a way to reduce toxic side effects. Gentamicin may be measured by several methods, including microbiologic assay and radioenzymatic assay. RIAs have been developed that show good correlation with the more tedious microbiologic assays.

DIGOXIN

RIA for clinical monitoring of serum levels of digitalis derivatives has been widely applied clinically. Several closely related digitalis derivatives can be conveniently measured by specific and sensitive RIAs. Digoxin is the most widely used digitalis preparation in current use.

Chemistry

Digoxin consists of a steroid end, which is the pharmacologically active part of the molecule, and a ribosyl residue, which is the portion of the molecule that enhances pharmacologic activity. The sugar residue for digoxin is termed digitoxose, whereas the steroid part is called digoxigenin. Digoxin and digitoxin differ by only a hydroxyl group at the seventeenth position on the steroid ring.

Pharmacodynamics

Whether administered orally, intravenously, or intramuscularly, digoxin requires a considerable period of time before equilibrium occurs between serum drug concentrations and tissue drug stores. Since it is the tissue stores that exert the pharmacologic effect, a serum level is not an accurate assessment of the therapeutically important drug concentration until this equilibrium period has occurred. For digoxin, a period of 4 hours or more is required after oral administration before equilibrium serum concentrations can be obtained.

Once the serum level has achieved equilibrium, there is a constant ratio between tissue and serum. For digoxin, this tissue:serum ratio approaches 30:1. Digitalis derivatives are eliminated by either the liver or the kidney. The specific derivative determines to a certain extent the site of degradation and excretion. Digoxin is excreted predominantly via the kidneys. Its half-life is about 33 hours for plasma clearance in the patient with normal renal function. In pa-

tients with renal failure, digoxin excretion may be markedly impaired. The degree of impairment correlates approximately with the degree of reduction of creatinine clearance.

The mechanism of action of digoxin relates to its effect on a sodium-, potassium-activated ATPase system located in the plasma membrane of heart muscle. The effect of the digoxin is improvement of the strength of myocardial contraction. In addition, digoxin has specific effects upon electrical conduction. Discussion of the full range of its known clinical effects is beyond the scope of this review. In view of the intimate relationship of digoxin action to sodium and potassium concentration, it is not surprising that the action of digoxin is markedly affected by the concentration of a variety of naturally occurring ionic constituents of extracellular fluids.

Method

Before the availability of RIA, chemical methods were developed that were useful for measurement of relatively large concentrations of cardiac glycosides. Colorimetric methods formed the basis for the standard USP assay for both digitoxin and digoxin. Double isotope derivative methods, gas liquid chromatography, inhibition of rubidium-86 red blood cell uptake, and inhibition of sodium-, potassium-activated ATPase have been employed. More recently, the sodium-potassium–ATPase enzymatic system has been used as a binder in a radioligand assay method. At present, however, these methods are used only in specialized circumstances, and RIA for digitalis derivatives is the dominant method for measurement of clinical levels of digoxin in serum.

As mentioned previously, cardiac glycosides are small molecules and are not inherently immunogenic. In order to produce specific antibodies, the cardiac glycoside itself must be used as a hapten coupled to a protein carrier. Butler and Chen prepared a bovine serum albumin conjugate of digoxin by periodate oxidation of the terminal glucose residue of the trisaccharide of the drug, with subsequent reaction to albumin. Oliver and associates (1968) used a similar method of preparation to create antisera to digitoxin. Because digoxin has become

---

DIGOXIN METHOD

Principle

Double antibody

$$R + [L + L^*] = [RL + RL^*] + [L + L^*]$$

Protocol

		Reagent	Volume
DAY 1	R	Rabbit antiserum to digoxin	$100\,\mu l$
	L*	Digoxin-BSA-^{125}I	$100\,\mu l$
	L	Standard: $0.25, 0.5, 1.0, 2.0, 4.0\,\mu g/liter$ in EDTA-plasma	$100\,\mu l$
		Sample: EDTA-plasma	

———————— *2 hours, 25° C* ————————

	Reagent	Volume
↓	Normal rabbit serum (1:25)	$100\,\mu l$
	Goat antiserum to rabbit IgG	$100\,\mu l$

———————— *1 hour, 25° C* ————————

	Volume
Add diluent	$500\,\mu l$
Centrifugation 2,500g, 15 minutes	
Decant supernatant	
Count precipitate for 1 minute	

Reagents

R — Rabbit antiserum to digoxin-BSA; cross-reaction to estradiol, estriol, and cortisol <0.002%, to progesterone and testosterone <0.01%, to Aldactone <0.01%

L* — Digoxin-BSA labeled with ^{125}I by lactoperoxidase (Appendix 17) Specific activity: $35\text{-}40\,\mu Ci/\mu g$; separation on Sephadex G-50 $T = 40,000\ cpm \approx 0.6\ ng$

L — EDTA-plasma Standards in EDTA-plasma

Diluent — Barbital-BSA (Appendix 34)

↓ — Appendix 28

Box 20-1

DIGOXIN METHOD, cont'd

Alternatives

| R | *Goat antiserum to digoxin*[22] |

| L* | *^{3}H-labeled digoxin*[1,3,6,18,22,30,40,48,51,59]
3-O-succinyl-digoxigenin-TME labeled with ^{125}I[24,27,67] |

| L | *Serum sample*[3,6,17,24,27,30,40,46,59,67] |

| Diluent | *Phosphate-BSA,*[6,22,51] *phosphate-HSA*[30] |

| ↓ | *Dextran-coated charcoal*[18,24,48,51,52,59,67]
Zinc-sulfate in alkali,[40] *polyethyelene glycol*[1]
Sephadex G-25,[6] *solid phase*[27]
Ammonium sulfate[17]
Antibody coupled to polymerized iron oxide[22,46]
Gel equilibrium method (molecule sieve)[19] |

Box 20-1

the most important drug clinically, this RIA is presented in detail.

Reagents

Digoxin has been coupled to a variety of substances in order to prepare immunogen for digoxin antisera. These substances include poly-L-lysine, human serum albumin and, most commonly, bovine serum albumin. Antibodies produced in rabbits have been primarily used, although goat antibodies also have been employed. The first radioligands used were tritiated digoxin preparations, but iodinated preparations are currently predominant.

Performance

A variety of separation techniques have been used, such as dextran-coated charcoal, polyethylene glycol, and double-antibody methods. Commercial preparations of digoxin RIAs have focused on solid phase separations, and a variety of well-characterized systems are available (from Kallestad Labs, Clinical Assays, Corning, Schwarz-Mann, and so forth). Among these various alternatives, coated charcoal has

perhaps been the most widely used. One disadvantage of this method is that the charcoal competes with the antibody for digoxin. The binding to the charcoal is quite sensitive to temperature and time of incubation. Careful standardization of assay conditions is necessary to permit reproducible testing.

Assay properties

Cross-reactivity of digoxin antisera with digitoxin may be a problem when a patient has taken both digitoxin and digoxin. Under most circumstances digoxin levels cannot be accurately determined in the presence of digitoxin.

See Box 20-1 for a detailed review of digoxin methodology.

Clinical applications

Pathophysiology: digitalis intoxication

Digitalis preparations all cause signs and symptoms of intoxication when given in high doses. The digitalis preparations have a very narrow margin of safety between an effective therapeutic zone and toxicity. Also, the toxicity itself can be life threatening.

The earliest indications of digitalis intoxication are gastrointestinal effects such as anorexia, nausea, and vomiting. Diarrhea and abdominal pain are commonly observed. These symptoms subside within a few days after the drug is stopped.

The most lethal effects of digitalis intoxication are the cardiac effects. A variety of arrhythmias are observed, including premature ventricular contractions and various degrees of atrioventricular block (with prolongation of the P-R interval). The appearance of ventricular arrhythmias is particularly ominous; ventricular fibrillation is the most common cause of death in digitalis intoxication.

RIA methods are helpful in making the diagnosis of digitalis intoxication, particularly if the value is clearly in the toxic range, or clearly in the nontoxic range. The values in toxic patients may overlap the therapeutic range, and the effect of digitalis is altered by a variety of influences (see list below). In particular, hypokalemia is a commonly associated finding and contributes to the digitalis effect.

FACTORS INCREASING SUSCEPTIBILITY TO DIGITALIS

Hypokalemia
Hypomagnesemia
Hypoxia
Alkalosis
Local myocardial ischemia
Hypercalcemia

Sampling

Samples for cardiac glycoside estimation should be collected as serum. Samples should be collected sufficiently long after administration of the dose so that equilibration between serum and tissue stores of the drug have occurred (4 hours or more after administration of an oral dose of digoxin). The best results are obtained by drawing the serum samples at a standard time, usually the morning before the patient has received a maintenance dose of the drug. Digoxin is relatively stable in serum but should be separated rapidly from the red blood cell component of the sample. If samples are to be kept for more than 24 hours before study, they should be frozen.

Reference values

Probable digitalis intoxication: >2 ng/ml
Therapeutic zone: 0.8-1.6 ng/ml

Interpretation of results

Proper interpretation of digoxin serum levels requires significant associated clinical information.

ELEVATED LEVELS. The mode of action of digoxin is complicated, and a variety of factors increase susceptibility to digitalis (see list opposite). Despite these influencing factors, the serum digitalis levels have been shown to be a reliable guide of digitalis intoxication. There is much individual variation in susceptibility to the toxic effects of digitalis; however, a few generalizations can be made regarding toxicity and serum concentration. Digitalis intoxication is very uncommon when the serum level is less than 1.5 ng/ml. The majority of patients with clearcut digitalis intoxication have serum levels greater than 2.0 ng/ml (Smith and associates, 1969).

DECREASED LEVELS. Serum digitalis levels are also useful in evaluating the degree of absorption of digoxin preparations. Poor absorption of the digoxin may be related either to limited bioavailability of digoxin in certain pill preparations or to small intestinal disorders. In patients with congestive heart failure, absorption of digoxin may be significantly impaired because of stasis of blood supply to the alimentary tract. In these situations serum levels will be low in comparison with that expected from the dose of the drug employed. Evaluation of plasma drug levels may be essential in these situations if the proper therapeutic response is to be achieved.

REFERENCES

1. Barret, M. J., and Cohen, P. S.: Radioimmunoassay of serum renin activity and digoxin concentrations, with use of polyethylene glycol to separate free and antibody-bound ligand, Clin. Chem. **18:**1339, 1972.
2. Beller, G. A., Smith, T. W., Abelmann, W. H., Haber, E., and Hood, W. B., Jr.: Digitalis intoxication; a prospective clinical study with serum level correlations, N. Engl. J. Med. **284:**989, 1971.
3. Berk, L. S., Lewis, J. L., and Nelson, J. C.: One-hour radioimmunoassay of serum drug concentrations, as exemplified by digoxin and gentamicin, Clin. Chem. **20:**1159, 1974.

4. Brooker, G., and Jelliffe, R. W.: Serum cardiac glycoside assay based upon displacement of ^{3}H-ouabain from Na-K 6 ATPase, Circulation **45**:20, 1972.

5. Broughton, A., and Strong, J. E.: Radioimmunoassay of bleomycin, Cancer Res. **36**:1418, 1976.

6. Bundgaard Christiansen, N. J., and Damkjaer Nielsen, M.: Digoxin radioimmunoassay; Sephadex separation of free from antibody-bound digoxin, Clin. Chim. Acta **42**:125, 1972.

7. Burnett, G. H., and Conklin, R. L.: The enzymatic assay of plasma digitoxin levels, J. Lab. Clin. Med. **71**:1040, 1968.

8. Butler, K. P., and Chen, J. P.: Digoxin-specific antibodies, Proc. Natl. Acad. Sci. USA **57**:71, 1969.

9. Cameron, E. H., Morris, S. E., and Nieuweboer, B.: Proceedings: Radioimmunoassay of norethisterone; a comparison of ^{3}H and ^{125}I-labelled radioligands, J. Endocrinol. **61**:39, 1974.

10. Catlin, D., Cleeland, R., and Grunberg, E.: A sensitive, rapid radioimmunoassay for morphine and immunologically related substances in urine and serum, Clin. Chem. **19**:216, 1973.

11. Churig, A., Kim, S. Y., Cheng, L. T., and Castro, A.: Phenobarbital specific antisera and radioimmunoassay, Experientia **29**:820, 1973.

12. Colburn, W. A.: Radioimmunoassay for prednisone, Steroids **24**:95, 1974.

13. Colburn, W. A.: Radioimmunoassay for fluoxymesterone (Halotestin), Steroids **25**:43, 1975.

14. Colburn, W. A., and Butler, R. H.: Radioimmunoassay for methylprednisolone (Medrol), Steroids **22**:687, 1973.

15. Cornette, J. C., Kirton, K. T., and Duncan, G. W.: Measurement of medroxyprogesterone acetate (Provera) by radioimmunoassay, J. Clin. Endocrinol. Metab. **33**:459, 1971.

16. Dixon, W. R., Early, J., and Poshna, E.: Radioimmunoassay of chlordiazepoxide in plasma, J. Pharm. Sci. **64**:937, 1975.

17. Drewes, P. A., and Pileggi, V. J.: Faster and easier radioimmunoassay of digoxin, Clin. Chem. **20**:343, 1974.

18. Evered, D. C., Chapman, C., and Hayter, C. J.: Measurement of plasma digoxine concentrations by radioimmunoassay, Br. Med. J. **3**:427, 1970.

19. Greenwood, H., Howard, M., and Landon, J.: A rapid, simple assay for digoxin, J. Clin. Pathol. **27**:490, 1974.

20. Haas, M. J., and Davies, J.: Enzymatic acetylation as a means of determining serum aminoglycoside concentrations, Antimicrob. Agents Chemother. **4**:497, 1973.

21. Heizer, W. D., Smith, T. W., and Goldfinger, S. E.: Absorption of digoxin; patients with malabsorption syndrome, N. Engl. J. Med. **285**:257, 1971.

22. Hersch, L. S., and Yaverbaum, S.: Magnetic solid-phase radioimmunoassay, Clin. Chim. Acta **63**:69, 1975.

23. Hickens, M., and Hogars, A. F.: Radioimmunoassay for dexamethasone in plasma, Clin. Chem. **20**:266, 1974.

24. Horgan, E. D., and Riley, E. D.: Radioimmunoassay of plasma digoxin with iodinated tracer, Clin. Chem. **19**:187, 1973.

25. Horowitz, P. E., and Spector, S.: Determination of serum d-tubocurarine concentration by radioimmunoassay, J. Pharmacol. Exp. Ther. **185**:94, 1973.

26. Jaton, J. C., Ungar-Waron, H.: Antibodies to folic acid and methotrexate obtained with conjugates of synthetic polypeptides, Arch. Biochem. Biophys. **122**:157, 1967.

27. Kuczala, J. Z., and Ahluwalia, G. S: Evaluation of two digoxin radioimmunoassay procedures in which ^{125}I-labelled digoxin is used, Clin. Chem. **22**:193, 1976.

28. Kundu, N.: Radioimmunoassay of contraceptive steroids. II. Synthesis of mestranol and ethinyl estradiol of high specific activity, Steroids **23**:155, 1974.

29. Landon, J., Moffat, A. C., and others: The radioimmunoassay of drugs. Analyst **101**:225, 1976.

30. Larbig, D., and Kochsiek, K.: Radioimmunchemische Bestimmungen von Digoxin im menschlichen Serum, Klin. Wochenschr. **49**:1031, 1971.

31. Larbig, D., Kochsiek, K., and Schrader, C.: Klinische Aspekte der radioimmunchemischen Bestimmung der Serum-Digoxinkozentration, Dtsch. Med. Wochenschr. **97**:139, 1972.

32. Lente, R. K., Ullman, E. F., Goldstein, A., and Herzenberg, L. A.: Spin immunoassay technique for determination of morphine, Nature (New Biol.) **236**:93, 1972.

33. Lewis, J. E., Nelson, J. C., and Elder, H. A.: Radioimmunoassay of an antibiotic; gentamicin, Nature (New Biol.) **239**:214, 1972.

34. Lindenbaum, J., Meuow, M. I. T., Blackstone, M. D., and Butler, V. P., Jr.: Variation in the biological availability of digoxin from four preparations, N. Engl. J. Med. **285**:1344, 1971.

35. Liu, C. T., and Adler, F. L.: Immunologic studies on drug addiction. I. Antibodies reactive with methadone and their use for detection of the drug, J. Immunol. **111**:472, 1973.

36. Lukas, D. S., and Peterson, R. E.: Double isotope dilution derivative assay of digitoxin in plasma, urine and stool of patients maintained on the drug, J. Clin. Invest. **45**:782, 1966.

37. Makou, W. A., Ezer, J., and Wilson, T. W.: Radioimmunoassay for measurement of gentamicin in blood, Antimicrob. Agents Chemother. **3**:585, 1973.

38. Manning, T., Bidorset, J. W., Cohen, S., and Lukash, L.: Evaluation of antiserum for methadone, J. Forensic Sci. **21**:112, 1976.

39. Marks, V., and others: Detection of cannabis products in urine by radioimmunoassay, Br. Med. J. **3**:348, 1975.

40. Meade, R. C., and Kleist, T. J.: Improved radioimmunoassay of digoxin and other sterol-like compounds using Somogyi precipitation, J. Lab. Clin. Med. **80**:748, 1972.

41. Minshew, B. H., Holmes, R. I. C., and Baxter, C. R.: Comparison of a radioimmunoassay with an enzymatic

assay for gentamicin, Antimicrob. Agents Chemother. **7:**107, 1975.

42. Morris, H. G., De Roche, G., and Caro, C. M.: detection of synthetic corticosteroid analogues by competitive protein binding radioassay, Steroids **22:**445, 1973.

43. Mule, S. J., Bastos, M. L., and Jukofsky, D.: Evaluation of immunoassay methods for detection in urine of drugs subject to abuse, Clin. Chem. **20:**243, 1974.

44. Mule, S. J., Whitlock, E., and Jukofsky, D.: Radioimmunoassay of drugs subject to abuse; critical evaluation of urinary morphine-barbiturate, morphine, barbiturate, and amphetamine assays, Clin. Chem. **21:** 81, 1975.

45. Noone, P., Pattison, J. R., and Samson, D.: Simple, rapid method for assay of aminoglycoside antibiotics, Lancet **2:**16, 1971.

46. Nye, L., Forrest, C. G., Greenwood, H., Gardner, J. S., Ray, R., Roberts, J. R., and Landon, J.: Solid-phase, magnetic particle radioimmunoassay, Clin. Chim. Acta **69:**387, 1976.

47. Nygren, K. G., and Johansson, E. D.: The effect of norethindrone and some other synthetic gestagens upon the peripheral plasma levels of progesterone and estradiol during early human pregnancy, Acta Obstet. Gynecol. Scand. **54:**57, 1975.

48. Oliver, G. C., Parker, B. M., and Parker, C. W.: Radioimmunoassay for digoxin; technic and clinical application, Am. J. Med. **51:**186, 1971.

49. Oliver, G. C., Jr., Parker, B. M., Brasfield, D. L., and Parker, C. W.: The measurement of digitoxin in human serum by radioimmunoassay, J. Clin. Invest. **47:** 1035, 1968.

50. Peskar, B., and Spector, S.: Quantitative determination of diazepam in blood by radioimmunoassay, J. Pharmacol. Exp. Ther. **186:**167, 1973.

51. Philips, A. P.: The improvement of specificity in radioimmunoassays, Clin. Chim. Acta **44:**333, 1973.

52. Ransom, J. P.: Practical competitive binding assay methods, St. Louis, 1976, The C. V. Mosby Co., pp. 76-77.

53. Robinson, J. D., Morris, B. A., Aherne, G. W., and Marks, V. J.: Proceedings; development of radioimmunoassays for anticonvulsant drugs, J. Endocrinol. **64:**7, 1975.

54. Sabath, L. D., Casey, J. I., Ruch, P. A., Stumpf, L. L., and Finland, M.: Rapid microassay of gentamicin, kanamycin, neomycin, streptomycin and vancomycin in serum or plasma, J. Lab. Clin. Med. **78:** 457, 1971.

55. Schatzmann, H. J.: Hertzglykoside als Hemmstoffe für den activen Kallurnund Narrceiurn-transport durch die Erythrocyten membran, Helv. Physiol. Pharmacol. Acta **11:**346, 1953.

56. Schwenk, R., Kelly, K., Tse, K. S., and Sehon, A. U.: A radioimmunoassay for isoniazid, Clin. Chem. **21:**1059, 1975.

57. Selden, R., and Smith, T. W.: Ouabain pharmacokinetics in dog and man; determination by radioimmunoassay, Circulation **45:**1176, 1972.

58. Smith, T. W.: Radioimmunoassay for serum digitoxin digitoxin concentration; methodology and clinical experience, J. Pharmacol. Exp. Ther. **175:**352, 1970.

59. Smith, T. W., Butler, V. P., Jr., and Haber, E.: Determination of therapeutic and toxic serum digoxin concentrations by radioimmunoassay, N. Engl. J. Med. **281:**1212, 1969.

60. Smith, T. W., and Haber, E.: Current techniques for serum or plasma digitalis assay and their potential clinical application, Am. J. Med. Sci. **259:**301, 1970.

61. Spector, S.: Development of antibodies to chlorpromazine. In Forrest, B. S., editor: The phenothiazines and structurally related drugs, New York, 1974, Raven Press, p. 363.

62. Spector, S.: Radioimmunoassay of drugs. In International Atomic Energy Agency: Radioimmunoassay and related procedures in medicine, vol. 2, Vienna, 1974, I.A.E.A., pp. 233-249.

63. Spector, S., Berkowitz, B., Flynn, E. J., and Peskar, B.: Antibodies to morphine, barbiturates and serotonin, Pharmacol. Rev. **25:**281, 1973.

64. Spector, S., and Flynn, E. J.: Barbiturates; radioimmunoassay, Science **174:**1036, 1971.

65. Spector, S., and Parker, C. W.: Morphine; radioimmunoassay, Science **168:**1347, 1970.

66. Stephens, P., Young, L. S., and Hewitt, W. L.: Radioimmunoassay, acetylating radioenzymatic assay and microbioassay of gentamicin; a comparative study, J. Lab. Clin. Med. **86:**349, 1975.

67. Taubert, K., and Shapiro, W.: Serum digoxin levels using an ^{125}I-labelled antigen; validation of method and observations on cardiac patients, Am. Heart J. **89:**79, 1975.

68. Taunton-Rigby, A., Sher, S. E., and Kelly, P. R.: Lysergic acid diethylamide; radioimmunoassay, Science **181:**165, 1973.

69. Tigelaar, R. E., Rapport, R. L. II, Inman, J. K., and Kupferberg, H. J.: A radioimmunoassay for diphenylhydantoin, Clin. Chem. Acta **43:**231, 1973.

70. Van Vunakis, H., Langone, J. J., Riceberg, L. J., and Levine, L.: Radioimmunoassays for Adriamycin and daunomycin, Cancer Res. **34:**25, 1974.

71. Warren, R. J., and Fotherby, K.: Radioimmunoassay of synthetic progestogens, norethisterone and norgestrel, J. Endocrinol. **62:**605, 1974.

72. Watson, E., and Kalmon, S. M.: Assay of digoxin in plasma by gas chromatography, J. Chromatogr. **56:** 209, 1971.

73. Williams, T. A., and Pittman, K. A.: Pentazocine radioimmunoassay, Res. Commun. Chem. Pathol. Pharmacol. **7:**119, 1974.

21 HEPATITIS B VIRUS

Radioimmunoassay (RIA) has been applied to only a few of the large number of clinically important viruses. One of these, however, RIA for hepatitis B surface antigen, is one of the most important clinical RIAs. Well over 6×10^6 RIA tests were performed in the United States alone in 1976, primarily as an aid to screening of donated blood to help prevent bloodborne hepatitis.

Hepatitis manifests itself in two clinical forms. Infectious hepatitis (also called hepatitis A) has high infectivity and relatively short incubation periods of about 30 days. Serum hepatitis (also called hepatitis B) has a long incubation period of up to 100+ days, with prolonged and usually more serious hepatic injury. In 1967 Krugman and associates showed that these two clinical forms were caused by infective agents that were clinically and immunologically distinct. Krugman named these two agents MS-1 and MS-2, respectively.

Allison and Bloomburg showed that multiply transfused patients had precipitating antibodies in their serum. These antibodies reacted with an antigenic component of serum from an Australian aborigine. This reactive antigen was first called "Australia antigen." Prince and Bloomburg subsequently demontrated that Australia antigen was identical to the MS-2 viral agent of Krugman and that these agents appeared in the blood of patients with serum hepatitis.

The preferred term for this viral agent is hepatitis B virus–associated antigen. Other previous designations (SH antigen, hepatitis antigen, hepatitis-associated antigen [HAA], Australia/SH antigen, and MS-2) are no longer used.

Chemistry

Hepatitis B virus is a small, stable, infective particle that is composed of a central core of nucleic acid and a surrounding protein capsid. The entire virus ("Dane particle") is about 45 nm in diameter. The nuclear core material has been found in the nucleus of patients with hepatitis and is about 23 nm in diameter. Associated with the nuclear core is an antigen, termed HB_c-Ag for hepatitis B core antigen. The antigen that is commonly detected in the RIA test is the protein capsid, HB_sAg (hepatitis B surface antigen). This particle is about 27 nm in diameter.

In Hb_sAg there are three distinct immunologic subgroups: *a, y,* and *d*. The *y* and *d* antigens are mutually exclusive. In addition, there are two immunologic subtypes: *w* and *r*. Thus for each virus there are four distinct immunologic subgroups: *ayw, ayr, adr,* and *adw*. The *ay* subgroup is most common in drug addicts; the *ad* subgroup occurs with greater frequency in asymptomatic carriers. The *y* and *r* subgroups are related to the country of origin of the infected patient. The subtype *adw* occurs in patients from Canada, China, Germany, and the West Indies; *adr* occurs only in patients from China.

Hepatitis B is an ether-stable particle that can survive at 60° C for 4 or more hours and may remain infective at $-10°$ to $-20°$ C for years. Infectivity is destroyed by heating at 100° C for 30 minutes, by ethylene oxide sterilization, and by tricresol treatment.

Physiology

Viruses are small obligatory intracellular parasites that use the enzymatic system of other cells to replicate. The virus structure includes a nucleic acid core (either RNA or DNA), a protein coat (capsid), and for more complex viruses an envelope that encloses the core and capsid. The entire virus is called a virion. Some enzymes, usually nucleic acid transcriptase, may also be part of the virion.

Viruses show considerable specificity for the cells that they infect. In the case of hepatitis B, mammalian liver cells (particularly primate liver cells) are the host.

Methods

A number of serologic techniques have been employed to detect HB_sAg in human serum. Insensitivity was a serious limitation of most of these methods, and new techniques were sought to overcome this problem. Walsh and associates introduced the first RIA procedure in 1970. Subsequent improvements made RIA procedures the "gold standard" against which the sensitivity of other methodologies is prepared.

The earliest RIA technique utilized purified HB_sAg labeled with ^{125}I as ligand. Hepatitis B antigen–specific rabbit antibody (HB_sAb) was incubated with radioligand and test serum for 3 days at 4° C. Separation of bound and unbound HB_sAg was achieved by chromatoelectrophoresis. Subsequently, several competitive RIAs were developed that differed only in detail. Most of these methods were more rapid and employed more generally applicable separation methods, including double-antibody precipitation and agar gel diffusion.

The first noncompetitive RIA was a one-site assay developed by Hollinger and associates. HB_sAg labeled with ^{125}I was used as radioligand. Polystyrene tubes were coated with HB_sAg (guinea pig), and incubation with serum was followed by subsequent addition of radioligand. The greater the concentration of HB_sAg in the serum, the less ^{125}I-labeled HB_sAg subsequently bound.

As a way to avoid handling of HB_sAg and the biologic hazard of iodinating a potentially infective agent, a two-site noncompetitive RIA was developed by Ling and Overby. HB_sAb labeled with ^{125}I was used as radioligand; polypropylene tubes were coated with HB_sAb (guinea pig), and serum containing Hb_sAg was incubated with it. After binding of the HB_sAg and

the HB_sAb attached to the solid phase, a second antibody labeled with ^{125}I-HB_sAb (guinea pig) was added. Wherever Hb_sAg had bound, the ^{125}I-Hb_sAb now bound. In this way, the HB_sAg was "sandwiched" between two antibodies.

A significant improvement was observed in the *sensitivity* of this technique over competitive RIA. However, the *specificity* of the early two-site assays was limited, partly because of the presence of guinea pig IgG-Ab (human) in the serum of a significant number of patients.

Employing ^{125}I-labeled HB_sAb (human) as the radioligand in the two-site RIA results in a significant improvement in specificity. An additional improvement in specificity is also noted if the assay is performed at 45° C.

Use of a kit system (Ausria) developed by Abbott Laboratories has become a dominant practice. Current methods (Ausria II) give about 1.5 times the number of confirmed positive results as counterelectrophoresis. With the use of human ^{125}I-labeled HB_sAb and 45° C as the incubation temperature, the problem of false positive results has been virtually eliminated. This method has been adopted by the Red Cross in the United States and is being used countrywide for screening blood samples for HB_sAg. This technique requires 3 hours to complete.

All methods for measurement of HB_sAg must take into account the frequent association of HB_sAb in the serum of infected patients. This is usually determined by the degree of HB_sAb binding of HB_sAg in the absence of antisera. The two-site method with its current modifications seems less sensitive to the effects of human HB_sAb.

Reagents

Guinea pig antibody coated to tubes or polystyrene beads are used as the first antibody. HB_sAb (human) labeled with ^{125}I is used as the radioligand.

Performance

The assay is usually performed at 45° C. Serum is first incubated with the solid phase HB_sAb (guinea pig). During the first step a 2-hour incubation procedure is performed, after which the beads are washed free of patient serum with deionized water. The ^{125}I-labeled HB_sAg (human) is added next, and the samples are incubated for 1 hour. The tubes are then counted and compared with a positive control.

Assay properties

Assay sensitivity is very good with this test, although not all of the infective blood units will give positive results. Thus some false negative results still occur. At the time of this writing, only about one third of the total cases of hepatitis and about half of the HB$_s$Ag-associated hepatitis cases will be detected by current methods (see Pathophysiology below).

Calculation of positive results

The detection of a positive result is a qualitative judgment, and the various methods have different techniques for setting the cutoff limit. The most widely used test (Ausria II-125, Abbott Laboratories) sets a limit as follows. Seven samples of negative patient sera are included as negative controls. The net count rate (sample − background) determined in each of these seven is averaged, and this average is multiplied by 2.1 to obtain the calculated cutoff limit. Patient samples with count rates higher than this limit are considered positive for HB$_s$Ag. These positive results are then usually subjected to further confirmation testing with the use of kits that contain human antisera to HB$_s$Ag to neutralize the reactivity.

A detailed overview of the Ausria II test for detecting HB$_s$Ag is given in Box 21-1.

In addition, a sensitive detection technique for antibody to HB$_s$Ag has been developed (Ausab, Abbott Laboratories). This method works as follows. Polyacrylamide beads are coated with HB$_s$Ag. The patient's serum is added to the kit, and any antibody present is fixed to the solid phase coupled antigen. HB$_s$Ag labeled with ^{125}I is then added, and the labeled antigen is bound to the immobilized antibody. (Details regarding the methodology of this technique are available from Abbott Laboratories, North Chicago, Illinois.)

Clinical applications
Pathophysiology

HB$_s$Ag is elaborated into the blood as part of the process of infection and subsequent multi-plication of hepatitis B viruses in human hepatocytes. HB$_s$Ag is itself probably noninfective, since it is only the protein coat of the virion. In association with nuclear core material (Hb$_c$Ag), however, the virion or infective virus particle is formed; for this reason HB$_s$Ag is a useful predictor of the presence of live hepatitis virus.

Hepatitis B virus is spread by blood and blood products during transfusion and may also be spread by menstrual discharge, the fecal/oral route, urine, or sexual intercourse, or it may be airborne. Spread is usually from human to human, although higher primates carry the virus, and spread of hepatitis B virus from chimpanzee to man has been documented.

After infection, during the preicteric and icteric phase of the disease, there is usually HB$_s$-Ag in the blood. By 5 to 8 weeks after infection, HB$_s$Ag is gone from the blood, and HB$_s$-Ab has appeared. In about 10% to 20% of adults and 35% of children, a chronic carrier state may develop. This persistence is particularly likely to develop in mild nonicteric hepatitis B infection and is associated with chronic hepatitis. Persistence also develops in patients with Down's syndrome and in immunosuppressed patients.

There are about 150,000 cases of hepatitis in the United States each year, with about 3,000 deaths. Hepatitis is particularly likely to occur in multiply transfused patients, drug addicts, and immunosuppressed patients, as well as in patients and staff of renal dialysis centers.

Very tiny amounts of virus can cause hepatitis, and none of the currently available methods can be relied on to totally prevent hepatitis B infection. Use of the most sensitive RIA will probably result in prevention of only an additional 29% of all transfusion-associated hepatitis and 45% of the HB$_s$Ag-associated hepatitis.

Of particular interest for the future is the possibility of an antigen test that may be specific for infection with hepatitis B, the so-called *e* antigen. This antigen has a molecular weight of about 300,000 and appears to be a soluble protein. This antigen is found only in the serum of patients who are HB$_s$Ag positive. The *e* antigen is apparently associated with continuing active liver disease. The presence of the antibody to *e* antigen, however, has been found only in the

---

HEPATITIS B SURFACE ANTIGEN METHOD†

Principle   Wash

$$S\text{-}R + L \rightarrow S\text{-}RL + R^* \rightarrow S\text{-}RLR^* + R^*$$

Protocol

		Reagent	Volume
DAY 1	S-R	*Guinea pig antisera to HB_sAg, bound to polystyrene beads*	*1 bead per sample*
	L { Control	*Negative and positive human control serum*	*200 μl*
	Sample	*Serum from patient*	*200 μl*

——————— *2 hours, 45° C* ———————

	↓	*Wash bead twice with distilled H_2O* *Aspirate H_2O from around bead*	*5 ml*
	R*	*^{125}I-labeled human antisera to HB_sAg*	*200 μl*

——————— *1 hour, 45° C* ———————

	↓	*Decant antibody solution* *Rinse with distilled H_2O twice* — *5 ml* *Count beads* *Positives identified as greater than 2.1 × negative counts*

Reagents

	R	*Guinea pig antiserum to HB_sAg, bound to polystyrene beads*
	L	*Serum; if plasma is used, it must be "recalcified" by addition of 0.1 ml $CaCl_2$ solution (2.77% calcium chloride in H_2O) to 0.9 ml of plasma and incubation at 37° C for 2 hours; serum obtained after centrifugation (3,000 rpm, 10 minutes)*
	L*	*Human antiserum to Hb_sAg, labeled with ^{125}I; this Ab is soluble*

†Ausria II-125, Abbott Laboratories.

Box 21-1

serum of patients who have recovered from the hepatic effect of the virus. Also, *e* antigen is associated with a risk of transmitting the HB_s-Ag-positive hepatitis. However, anti-*e* is protective and apparently prevents this transmission. This is at least the situation apparently as far as vertical transmission from mother to offspring is concerned.

HB_sAb develops after 3 to 4 weeks in patients with hepatitis B infection. HB_sAb can be easily detected by methods similar to those for HB_sAg.

Current status of viral detection methods

Application of radioligand methods to viral detection is still in an early stage of development. Even with respect to transfusion-associated hepatitis, the best studied from a methodologic point of view, there are major gaps in our ability to detect the causative agents in infected blood. In addition to the problem of specificity, other viruses may be present (such as the hepatitis C virus postulated by Prince). The role of HB_cAg and HB_cAb has not been well studied. Even with these limitations, many patients have already benefited from the sensitivity of RIA techniques.

REFERENCES

1. Aach, R. D., Grisham, M. W., and Parker, C. W.: Detection of Australia antigen by radioimmunoassay, Proc. Natl. Acad. Sci. USA **68:**1056, 1971.
2. Allison, A. C., and Blumberg, B. S.: An isoprecipitation reaction distinguishing human serum protein types, Lancet **1:**632, 1961.
3. Blumberg, B. S.: Polymorphisms of serum proteins in the development of isoprecipitins in transfused patients, Bull. N.Y. Acad. Med. **40:**377, 1964.
4. Coller, J. A., Millman, I., Halberr, T. C., and Blumberg, B. S.: Radioimmunoprecipitation assay for Australia antigen, antibody and antigen-antibody complexes, Proc. Soc. Exp. Biol. Med. **138:**249, 1971.
5. Dane, D. S., Cameron, C. H., and Briggs, M.: Virus-like particles in serum of patients with Australia-antigen-associated hepatitis, Lancet **1:**695, 1970.
6. Ginsberg, A. L., Bancroft, W. H., and Conrad, M. E.: Simplified and sensitive detection of subtypes of Australia antigen (HBAg) using a solid phase radioimmune assay, J. Lab. Clin. Med. **80:**291, 1972.
7. Hollinger, F. B., Voradain, V., and Dreesman, G. R.: Assay of Australia antigen and antibody employing double antibody and solid phase radioimmunoassay techniques and comparison with the passive hemagglutination methods, J. Immunol. **107:**1099, 1971.
8. Huang, S.: Hepatitis associated antigen hepatitis, Am. J. Pathol. **64:**483, 1971.
9. Krugman, S., Giles, J. P., and Hammond, J.: Infectious hepatitis; evidence for two distinctive clinical, epidemiological and immunological types of infections, J.A.M.A. **200:**365, 1967.
10. Ling, C. M., Ivace, H., Decker, R., and Overby, L. R.: Hepatitis B virus antigen; validation and immunologic characterization of low titer serums with I^{125} antibody, Science **180:**203, 1973.
11. Ling, C. M., and Overby, L. R.: Prevalence of hepatitis B virus antigen as revealed by direct radioimmune assay with I^{125} antibody, J. Immunol. **109:**834, 1972.
12. Miller, J. P., and Overby, L. R.: Australia antigen. In Rothfeld, B., editor: Nuclear medicine in-vitro, Philadelphia, 1975, J. B. Lippincott Co., p. 365.
13. Prince, A. M.: An antigen detected in the blood during the incubation period of serum hepatitis, Proc. Natl. Acad. Sci. USA **60:**814, 1968.
14. Sutnick, A. I., London, W. T., Genstley, B. J., Cronlund, M. M., and Blumberg, B. S.: Anicteric hepatitis associated with Australia antigen, J.A.M.A. **205:**670, 1968.
15. Taswell, H. F., Nicholson, L., Cochran, M., and Tauze, W. N.: A rapid, safe method for the detection of hepatitis B antigen by radioimmunoassay (abstract from the twenty-sixth annual meeting of the American Association of Blood Banks, Miami), Nov. 1973, p. 80.
16. Tilden, R. L., and DeLand, F. H.: Electro-osmophoretic radioimmunoassay; application to hepatitis-associated antigen, J. Nucl. Med. **13:**599, 1972.
17. Walsh, J. H., Yalow, R., and Berson, S. A.: Detection of Australia antigen and antibody by means of radioimmunoassay techniques, J. Infect. Dis. **121:**550, 1970.

Appendixes

1/Preparation of immunogen-adjuvant mixture

PRINCIPLE

A stable emulsion is prepared between the immunogen in a water solution and paraffin oil, with mannide mono-oleate as emulsifier.

MATERIALS

1. Immunogen dissolved in phosphate buffer (0.05-0.5 mg/ml, depending on the dose to be used)
2. Freund complete adjuvant (Difco): contains Arlacel A, (mannide mono-oleate), Bayol F (paraffin oil), and killed *Mycobacterium butyricum*
3. Mixer: this may be a high-speed rotating homogenizer such as Virtis or Polytron; of similar efficiency or better (but much less expensive) are two 5-ml glass syringes connected to each other by two cannulas (1-mm opening) that are cut off and soldered together, the contents can be pressed back and forth through the small opening of the cannula (see figure below).

PERFORMANCE

1. Draw equal volumes (for example, 1 ml) of protein solution and adjuvant per rabbit to be immunized, by means of a heavy cannula (1 ml of each into one of the syringes).

2. Mount the syringes against each other via the connecting piece. Pump the contents back and forth between the syringes until the mixture is thick. It should be very thick—at least as thick as whipped cream—or else the emulsion will not be stable. Since the plunger will become difficult to press (into the syringe) when the emulsion begins to thicken, press the plunger against the surface of a laboratory bench for increased power. It takes 1-5 minutes of pumping to achieve a good emulsion.
3. To test the stability of the emulsion put a drop on a glass plate or float a drop on lukewarm water, and let it remain there for at least 5 minutes to be certain that the oil and water phases do not separate. An unstable emulsion gives a poor immunogenic stimulus, since the water-soluble immunogens are resorbed rapidly. In the case of immunogens with high biologic activity, this may even hurt the animals. For example, many guinea pigs may be lost because of hypoglycemia when one immunizes against insulin if the emulsion is not stable.
4. Two milliliters of this solution (= 100μg immunogen if the starting immunogen solution contained 0.1 mg/ml) are injected per rabbit, 0.5-2 ml per guinea pig, and 10 ml per goat or other large animal.

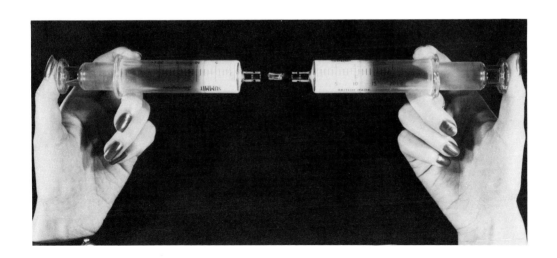

2/Preparation of 3,5,3′-triiodothyronine conjugates to human serum albumin

PRINCIPLE

Carbodiimide is used as a coupling reagent to induce peptide bond between T_3 (the carboxyl group) and primarily lysine residues (amino group) of HSA (compare Fig. 2-6). The same principle may be employed to couple any polypeptide to a protein containing free amino groups.

MATERIALS

1. T_3
2. Human serum albumin
3. "Morpho CDI": 1-cyclohexyl-3(2-morpholinoethyl)-carbodiimide metho-*p*-toluene sulfonate (Aldrich Chemical Co., Milwaukee, Wisconsin)
4. Dimethylformamide

PERFORMANCE

1. Twenty milligrams of T_3 are dissolved in 5 ml of dimethylformamide.
2. Fifty milligrams of HSA are dissolved in 25 ml of distilled water.
3. Thirty milligrams of "morpho CDI" are added to the albumin solution.
4. The T_3 solution is mixed dropwise with the albumin solution with continuous stirring. The pH of the mixture is maintained at 5.5 by continuous monitoring with a pH meter and adjustment of pH as necessary with 0.01 M NaOH or 0.01 M HCl.
5. After 10 minutes of incubation at room temperature an additional 10 mg of "morpho CDI" is added to the incubation mixture, which is kept at room temperature in the dark for 18 hours.
6. The reaction mixture is then dialyzed against continuously running distilled water for 72 hours in the dark.
7. After dialysis, the T_3-HSA conjugate is lyophilized.

REFERENCES

Chopra, I. J., Nelson, J. C., Solomon, D. C., and Beall, G. N.: Production of antibodies specifically binding triiodothyronine and thyroxine, J. Clin. Endocrinol. Metab. **32**:299, 1971.
Gharib, H., Ryan, R. J., Mayberry, W. E., and Hackert, T.: Radioimmunoassay for triiodothyronine (T_3) I. Affinity and specificity of the antibody for T_3, J. Clin. Endocrinol. Metab. **33**:509, 1971.
Goodfriend, T. L., Levine, L., and Fasman, G.: Antibodies to bradykinin and angiotensin; a use of carbodiimides in immunology, Science **143**:1344, 1964.
Sheehan, J. C., Cruickshank, P. A., and Boschart, C. L.: A convenient synthesis of water-soluble carbodiimides, J. Org. Chem. **26**:2525, 1961.
Sheehan, J. C., and Hlavka, J. S.: The use of water-soluble and basic carbodiimides in peptide synthesis, J. Org. Chem. **21**:439, 1956.
Young, J. D., Byrnes, D. J., Chisholm, D. J., Griffiths, F. B., and Lazarus, L.: Radioimmunoassay of gastrin in human serum; J. Nucl. Med. **10**:746, 1969.

3/Preparation of progesterone-11α-hemisuccinate

PRINCIPLE

The hydroxyl group of 11α-hydroxyprogesterone is reacted with succinic anhydride to form the stable progesterone-hemisuccinate for later conjugation with proteins and other compounds containing free amino groups (compare Table 2-1). The same method may be used for the activation of other steroids with one hydroxyl group.

MATERIALS

1. 11α-Hydroxyprogesterone
2. Succinic anhydride
3. Pyridine (water-free)
4. Ethyl acetate
5. 5% NaOH
6. 1 M HCl
7. Magnesium sulfate (anhydrous)
8. Benzene
9. Hexane
10. Acetone
11. Methanol
12. Thin-layer chromatography plates (Silica gel 60, Merck A.G., Darmstadt, West Germany)

PERFORMANCE

1. Two grams (6.1 mmol) 11α-hydroxyproges-
   terone and 2.0 g (20 mmol) succinic anhydride
   are dissolved in 20 ml of water-free pyridine.
2. The reaction solution is heated under reflux for
   4.5 hours with a drying tube at the top of the
   condenser.
3. The reaction mixture is evaporated in a vacuum
   evaporator. The residue is dissolved in ethyl
   acetate. The solution is then washed three
   times with 10 ml of distilled water and then
   extracted three times with 25 ml of 5% NaOH.
4. The collected alkaline extract is washed twice
   with 50 ml of ethyl acetate. The water phase
   is acidified with 1 M HCl, and the pH is adjusted to 2. At this point, the progesterone-
   11α-hemisuccinate precipitates. The proges-
   terone-11α-hemisuccinate is extracted with
   100 ml of ethyl acetate.
5. The ethyl acetate solution is dried over $MgSO_4$

and evaporated to dryness in a rotary vacuum
evaporator.

6. The substance is recrystallized from benzene
   and hexane (1:1).
7. The melting point is analyzed to ascertain
   purity. The melting point should be 150°-
   155° C. Thin-layer chromatography may also
   be performed to evaluate purity. A spot with
   an R_f value of 0.43 should be observed when
   benzene, acetone, and methanol (5:5:2) are
   used as the developing solvents on Silica gel
   60.

REFERENCE

Erlanger, B. F., Borek, F., Beiser, S. M., and Lieberman,
S.: Steroid-protein conjugates. II. Preparation and characterization of conjugates of bovine serum albumin with
progesterone, deoxycorticosterone and estrone, J. Biol.
Chem. **234:**1090, 1959.

4 / Preparation of testosterone-3-(O-carboxymethyl)-oxime

PRINCIPLE

The 3-ketone group of testosterone reacts with the
amino group of aminooxyacetic acid, forming a carboxymethyloxime. This reactive group is used in the
conjugation of testosterone to a protein. The same
method may be used for the activation of other steroids with one ketone group.

MATERIALS

1. Testosterone
2. Methanol and water (80:20)
3. Aminooxyacetic acid (hemihydrochloride)
4. Ethyl acetate
5. Sodium sulfate (anhydrous)
6. Dioxane
7. Ligroin (Bensoline, refined solvent naphtha)
8. Chloroform
9. Sodium acetate
10. 2 M NaOH
11. 1 M HCl
12. Thin-layer chromatography plates (Silica gel
    60, Merck A.G., Darmstadt, West Germany)

PERFORMANCE

1. Testosterone, 1.7 mmol (490 mg), is dissolved
   in 60 ml methanol/water (80:20).
2. Aminooxyacetic acid (hemihydrochloride),

600 mg, is dissolved in 40 ml 1 M sodium acetate.

3. The solutions from steps 1 and 2 are mixed together and stirred at room temperature for 24
   hours. The volume is reduced to 50 ml in a
   rotary vacuum evaporator.
4. Distilled water is then added to bring the total
   volume to 200 ml. The pH is adjusted to 8.5
   with 2 M NaOH.
5. The resulting solution is then extracted four
   times with 100 ml of ethyl acetate each time to
   remove unreacted steroid. The water phase is
   then acidified with 1 M HCl to pH 3.0 and extracted four times with 200 ml ethyl acetate.
6. The collected extracts are washed twice with
   300 ml distilled water. The extract is then dried
   over anhydrous sodium sulfate. The solution is
   taken to dryness in a rotary vacuum evaporator. The yield is normally 60% of the maximum theoretical yield.
7. The impure product is dissolved in the smallest
   possible volume of dioxane. The testosterone-
   3-(O-carboxymethyl)-oxime is precipitated by
   the addition of ligroin. The crystalline precipitate is separated and dried over silica gel in a
   vacuum desiccator. The melting point of the
   material is checked; it should be 179°-182° C.

Thin-layer chromatography may also be used to evaluate purity. A spot with an R_f value of 0.10 should be observed when the developing solvents chloroform, methanol, and water (90:10:1) are used. Precoated plates (Silicia gel 60, Merck A. G.) are used.

REFERENCES

Dean, P. D. G., Exley, D., and Johnson, M. W.: Preparation of 17β-oestradiol-6-(O-carboxymethyl)-oxime–bovine serum albumin conjugate, Steroids **18**:593, 1971.

Erlanger, B. F., Borek, F., Beiser, S. M., and Lieberman, S.: Steroid-protein conjugates. I. Preparation and characterization of conjugates of bovine serum albumin with testosterone and with cortisone, J. Biol. Chem. **228**:713, 1957.

5 / Conjugation of testosterone-3-(O-carboxymethyl)-oxime to bovine serum albumin

PRINCIPLE

Testosterone-3-(O-carboxymethyl)-oxime reacts with isobutyl chloroformate in water-free dioxane to form a mixed anhydride. The mixed anhydride reacts with the primary amino groups of the albumin in a dioxane water solution to form a stable conjugate (compare Table 2-1). The same method may be used for conjugation of other steroid-oxime compounds.

MATERIALS

1. Testosterone-3-(O-carboxymethyl)-oxime (see Appendix 4)
2. Tributylamine
3. Dioxane
4. Isobutyl chloroformate
5. BSA
6. 1 M sodium hydroxide
7. 5% sodium bicarbonate in water

PERFORMANCE

1. Three-tenths millimole (110 mg) testosterone-3-(O-carboxymethyl)-oxime and 75μl (0.3 mmol) tributylamine are dissolved in 5 ml dioxane. The solution is then chilled to 11° C.
2. Forty microliters (0.3 mmol) isobutyl chloroformate are added, and the mixture is incubated at 4° C for 20 minutes.
3. The solution is then mixed with a BSA solution containing 420 mg (6×10^{-3} mmol) BSA in 20 ml of a dioxane/water solution (1:1) (The dioxane/water solution should previously have been chilled to 4° C and the pH adjusted to 9.0 with 1 M NaOH).
4. The pH of the mixture is continuously monitored with a pH meter, and the pH is maintained between 8 and 9 with 1 M NaOH. The solution is continuously stirred at 4° C for 4 hours.
5. After 4 hours of incubation, the reaction mixture is dialyzed against continuously running distilled water overnight. The pH is adjusted to 4.5 with 1 M HCl, and the mixture is kept at 4° C for 4 days, during which time the steroid-protein conjugate will precipitate.
6. The mixture is centrifuged at 4° C (2,500g) for 15 minutes; the water phase is decanted, and the precipitate is suspended in 5 ml of distilled water. The precipitate is dissolved by the addition of 1 ml of 5% NaHCO$_3$.
7. The solution is then dialyzed against running distilled water for another 4 hours, after which the testosterone-(3-O-carboxymethyl-oxime–BSA conjugate is lyophilized and weighed.
8. The number of testosterone molecules per molecule of albumin can be determined by measuring the absorbance at 254 nm.

REFERENCES

Erlanger, B. F., Borek, F., Beiser, S. M., and Lieberman, S.: Steroid-protein conjugates. I. Preparation and characterization of conjugates of bovine serum albumin with testosterone and with cortisone, J. Biol. Chem. **228**:713, 1957.

Erlanger, B. F., Borek, F., Beiser, S. M., and Lieberman, S.: Steroid-protein conjugates. II. Preparation and characterization of conjugates of bovine serum albumin with progesterone, deoxycorticosterone and estrone, J. Biol. Chem. **234**:1090, 1959.

6/Conjugation of progesterone-11α-hemisuccinate to bovine serum albumin

PRINCIPLE

Progesterone-11α-hemisuccinate reacts with iso-butyl chloroformate in water-free dioxane to form a mixed anhydride. The mixed anhydride reacts with the primary amino group of the albumin in a dioxane/water solution to form a stable conjugate (compare Fig. 2-7). The same method may be used for other steroid-hemisuccinate compounds.

MATERIALS

1. Progesterone-11α-hemisuccinate (see Appendix 3)
2. BSA
3. Tributylamine
4. Isobutyl chloroformate
5. Water-free dioxane
6. 1 M NaOH
7. 1 M HCl
8. 5% NaHCO$_3$ in water

PERFORMANCE

1. Progesterone-11α-hemisuccinate, 130 mg (0.30 mmol) is dissolved in 5 ml of dioxane. Tributylamine, 75μl (0.30 mmol), is added. The solution is chilled to 11° C.
2. Forty microliters (0.30 mmol) of isobutyl chloroformate are added, and the solution is kept for 20 minutes at 4° C. The mixture is then poured into a well-chilled solution of 420 mg (6.0 μmol) BSA in 20 ml dioxane/water (1:1), pH 8.5.

3. The solution is stirred continuously for 4 hours at 4° C. The pH is monitored with a pH meter and kept at 8 to 9 by addition of 1 M NaOH.
4. The solution is dialyzed for 24 hours against slowly running distilled water. The solution is then acidified to pH 4.5 and allowed to stand at 4° C for 4 days.
5. The precipitate that forms is separated by centrifugation (15 minutes at 2,500g). After the supernatant is decanted, the precipitate is suspended in 5 ml of distilled water and then dissolved by adding the smallest possible amount (about 1 ml) of 5% NaHCO$_3$. The solution is dialyzed 4 hours against running distilled water.
6. The progesterone-11α-hemisuccinate–BSA conjugate is freeze-dried. The number of progesterone molecules per albumin molecule can be determined by measuring the absorbance at 250 nm.

REFERENCES

Erlanger, B. F., Borek, F., Beiser, S. M., and Lieberman, S.: Steroid-protein conjugates. I. Preparation and characterization of conjugates of bovine serum albumin with testosterone and with cortisone, J. Biol. Chem. **238:**713, 1957.

Erlanger, B. F., Borek, F., Beiser, S. M., and Lieberman, S.: Steroid-protein conjugates. II. Preparation and characterization of conjugates of bovine serum albumin with progesterone, deoxycorticosterone and estrone, J. Biol. Chem. **234:**1090, 1959.

7/Preparation of cortisol-21-hemisuccinate thyroglobulin

PRINCIPLE

Cortisol-21-hemisuccinate reacts with isobutyl chloroformate in water-free dioxane to form a mixed anhydride. The mixed anhydride reacts with primary amino groups of thyroglobulin in dioxane/water to form a stable conjugate.

MATERIALS

1. Cortisol-21-hemisuccinate (commercially available)
2. Bovine thyroglobulin
3. Tributylamine
4. Isobutyl chloroformate

5. Dioxane (water-free)
6. 1 M NaOH
7. 1 M HCl
8. 5% NaHCO$_3$ in water

PERFORMANCE

1. Cortisol-21-hemisuccinate, 46 mg (0.1 mmol), is dissolved in 5 ml dioxane. Tributylamine, 25μl (0.1 mmol), is added, and the solution is chilled to 11° C.
2. Fifteen microliters (0.1 mmol) of isobutyl chloroformate are added, and the solution is incubated for 20 minutes at 5°-10° C.

3. Thyroglobulin, 68 mg, is dissolved in 6.0 ml distilled water, and 4.0 ml dioxane (pH adjusted to 8-9 with 1 M NaOH) are added. The reaction solution is continuously stirred for 4 hours at 4° C. The pH is maintained at 8 to 9 with 1 M NaOH.
4. The solution is dialyzed for 24 hours against slowly running distilled water. Then the reaction solution is acidified to pH 4.5 with 1 M HCl. The solution is stored at 4° C for 4 days.
5. The precipitate that forms in the cold is separated by centrifugation. The precipitate is suspended in 5 ml of distilled water and dissolved by the addition of the least amount necessary of 5% $NaHCO_3$.
6. The resulting solution is dialyzed again for 4 hours against running distilled water.
7. The cortisol-21-hemisuccinate–thyroglobulin conjugate is then freeze-dried.

8. The number of cortisol molecules per molecule of thyroglobulin can be determined by measuring the absorbance at 248 nm.

REFERENCES

Dean, P. D. G., Exley, D., and Johnsson, M. W.: Preparation of 17β-oestradiol-6-(O-carboxymethyl)-oxime–bovine serum albumin conjugate, Steroids **18**:5, 593, 1971.

Erlanger, B. F., Borek, F., Beiser, S. M., and Lieberman, S.: Steroid-protein conjugates. I. Preparation and characterization of conjugates of bovine serum albumin with testosterone and with cortisone, J. Biol. Chem. **228**:713, 1957.

Erlanger, B. F., Borek, F., Beiser, S. M., and Lieberman, S.: Steroid-protein conjugates. II. Preparation and characterization of conjugates of bovine serum albumin with progesterone, deoxycorticosterone and estrone, J. Biol. Chem. **234**:1090, 1959.

8/Protocol for antibody testing

Antibody concentration (titer) illustrated with a TSH antiserum

MATERIALS

PB-BSA
Antiserum (rabbit)
^{125}I-TSH
Normal rabbit serum diluted 1:200 with PB-BSA (NRS)
Goat antiserum to rabbit IgG diluted 1:10 (GAR)

DOUBLE-ANTIBODY PRECIPITATION METHOD

This method must, from previous studies, be known to produce adequate precipitation. Other alternatives for isolation of antibody-bound activity are given in Chapter 4.

PERFORMANCE

1. Make a 1:2 dilution series of TSH antiserum with PB-BSA. If the amount of antiserum available is limited, an initial testing with 1:10 dilution steps could be performed. Since dilutions of less than 1:100 usually are not suitable for RIAs the dilution series could be restricted to 1:128–1:242,000 or to 1:100–1:1,000,000. If there is reason to believe that the titer does not vary to this extent, a narrower range should be tested.
2. Pipette 400μl out of each tube of the dilution series to a new series of tubes. (Start all

pipetting from the tubes with the highest dilution to avoid contamination.)
3. Add 100μl of ^{125}I-TSH (diluted to give about 10,000 cpm/100μl) to each tube. Make a blank tube that contains PB-BSA (400μl) and ^{125}I-TSH but no antibody. Also, add ^{125}I-TSH to two empty tubes that are stoppered and set aside. These are used as total count controls (C_{TC}) and are excluded from all procedures until the radioactivity is counted.
4. Mix contents in tubes (vortex).
5. Incubate at 4° C overnight.
6. To perform antibody precipitation: add 100μl diluted GAR; add 100μl diluted NRS.
7. Mix.
8. Incubate at room temperature for 4 hours (or the period necessary to give adequate precipitation).
9. Centrifuge (3,000 rpm or approximately 2,000g) for 15 minutes.
10. Decant supernatant, and count precipitate in all tubes and the two C_{TC} tubes.
11. Subtract activity in precipitate in blank tubes from all tubes before calculating the percentage bound.
12. Plot the results as bound activity in percent of C_{TC} (mean of the two C_{TC} tubes). Typical results are shown in Fig. 2-9.

9/Protocol for antibody testing

Antibody avidity (sensitivity) illustrated with a TSH antiserum

MATERIALS

Antiserum (rabbit anti-TSH)

^{125}I-TSH

Normal rabbit serum (NRS) at appropriate dilution

Goat anti-rabbit serum (GAR) at appropriate dilution

0.05 M phosphate buffer, pH 7.5, with 0.25% BSA

TSH standards. The concentration of the standards should cover the expected range of concentrations of TSH that may be found in the unknown sample. It is usually convenient to use them at logarithmically increasing concentrations. The lowest standard concentration used should be below the lowest concentration of TSH anticipated in the sample. In the case of TSH, the concentrations selected are 0, 1.25, 2.5, 5, 10, 20, 40, and 80μU/ml.

For the preliminary test an abbreviated series (for example, 0, 5, and 40μU/ml) may be used.

PRELIMINARY TEST

Use antisera dilutions giving 80%-20% bound activity. These dilutions were selected from the titer testing (Appendix 8; see also Fig. 2-9). The dilutions $1:12,500-1:100,000$ were included. Hence four different antisera dilutions are tested. In the preliminary test only three standards are used (0, 5, and 40μU/ml). The 0μU-40μU/ml of TSH is located in the midportion of the standard curve and gives an estimate of its average slope. The 5μU-0μU/ml is a concentration that must be possible to measure and is well above the sensitivity desired.

PERFORMANCE

1. Set up 4×2 tubes for each antiserum dilution (all concentrations are made up in duplicate). Extra 2×2 tubes are added for total-control counts (C_{TC}) and for blanks (C_{NA}, control–no antibody).
2. Pipette 100μl ^{125}I-TSH (approximately

10,000 cpm/100μl = 0.05 ng TSH/100μl) in all tubes. The C_{TC} tubes are stoppered and set aside and excluded from all procedures until counted.

3. Pipette 100μl of standards to tubes 3 and 4 (7.5μU/ml), 5 and 6 (30μU/ml), and 7 and 8 (120μU/ml) of each antiserum dilution.
4. Pipette 100μl PB-BSA to tubes 1 and 2 of each antiserum dilution (= standard 0μU/ml).
5. Pipette 300μl antiserum to all tubes except controls.
6. Pipette 400μl PB-BSA into C_{NA}.
7. Mix.
8. Incubate overnight at 4° C.
9. Add 100μl NRS and 100μl GAR to all tubes except C_{TC}.
10. Incubate 4 hours at room temperature.
11. Centrifuge (3,000 rpm or approximately $2,500g$) for 15 minutes.
12. Decant supernatant, and count precipitate. Counts found in the precipitate of the C_{NA} tube (mean) are subtracted from counts in all other tubes.
13. Plot results.

FINAL TEST

The procedure is repeated with the antiserum dilution that was most promising ($1:50,000$ in the example in Fig. 2-8), but now a complete standard curve with all standard concentrations is included. If the initial testing indicates that some intermediate dilution of the antiserum rather than those selected for the initial testing (for example $1:62,000$) would give a better standard curve in terms of the range and sensitivity needed, it may be worth testing several complete standard curves with small differences in antiserum dilution (such as $1:50,000$, $1:62,000$, and $1:75,000$).

10/Protocol for calculation of "true" count rate from ^{125}I and ^{131}I in mixtures containing both isotopes

PRINCIPLE

In order to get a true count for ^{125}I in a mixture with ^{131}I counted with a crystal sodium iodide (thallium-activated) detector system, a correction must be made for the Compton-scattered radiation of the ^{131}I, which falls on the photopeak of ^{125}I. This is done by counting the appropriate standard of ^{131}I with energy settings ("windows") on the gamma counter that enables one to simultaneously determine the photopeak counts of ^{131}I and the down-scattered counts that fall into the ^{125}I window. A correction factor can be calculated that expresses the relationship of ^{131}I counts that appear in the ^{125}I photopeak window to the number of ^{131}I counts that appear in its own photopeak window. This permits determination of the true ^{125}I count in the ^{125}I window. The counts in the upper (^{131}I photopeak) window represent only ^{131}I photons.

MATERIALS

1. Pure standard of ^{131}I
2. Pure standard of ^{125}I
3. Mixture of ^{131}I and ^{125}I (it is important that this mixture be of the same volume as that of the pure standards)
4. Dual channel gamma spectrometer

PERFORMANCE

1. Two windows are set on the gamma spectrometer (A for ^{125}I and B for ^{131}I). A is centered near the photopeak of ^{125}I (27-35 keV), and B is centered near the photopeak of ^{131}I (364 keV). The window width is arbitrary but is usually about 40 keV for ^{131}I and 20 keV for ^{125}I.
2. The pure ^{131}I standard is counted, and the counts in the A window and the B window are recorded. A correction factor K is calculated as $K = A/B$ for ^{131}I counts that appear in the ^{125}I window.
3. A mixture of ^{131}I and ^{125}I is then counted. Counts in window A ("a") and counts in window B ("b") are recorded.
4. The true count for ^{131}I is b, because ^{125}I does not contribute to counts in the ^{131}I window.
5. The true count for ^{125}I will be a minus the fraction of ^{131}I counts from ^{131}I Compton photons, counted in window A. This is $K \times b$.
6. True ^{125}I counts are thus equal to $a - (K \times b)$.

11/Trichloroacetic acid precipitation for estimating yield of iodination (labeling) reactions

PRINCIPLE

The labeled protein is precipitated with trichloroacetic acid (TCA). Iodide not bound to the protein will remain in solution. The precipitable fraction represents the iodide that has been incorporated into the protein.

MATERIALS

1. TCA (30%) in distilled water (weight/volume)
2. Bovine serum albumin, 1 mg/ml, in 0.9% sodium chloride (human serum albumin may also be used)
3. The radioactive material to be tested

PERFORMANCE

1. An aliquot ($1 \mu l$-$10 \mu l$, depending on the count rate; usually the smallest amount that can be pipetted is more than enough) of the iodination mixture is pipetted into a small plastic tube.
2. One milliliter of BSA solution is added and mixed well with the iodination mixture.
3. The radioactivity of the contents is counted. Note that the high activity used may be well above the maximal count rate capacity of the well detector. In this case the tube is counted at a fixed distance from the detector.
4. The labeled protein is precipitated together

with the added albumin by adding 1.0 ml of 30% TCA (15% final concentration).

5. After mixing, the tube is centrifuged at 2,500*g* for a few minutes.
6. The supernatant is decanted.
7. The radioactivity of the precipitate (protein-bound activity) is measured and compared with the radioactivity of the original iodination mixture. The yield of the iodination is calculated as the quotient between these values. This method is adequate for high yields. At low yields the coprecipitation of unbound iodide may falsely increase the apparent yield.

12/Preparation of progesterone-11α-hemisuccinate–tyrosine methyl ester derivative

PRINCIPLE

The progesterone-11α-hemisuccinate is converted to a mixed acid anhydride and then reacted in an aqueous dioxane solution with the amino group of tyrosine methyl ester (TME).

MATERIALS

1. Progesterone-11α-hemisuccinate (see Appendix 3)
2. Tributylamine
3. Isobutyl chloroformate
4. Tyrosine methyl ester hydrochloride
5. Dioxane
6. 1 M NaOH
7. 1 M HCl
8. 1 M NaHCO₃
9. Benzene/acetone/methanol (5:5:2)
10. Thin-layer chromatography plates (Silica gel 60, Merck A.G., Darmstadt, West Germany)

PERFORMANCE

1. Progesterone-11α-hemisuccinate, 0.3 mmol (130 mg), is dissolved in 5 ml water-free dioxane. Tributylamine, 0.30 mmol (75μl), is added, and the mixture is chilled to 11° C.
2. Isobutyl chloroformate, 0.30 mmol (40μl), is added, and the solution is incubated for 20 minutes at 4° C.
3. To the reaction mixture 0.30 mmol (69 mg) TME in 20 ml dioxane/distilled water (1:1), pH 8.5, is added.

4. The reaction mixture is stirred continuously at 4° C for 4 hours. The pH is maintained at 7 to 8 by addition of 1 M NaOH.
5. The reaction mixture is poured into 150 ml of ice-cold distilled water, and the progesterone-11α-hemisuccinate precipitates. The precipitate is spun down at 14,000 rpm in a refrigerated centrifuge.
6. The precipitate is washed sequentially with the following solutions: 30 ml distilled water, 30 ml 1 M HCl, 40 ml 1 M NaHCO₃, and finally with 40 ml distilled water.
7. The substance is dried over blue gel in a vacuum desiccator.
8. To test the purity of this compound, thin-layer chromatography may be used. When benzene/acetone/methanol (5:5:2) is used as the developing solvent with Silica gel 60 (Merck A.G.) thin-layer chromatography plates, a single spot with $R_f = 0.72$ should be observed.

REFERENCES

Barbieri, U., Massaglia, A., Zannino, M., and Rosa, U.: Thin-layer chromatography of steroid derivatives for radioimmunoassay, J. Chromatogr. **69:**151, 1972.

Oliver, G. C., Parker, M. B., Brasfield, D. L., and Parker, C. W.: The measurement of digitoxin in human serum by radioimmunoassay, J. Clin. Invest. **47:**1035, 1968.

13/Iodination (labeling) of progesterone-11α-hemisuccinate–tyrosine methyl ester derivative

PRINCIPLE

A steroid conjugated to TME is iodinated within the tyrosine residue by means of lactoperoxidase. The iodinated product is purified by thin-layer chromatography.

MATERIALS

1. Progesterone-11α-hemisuccinate–TME for labeling is obtained as in Appendix 12. 1 mg of the material is dissolved in 2.0 ml of methanol; the solution may be kept at −20° C for up to 6 months
2. LPO, 2.0 mg/ml, in 0.05 M phosphate buffer at pH 7.5
3. Na ^{125}I specified as carrier-free and free from reducing agents, 100 mCi/ml
4. Hydrogen peroxide, 30% solution; for labeling dilute 1:10,000 with distilled water (0.03 mg/ml)
5. 0.05 M phosphate buffer, pH 7.5
6. Benzene
7. Methanol
8. Ethanol, 99.5%
9. Thin-layer chromatography plates (Silica gel 60, Merck A.G., Darmstadt, West Germany)

PERFORMANCE

1. The procedure is carried out at room temperature. The following volumes and amounts of reagent are pipetted in the order stated into a 11 × 55 mm glass tube with continuous stirring.

a. 1.0 mCi ^{125}I-NaI (10μl-15μl)
b. 50μl phosphate buffer
c. 5μl progesterone-11α-hemisuccinate–TME, 0.5 mg/ml (2.5μg)
d. 2μl LPO, 2 mg/ml (4μg)
e. 1μl H_2O_2, 0.03 mg/ml (0.03μg)

The reaction mixture is stirred for 1 minute. Then a thin-layer chromatography purification is immediately performed.

2. Thirty microliters of the reaction solution are applied to a thin-layer chromatography plate (Silica gel 60, Merck A.G.). The chromatogram is developed with chloroform/methanol/water (90:10:1). After drying, radioactive spots are localized with autoradiography: The thin-layer plate is laid on an x-ray film in the dark and exposed for 5 minutes. The film is developed immediately. The ^{125}I-labeled progesterone-α-hemisuccinate–TME spot is scraped off the plate and extracted from the powder with two 5-ml portions of 99.5% ethanol. The ethanol solution is then stored at −20° C.

REFERENCES

Barbieri, U., Massaglia, A., Zannino, M., and Rosa, U.: Thin-layer chromatography of steroid derivatives for radioimmunoassay, J. Chromatogr. **69**:151, 1972.

Thorell, J. I., and Johansson, B. G.: Enzymatic iodination of polypeptides with ^{125}I to high specific activity, Biochim. Biophys. Acta **251**:363, 1971.

14/Labeling (iodination) of proteins with a conjugation method

Bolton-Hunter technique

PRINCIPLE

N-succinimidyl-3-(4-hydroxyphenyl)-propionate is iodinated by means of chloramine-T, and the ^{125}I-(or ^{131}I-) labeled N-succinimidyl-3-(4-hydroxyphenyl)-propionate is separated from other products of the iodination by benzene extraction. The iodinated N-succinimidyl-3-(4-hydroxyphenyl)-propionate is reacting with free amino groups in the protein molecule, producing amide bonds.

MATERIALS

1. N-Succinimidyl-3-(4-hydroxyphenyl)-propionate
2. ^{125}I-NaI specified as carrier-free and free from reducing agents, 100 mCi/ml
3. Chloramine-T, 5 mg/ml in 0.25 M phosphate buffer at pH 7.5
4. Sodium metabisulfite, 12 mg/ml in 0.05 M phosphate buffer (pH 7.5)

5. Potassium iodide, 20 mg/ml in 0.05 M phosphate buffer (pH 7.5)
6. Dimethylformamide
7. Benzene, water-free
8. 0.05 M and 0.25 M phosphate buffer (pH 7.5)
9. 0.1 M borate buffer, pH 8.5

PERFORMANCE

1. *N*-Succinimidyl-3-(4-hydroxyphenyl)-propionate, 2.0 mg, is dissolved in 50 ml of benzene. Five microliters of this solution is pipetted into an 11 × 55 mm glass tube.
2. The benzene is evaporated under a continuous flow of nitrogen. The remaining reagents are rapidly added to the reaction tube with continuous stirring in the following order in the amounts stated.
   a. 2 mCi ^{125}I-NaI (20μl)
   b. 10μl chloramine-T, 5 mg/ml (50μg)
   c. 10μl sodium metabisulfite, 12 mg/ml (120 μg)
   d. 10μl KI, 20 mg/ml (200μg)
   e. 5μl dimethylformamide
   f. 250μl benzene for extraction of the iodinated product
3. After addition of benzene the mixture is immediately shaken (vortex) and the phases are allowed to separate. The benzene phase is transferred to another glass tube (11 × 55 mm). The reaction mixture is extracted with another 250μl of benzene in the same way.

The benzene solution is evaporated to dryness by passing a stream of nitrogen gas over the surface of the benzene. *Note:* Volatile radioactive material may be released during evaporation.

The time from the addition of the ^{125}I-NaI to the benzene extraction of the iodinated product must not exceed 20 s.

4. The protein (5μg) is dissolved in 10μl 0.1 M borate buffer, pH 8.5, and added to the dried iodinated *N*-succinimidyl-3-(4-hydroxyphenyl)-propionate. The reaction mixture is stirred for 15 minutes at 0° C.
5. In order to avoid possible later conjugation of the unreacted iodinated ester to carrier protein, 0.5 ml of 0.2 M glycine in borate buffer, pH 8.5, is added with stirring at 0° C for 5 minutes.
6. The labeled product is separated from unconjugated labeled product by gel filtration.

REFERENCE

Bolton, A. E., and Hunter, W. M.: The labelling of proteins to high specific radioactivities by conjugation to a ^{125}I-containing acylating agent, Biochemistry **133:**529, 1973.

15 / Labeling of testosterone-3-(O-carboxymethyl)-oxime by conjugation with ^{125}I-labeled histamine

Nars-Hunter technique

PRINCIPLE

Testosterone-3-(O-carboxymethyl)-oxime is reacted with isobutyl chloroformate to form a mixed anhydride. Histamine is iodinated with a chloramine-T method and then reacted with the mixed anhydride. The amino group of histamine forms an amide bond with the carboxyl group in testosterone-3-(O-carboxymethyl)-oxime.

MATERIALS

1. Testosterone-3-(O-carboxymethyl)-oxime (testosterone-3-CMO)
2. Isobutyl chloroformate, 10% (vol.) in dioxane
3. Tributylamine, 20% (vol.) dioxane
4. Dioxane (water-free)
5. Chloramine-T, 5.0 mg/ml, in distilled water
6. Sodium metabisulfite (sodium disulfite), 30 mg/ml, in distilled water
7. ^{125}I-NaI, 100 mCi/ml, specified as carrier-free and without reducing agents
8. Histamine, 22.2μg/ml, in 0.5 M phosphate buffer (pH 8.0)
9. Sodium metabisulfite 1.0 mg/ml, in 0.5 M phosphate (pH 7.0)
10. Toluene
11. 0.5 M phosphate buffer (pH 7.0)
12. 0.5 M phosphate buffer (pH 8.0)
13. 0.2 M NaOH
14. 0.1 M NaOH
15. 0.1 M HCl
16. Benzene
17. Ethanol, 99.5%

18. TLC plate (Silica gel 60, Merck A.G., Darmstadt, West Germany)

PERFORMANCE

1. In an 11 × 55 glass tube, mix:
   a. 2.0 mg testosterone-3-CMO dissolved in 50µl dioxane
   b. 10µl tributylamine, 20%, in dioxane
   c. 10µl isobutyl chloroformate, 10%, in dioxane
2. The solution is incubated for 20 minutes in a refrigerator. Then it is diluted to 2.8 ml total volume with dioxane.
3. Into an 11 × 55 mm glass tube pipette the following reagents with continuous stirring:
   a. 2 mCi ^{125}I-NaI (20µl-30µl)
   b. 10µl histamine, 22.2µg/ml (0.222µg)
   c. 10µl chloramine-T, 5 mg/ml (50µg)
   d. 10µl sodium metabisulfite, 30 mg/ml (300µg)

Note: The iodination of histamine and the activation of testosterone-3-CMO must be carefully timed so that the coupling to the previously activated testosterone-3-CMO can be performed immediately after the histamine is labeled.

4. Immediately after iodination, 50µl of the testosterone-3-CMO (36µg) solution are added to the iodinated histamine solution.
5. Ten microliters of 0.2 M NaOH are added, and the mixture is incubated for 60 minutes in a refrigerator with continuous stirring. Then an additional 10µl 0.2 M NaOH is added, and the incubation is continued for another 60 minutes.

6. Nine-tenths milliliter of 0.1 M HCl is added, and the reaction solution is washed with 1 ml of toluene. The toluene phase is removed and saved for later counting.
7. NaOH, 0.90 ml, 0.1 M, and 1.0 mg sodium metabisulfite in 1.0 ml 0.5 M phosphate buffer at pH 7.0 are added to the water phase. The labeled product is then extracted with 0.5 ml toluene. After forceful shaking and phase separation, 0.25 ml of the toluene phase is removed, and the activity distribution is determined in the water phase, the toluene wash (6), and the toluene extract (7).
8. Two hundred microliters of the toluene extract are placed on a thin-layer chromatography plate (Silica gel 60, Merck A.G.) as a band 5 cm wide. The chromatogram is developed using benzene/ethanol/acetic acid (75:24:1 by volume).
9. When the solvent front has migrated 15 cm, the plate is air-dried. The radioactive band is detected with autoradiography. The thin-layer plate is placed on x-ray film for 5 minutes. Development of the film is performed immediately thereafter.
10. Testosterone-3-CMO–^{125}I-labeled histamine (R_f value = 0.35-0.40) is scraped off, and the powdered silica gel is extracted with 5 ml 99.5% ethanol. The ethanol extract is stored at −20° C.

REFERENCE

Nars, P. W., and Hunter, W. M.: A method for labelling oestradiol-17 with radioiodine for radioimmunoassays, J. Endocrinol. **57:**xlvii, 1973.

16/Labeling of proteins or polypeptides with chloramine-T method

PRINCIPLE

I$^-$ is oxidized to the reactive species I$^+$ by chloramine-T, after which the reaction is stopped by addition of the reducing agent sodium metabisulfite.

MATERIALS

1. Chloramine-T
2. Sodium metabisulfite, $Na_2S_2O_5$
3. 0.05 M phosphate buffer, pH 7.5
4. ^{125}I-NaI, specified as carrier-free and free from reducing agents
5. The protein to be labeled

PERFORMANCE

1. The protein or polypeptide to be labeled is dissolved in 0.05 M phosphate buffer, pH 7.5 (≥ 0.2 mg/ml).
2. Chloramine-T, 20 mg, is dissolved in 10.0 ml 0.05 M phosphate buffer, pH 7.5 (2.0 mg/ml). The solution is freshly prepared on the day of use.
3. Sodium bisulfite, 10 mg, is dissolved in 10 ml 0.05 M phosphate buffer, pH 7.5 (1.0 mg/ml). The solution should be freshly prepared on the day of use.

4. The iodination procedure is carried out at room temperature in an 11 × 55 mm polystyrene or glass tube. The reactants are stirred with the aid of a very small magnetic stirrer.

5. The reactants are mixed in the following order and amounts:

   a. 1.0 mCi ^{125}I-NaI (10μl-15μl)
   b. 25μl protein solution (≥ 5μg)
   c. 20μl chloramine-T (40μg)

   After a reaction time of 2-60 seconds, the reaction is stopped by the addition of:

   d. 100μl sodium metabisulfite (100μg)

6. Unreacted iodide is separated from the iodinated protein by the appropriate method (gel filtration, adsorption chromatography, dialysis; see Appendixes 19-21).

REFERENCES

Greenwood, F. C., Hunter, W. M., and Glover, J. S.: The preparation of ^{131}I-labelled human growth hormone of high specific radioactivity, Biochem. J. **89:**114, 1963.

17 / Iodination (labeling) of proteins or polypeptides with lactoperoxidase method

PRINCIPLE

Oxidation of I$^-$ to the reactive species I$^+$ is achieved by the enzyme lactoperoxidase (LPO)

MATERIALS

1. LPO, bovine; absorbance (O.D.) at 412 nm/ absorbance at 280 nm ≥ 0.8; for labeling, 2.0 mg/ml in 0.05 M phosphate buffer (pH 7.5); the mixture may be thawed and frozen several times if necessary

2. ^{125}I-NaI, specified as carrier-free and without any reducing agents, ≥ 50 mCi/ml

3. Hydrogen peroxide, 30% solution; for use in the iodination procedure dilute 1:10,000 with distilled water (0.9 mmol/liter)

4. 0.05 M phosphate buffer (pH 7.5) is used to make up the solution of the protein or polypeptide that is to be labeled

5. The protein to be labeled

PERFORMANCE

1. The protein or polypeptide to be labeled is dissolved in 0.05 M phosphate buffer at pH 7.5 (≥ 0.2 mg/ml).

2. The iodination is carried out in an 11 × 55 mm polystyrene or glass tube. The reagents are continuously mixed with a small magnet. This can be conveniently made from by cutting 1-mm pieces from a common paper clip.

3. The reagents are then added in the following order and concentrations:

   a. 1.0 mCi ^{125}I-NaI (5μl-20μl)
   b. 25μl of protein solution, ≥ 0.2 mg/ml (≥ 5μg)
   c. 2μl LPO, 2.0 mg/ml (4μg)
   d. 1μl H$_2$O$_2$, 0.03 mg/ml (0.03μg)

4. After a reaction time of only 10 s, 500μl of 0.05 M phosphate buffer (pH 7.5) is added to stop the reaction.

5. Unreacted iodide is removed from the reaction mixture by any one of a number of separation methods, such as gel filtration, dialysis, or adsorption chromatography.

6. The reaction yield is calculated by dividing the activity in the protein fraction by the total activity eluted from the column. For example, if a gel column is used to obtain a separation of a protein and a iodide fraction, the yield in the protein peak is computed by summing all the activity in the protein peak and dividing by the total activity coming from the column × 100 (%).

REFERENCES

Marchalonis, J. J.: An enzymatic method for the trace iodination of immunoglobulins and other proteins, Biochem. J. **113:**299, 1969.

Thorell, J. I., and Johansson, B. G.: Enzymatic iodination of polypeptides with ^{125}I to high specific activity, Biochim. Biophys. Acta **251:**363, 1971.

Thorell, J. I., and Johansson, B. G.: High-specific activity labelling of glycoprotein hormones by means of lactoperoxidase (LPO). In Margoulis, M., and Greenwood, F. C.: Excerpta Med. ICS **241:**531, 1972.

Von Schenck, H., Larsson, I., and Thorell, J. I.: Improved radioiodination of glucagon with the lactoperoxidase method; influence of pH on iodine substitution, Clin. Chim. Acta **69:**225, 1976.

18 / Iodination by means of polyacrylamide-coupled lactoperoxidase (solid phase enzyme)

PRINCIPLE

The enzyme lactoperoxidase is made insoluble by coupling to polyacrylamide beads. This solid phase enzyme is utilized to activate I^- to I^+ in the iodination reaction.

MATERIALS

1. LPO, absorbance at 412 nm/absorbance at 280 nm $\geq$ 0.8; 5 mg lyophilized or dissolved in 1 ml 0.1 M phosphate buffer, pH 7.7; commercially available from Sigma Chemical Co., St. Louis, Mo., or Calbiochem, La Jolla, Calif.
2. Biogel P-200, 100-200 mesh
3. Glutaraldehyde (British Drug Houses Ltd., London, England), 25% in water
4. ^{125}I-NaI, specified as carrier-free and free from reducing agents, $\geq$ 50 mCi/ml
5. Hydrogen peroxide, 30%; for use in the labeling procedure dilute 1 : 10,000 with distilled water (0.9 mmol/liter)
6. 0.1 M sodium phosphate buffers, pH 6.9 and 7.7
7. 0.05 M sodium phosphate buffer, pH 7.5

PERFORMANCE

Preparation of the insoluble peroxidase; PA-coupled LPO (PA-LPO)
1. Biogel P-200, 0.5 g, is allowed to swell in 0.1 M phosphate buffer, pH 6.9, for 24 hours (final volume of 23 ml). Then 2.8 ml 25% glutaraldehyde are added, and the mixture is allowed to react for 48 hours at 37° C in a closed vessel.
2. The gel is then washed five times with 100 ml 0.1 M phosphate buffer, pH 6.9, and ten times with 0.1 M phosphate buffer, pH 7.7, to remove all unreacted glutaraldehyde.
3. To 5.0 ml of the washed gel in a 10-ml centrifuge tube 5.0 mg LPO are added. The mixture is allowed to react for 24 hours at 4° C using any type of movement that keeps the particles in suspension, for example, vertical rotation.
4. The amount of LPO coupled to the gel is determined from the absorbance at 280 nm of the LPO solution before and after reaction with the

gel. The unreacted LPO is removed by repeated washing with 0.05 M phosphate buffer, pH 7.5. The PA-LPO is stored in 0.05 M phosphate buffer, pH 7.5, at 2°-4° C. The gel settles on the bottom of the tube. Before use, the buffer above the gel is decanted. The remaining gel has an approximate concentration of 0.02 g dry gel per milliliter.

Iodination (labeling) procedure
1. The protein to be labeled is dissolved in 0.05 M phosphate buffer, pH 7.5 ($\geq$ 0.2 mg/ml). The procedure is performed at room temperature in an 11 $\times$ 55 mm polystyrene or glass tube. The reagents are mixed continuously with a very small magnetic stirrer.
2. The reagents are added in the following order and amounts:
   a. 1.0 mCi ^{125}I-NaI (5μl-20μl)
   b. 25μl of the polypeptide or protein to be labeled ($\geq$ 5μg)
   c. 10μl PA-LPO
   d. 1μl 0.9 mM H_2O_2 (0.03μg)
3. After 60 s the reaction is stopped by addition of 500μl 0.05 M phosphate buffer. To separate the solid phase from the reaction mixture, the tube is centrifuged at 2,000g for 5 minutes. The clear solution containing the labeled protein and unreacted iodide is decanted. The unreacted iodide is removed either by dialysis or by gel filtration. To estimate the loss of activity on the PA-LPO, it is washed twice with 1 ml 0.05 M phosphate buffer, pH 7.5. The residual activity is determined, and the loss to the PA-LPO is calculated as the quotient between the residual activity and the total activity added to the reaction mixture. The yield of the iodination is calculated from the activity distribution in dialysis or gel filtration and the loss of activity retained by the PA-LPO.

REFERENCE

Thorell, J. I., and Larsson, I.: Lactoperoxidase coupled to polyacrylamide for radio-iodination of proteins to high specific activity, Immunochemistry **11**:203, 1974.

19/Separation of iodinated products from unreacted iodide using gel filtration

PRINCIPLE

Gel filtration by Sephadex G-25 may be used to separate molecules on the basis of their size. Large molecules (such as proteins) pass rapidly through the column, and small molecules (such as iodide) pass more slowly.

MATERIALS

1. Sephadex G-25 (fine) (Pharmacia, Uppsala, Sweden)
2. Barbital buffer, 0.075 M (pH 8.6), containing 0.05% sodium azide (which serves as a preservative); any common buffer of midrange pH may be used
3. Bovine serum albumin, 2%, in barbital buffer

PERFORMANCE

1. Sephadex G-25 (fine), 3 g, is preswollen overnight in 25 ml 0.075 M barbital buffer. A 15 × 1 cm gel column is packed inside a 30 × 1 cm chromatography column.
2. One milliliter 2% BSA in barbital buffer is passed over the column in order to minimize adsorption of the labeled substance to the column. The excess albumin is washed from the column with 4 × 10 ml barbital buffer.
3. After the last wash has gone into the gel, the reaction solution, containing the iodinated material and unreacted iodide, is placed on top of the gel bed. When it has sunk into the gel, the column is carefully filled with barbital buffer, which will elute the material from the column. Additional buffer is added if necessary.
4. One-milliliter fractions are collected in 11 × 55 mm test tubes to which 1.0-ml aliquots of 2% BSA in barbital buffer have been previously added. About 25 fractions are collected.
5. The relative distribution of activity in the fractions is measured by counting at an appropriate distance from the crystal of a gamma counter. Because the radioactivity is relatively high, this may be readily accomplished with a simple probe-type counter positioned at some distance from the sample to be measured.
6. The yield of the iodination reaction may be calculated from the activity in the protein peak (the first eluted peak) and the activity in the iodide peak (the last eluted peak). This gives a relative estimate of yield that is adequate for most purposes. The absolute amount of eluted activity may be measured by counting a measured aliquot of the fractions in a gamma counter of known efficiency.

20/Separation of iodinated products from iodide using adsorption chromatography with cellulose

PRINCIPLE

Certain polypeptides have a very high affinity for cellulose. This property can be used for separation and purification of reaction products after radioiodination. The reaction solution is applied to a cellulose column to which the reactive polypeptide adsorbs. Unreacted iodide is not adsorbed and is washed out with buffer. Weakly adsorbed, denatured polypeptide is eluted from the column with 0.1% albumin. The purified iodinated product is eluted with a 1% albumin and 20% acetone solution.

MATERIALS

1. Cellulose powder, Whatman CF 11

2. 0.075 M barbital buffer (pH 8.6) with 0.05% sodium azide
3. 0.075 M barbital buffer (pH 8.6) with 0.05% sodium azide and 0.1% bovine serum albumin
4. 0.075 M barbital buffer (pH 8.6) with 0.05% sodium azide, 1% BSA, and 20% acetone

PERFORMANCE

1. A 2 × 1 cm column is packed with dry cellulose powder. A disposable 5-ml syringe with a small pad of glass fiber placed above the outlet can be used as the column.
2. Four milliliters of barbital buffer are passed

through the column. The reaction solution is then placed on the column.

3. Elution of the column is thereafter performed as follows:

   a. 3 × 4.0 ml 0.075 M barbital buffer with 0.05% sodium azide is passed through the column; this eluate is collected in one volume (fraction I)

   b. 3 × 4.0 ml 0.075 M barbital buffer with 0.05% sodium azide and 0.1% BSA is passed through the column; this eluate is fraction II.

   c. 2 × 2 ml 0.075 M barbital buffer with 0.05% sodium azide, 1% BSA, and 20% acetone are passed over the column; the eluate is collected in two fractions of 2 ml each (III and IV).

   d. The distribution of activity is measured in fractions I, II, III, and IV. Fraction IV contains the most pure and undegraded radioiodinated polypeptide. Store at −20° C.

21 / Separation of iodinated products from iodide by dialysis

PRINCIPLE

The mixture of iodinated material and unreacted iodide is placed within a dialysis membrane in contact with buffer. The iodide follows a diffusion gradient out of the dialysis bag, but the larger iodinated molecules cannot penetrate the pores of the membrane and thus are retained within the bag.

MATERIALS

1. Dialysis tubing (Visking), 20-mm width, 24-Å pore diameter
2. 0.05 M phosphate buffer, pH 7.5
3. Anion exchange resin (Amberlite IRA 401)

PERFORMANCE

1. A 15-cm long dialysis tube is soaked in 0.05 M phosphate buffer (pH 7.5) for 1 hour. One end is closed with a knot. The other end is closed by inserting a 10-mm diameter rubber stopper through which a cannula is placed. The tubing is tied to the stopper with a string. A string is fastened to the upper end that will later be used to suspend the bag within the beaker.

A small weight may be needed at the lower end.

2. The solution to be dialyzed is taken up into a 1-ml disposable syringe (Mantoux type) and injected via the cannula into the dialysis bag.

3. The dialysis bag is immersed into 1,000 ml of 0.05 M phosphate buffer (pH 7.5) containing about 1 g of Amberlite IRA 401. The buffer is continuously stirred for 30 minutes. The ion exchanger will take up the iodide passing out of the bag and thus maintain a high concentration gradient of iodide over the membrane.

4. The dialysis buffer is changed after 30 and 60 minutes.

5. The dialysis is almost completed after 2 hours; thus any additional effect of a more extended dialysis is small.

6. Calculation of the yield is determined by measuring the activity in the dialysis bag before and after dialysis. The dialyzed labeled substance is removed from the dialysis bag with a 1-ml syringe.

22/Purification of radioiodinated material on QUSO G-32

PRINCIPLE

Some polypeptides (such as calcitonin) have a very high affinity for QUSO silica G-32 and adsorb in the presence of whole serum. Denatured calcitonin is not adsorbed but is bound to serum albumin. After labeled calcitonin is adsorbed to QUSO and denatured material is washed away, the ^{125}I-calcitonin is extracted with a hydrochloric acid/acetone solution.

MATERIALS

1. QUSO silica G-32 (Philadelphia Quartz Co.)
2. Normal human serum
3. 0.01 M HCl with 10% acetone

PERFORMANCE

1. ^{125}I-calcitonin solution (which may have been prepurified by separation on Sephadex G-25),

200μl, is mixed with 1.0 ml normal human serum.
2. QUSO, 40 mg, is added, and the mixture is agitated. The solution is centrifuged and decanted (the supernatant is discarded).
3. The absorbent is washed with 2.0 ml distilled water. ^{125}I-calcitonin is then extracted from the QUSO with 1.0 ml 0.01 M HCl with 10% acetone.
4. The extract is diluted with the buffer used in the RIA system and stored at $-20°$ C.

REFERENCE

Yalow, R. S., and Berson, S. A.: Purification of ^{131}I parathyroid hormone with microfine granules of precipitated silica, Nature **212:**357, 1966.

23/Purification of monoiodoangiotensin

PRINCIPLE

The difference in pK_a between tyrosine, monoiodotyrosine, and diiodotyrosine in the angiotensin peptide chain gives the angiotensin, monoiodoangiotensin, and diiodoangiotensin different affinities for an anion exchanger. At the appropriate pH they may be eluted in the order mentioned from a DEAE Sephadex column.

MATERIALS

1. DEAE Sephadex A-25
2. Phosphate buffer, 0.1 M, pH 8.0
3. Human serum albumin
4. 0.05 M phosphate buffer, pH 7.4, with 0.5% HSA and 0.25% EDTA
5. Chromatography column, 40 × 1 cm (pump and fraction collector facilitates the separation)

PERFORMANCE

1. DEAE Sephadex A-25, 10 g, is permitted to swell overnight in 0.1 M phosphate buffer, pH 8.0, and is equilibrated with this buffer.

2. It is packed into a 25 × 1 cm column. A flow of 1 ml/min of the same buffer is applied.
3. The mixture of angiotensin and iodoangiotensin is applied to the column. Angiotensin I is iodinated with an excess of angiotensin— 50μg of angiotensin instead of the 5μg of protein as given in the Method section of Chapter 13.
4. The material is eluted with 0.1 M phosphate buffer, pH 8.0; 1-ml fractions are collected in tubes containing the phosphate buffer HSA-EDTA solution. The unlabeled angiotensin comes first out of the column. The first radioactive peak eluted (approximately fractions 30-40) contains monoiodinated angiotensin I.

REFERENCE

Nielsen, M. D., Jörgensen, M., and Giese, J.: ^{125}I-labelling of angiotensin I and II, Acta Endocrinol. **67:**104, 1971.

24/Ethanol precipitation of antibody-bound radioactivity applied to an insulin assay

PRINCIPLE

The immunoglobulins are precipitated with 70% ethanol. To achieve identical protein concentrations in all tubes, plasma is added to standard tubes.

MATERIALS

1. Same reagents as in the primary step of the insulin assay (see Box 15-1), distributed in tubes that have been incubated in a refrigerator overnight to achieve a distribution of ^{125}I-insulin between antibody-bound and free forms
2. 99% ethanol

PERFORMANCE

1. Pipette 0.1 ml of a plasma pool (low insulin concentration) into all standard tubes.
2. To compensate for the increase in volume, pipette 0.1 ml of the buffer-diluent used (barbital buffer) into all sample tubes.
3. Rapidly pipette 1.5 ml ethanol into all tubes

(Cornwall-type syringe). The ethanol should be added forcefully so that it mixes immediately with the incubate.
4. Cap tubes.
5. Mix contents in a vortex mixer.
6. Centrifuge at 2,000g for 15 minutes.
7. Decant supernatant carefully.
8. Count tubes with precipitate.

REFERENCES

Chard, T., Martin, M., and Landon, J.: The separation of antibody bound from free peptides using ammonium sulphate and ethanol. In Kirkham, K. E., and Hunter, W. M. editors: Radioimmunoassay methods, Edinburgh, 1971, Churchill Livingstone, pp. 257-266.

Heding, L. G.: A simplified insulin radioimmunoassay method. In Danato, L., Milhaud, G., and Sirchis, J., editors: Labelled proteins in tracer studies (proceedings of the conference held at Pisa, January 17-19, 1966, European Atomic Energy), Brussels, 1966, Eurotom, pp. 345-350.

25/Ammonium sulfate precipitation of antibody-bound radioactivity applied to a testosterone assay

PRINCIPLE

IgG with bound radioligand is precipitated with 50% ammonium sulfate.

MATERIALS

1. Same as in the primary step of the testosterone assay (see Box 10-5), distributed in tubes that have been incubated in refrigerator to achieve distribution of testosterone-3-^{125}I-histamine between bound and free forms (PBS-BSA, 0.1%, is used as diluent instead of PBS-gelatin, 0.1%)
2. Ammonium sulfate (saturated solution in water)

PERFORMANCE

1. Pipette 500μl ammonium sulfate solution into all tubes.

2. Mix contents in a vortex mixer.
3. Incubate all tubes 10 minutes at 4° C.
4. Centrifuge at 2,500g for 15 minutes at 4° C.
5. Decant supernatant into a new series of tubes.
6. Count tubes with supernatant.

REFERENCES

Castro, A., Shih, H., and Chung, A.: A direct plasma testosterone radioimmunoassay, Experientia **29:**1447, 1973.

Chard, T., Martin, M., and Landon, J.: The separation of antibody-bound from free peptides using ammonium sulphate and ethanol. In Kirkham, K. E., and Hunter, W. M. editors: Radioimmunoassay methods, Edinburgh, 1971, Churchill Livingstone, pp. 257-266.

Forti, G., Pazzagli, M., Calabresi, E., Fiorelli, G., and Serio, M.: Radioimmunoassay of plasma testosterone, J. Clin. Endocrinol. Metab. **3:**5, 1974.

26/Polyethylene glycol precipitation of antibody-bound radioactivity applied to a thyroxine assay

PRINCIPLE

IgG is precipitated with 15% polyethylene glycol.

MATERIALS

1. Reagents used in the primary step of the thyroxine assay (see Box 8-2), distributed in tubes that have been incubated in the refrigerator overnight to achieve distribution of ^{125}I-thyroxine between antibody-bound and free forms
2. Polyethylene glycol 6000, 21.7% (v/v) in water

PERFORMANCE

1. Pipette 1 ml polyethylene glycol into all tubes (fixed-volume manual pipette, Eppendorf type).

2. Mix contents in a vortex mixer.
3. Centrifuge at 2,500g, 4° C, for 15 minutes.
4. Decant supernatant carefully.
5. Count tubes with precipitate.

REFERENCES

Cheung, M. C., and Slaunwhite, W. R.: Use of polyethylene glycol in separating bound from unbound ligand in radioimmunoassay of thyroxine, Clin. Chem. **22**:299, 1976.

Desbuquois, B., and Aurbach, G. D.: Use of polyethylene glycol to separate free and antibody-bound peptide hormones in radioimmunoassays, J. Clin. Endocrinol. Metab. **33**:732, 1971.

27/Dextran-coated charcoal adsorption of free radioactivity applied to an estradiol assay or a T$_4$ assay

PRINCIPLE

Free estradiol is adsorbed to dextran-coated charcoal, whereas antibody-bound estradiol remains in solution.

MATERIALS

1. Same as in the primary step of the estradiol assay (see Box 10-3), distributed in tubes that have been incubated to achieve distribution of estradiol-6-^{125}I-histamine between antibody-bound and free forms
2. Dextran, 0.25 mg/ml, and charcoal, 2.5 mg/ml, in phosphate-gelatin buffer (for estradiol assay) or dextran, 0.6 mg/ml, and charcoal, 6 mg/ml, in barbital-BSA (for T$_4$ assay)

PERFORMANCE

1. Pipette 0.5 ml cold dextran-charcoal suspension into all tubes (with a manual fixed-volume Eppendorf-type pipette). The dextran-charcoal solution must be continuously stirred with a magnetic stirrer. The time elapsed between the

addition to the first and the last tube of the series should not exceed 10 minutes.
2. Mix contents in a vortex mixer.
3. Incubate all tubes 10 minutes at 4° C.
4. Centrifuge at 2,500g, 4° C for 15 minutes.
5. Decant supernatant into other tubes (disposable plastic tubes).
6. Count tubes with supernatant.

The following modifications are necessary when the method is applied to a T$_4$ assay:

1. Pipette 1 ml dextran-charcoal into all tubes.
2. Incubate tubes for 10-60 min at 4° C. (These two steps are frequently modified in relation to the properties of the charcoal-ligand interaction of other ligands.) It is important that all the tubes be incubated for the same time period.

REFERENCE

Herbert, V., Lau, K. S., Gottlieb, C. W., and Bleicher, S. J.: Coated charcoal immunoassay of insulin, J. Clin. Endocrinol. Metab. **25**:1375, 1965.

28/ Second-antibody precipitation of antibody-bound radioactivity applied to an hLH assay

PRINCIPLE

Rabbit IgG is precipitated with goat antiserum to rabbit IgG. This antiserum is sensitive to the effect of plasma; thus plasma is added to all standards.

MATERIALS

1. Same as in the primary step of the hLH assay (see Box 10-2), distributed in tubes that have been incubated (in the refrigerator for 3 days) to achieve distribution of ^{125}I-hLH between antibody-bound and free forms
2. Barbital buffer with 0.25% BSA, or any other common buffer at midrange pH
3. Normal human plasma
4. Normal rabbit serum (NRS, 1:250 in barbital-BSA)
5. Goat antiserum to rabbit IgG (1:10 in barbital-BSA)

PERFORMANCE

1. Pipette 0.1 ml normal human plasma into all standard tubes.
2. To compensate for the increase in volume of the standards, pipette 0.1 ml barbital-BSA into all sample tubes.
3. Pipette 0.05 ml NRS (1:250) and 0.05 ml goat antiserum to rabbit IgG (1:10) into all tubes. An alternative is to use NRS (1:250) and goat antiserum to rabbit IgG (1:10) in 1:1 proportions. Pipette 0.1 ml of this mixture into all tubes. We have found that the precipitate develops so slowly that the antiserum and the NRS may be mixed before if the assay series is not too long, which saves one pipetting operation. However, possible effects of this simplification should be tested in the individual assay system.
4. Incubate tubes overnight at 4° C.
5. Add 0.5 ml barbital-BSA (with semiautomated dispenser syringe Cornwall type).
6. Centrifuge at 2,500g 4° C, for 15 minutes.
7. Decant supernatant carefully.
8. Count tubes with precipitate.

REFERENCES

Hales, C. N., and Randle, P. J.: Immunoassay of insulin with insulin antibody precipitate, Biochem. J. **88**:137, 1963.

Morgan, C. R., and Lazarow, A.: Immunoassay of insulin using a two-antibody system, Proc. Soc. Exp. Biol. Med. **110**:29, 1962.

29/ Double-antibody production and testing

PRINCIPLE

Rabbit IgG is isolated by anion exchange chromatography. IgG is emulsified with Freund's adjuvant and injected monthly into goats. The precipitation capability of the antiserum is tested with a rabbit FSH antiserum that has been preincubated with ^{125}I-FSH.

MATERIALS

For immunization

1. Rabbit IgG prepared according to Appendix 33; the IgG solution in 0.02 M phosphate buffer, pH 6.6, from the DEAE Sephadex column may be used directly; 10 mg IgG are needed for each immunization
2. Freund complete adjuvant (Difco)

For testing antiserum

1. Normal rabbit serum (used to increase the concentration of rabbit IgG to an optimal level when the primary antiserum is highly diluted)
2. Rabbit antiserum to hFSH
3. ^{125}I-hFSH, $120\mu Ci$-$160\mu Ci/\mu g$
4. Barbital buffer, 0.075 M, pH 8.6, containing 0.25% BSA and 0.05% sodium azide (BBSA)
5. Barbital buffer, 0.075 M, pH 8.6, containing 0.25% BSA, 0.05% sodium azide, and 0.25% EDTA (BBSA-EDTA)
6. Normal human EDTA-plasma

PERFORMANCE

Immunization

1. Rabbit IgG, 10 mg, in 2-3 ml phosphate buffer

is emulsified with an equal volume of Freund complete adjuvant. A very thick emulsion may be prepared by using two 10-ml glass syringes as described in Appendix 1. The contents are pumped back and forth until the mixture is very thick. It takes about 5 minutes to achieve a good emulsion.

2. The emulsion is injected subcutaneously in four to six places on the back of the goat.
3. The immunization is repeated monthly until the goat produces an antiserum that, according to the testing procedure, can be diluted at least 1:10 in a double-antibody RIA.

Collecting antisera

1. Whole blood, 300 ml, is taken at 2-week intervals without any additives. The serum is separated and frozen.

Testing antiserum

The precipitation capability of the antiserum is tested by using a standard RIA system, exemplified here by an assay for hFSH (any working RIA system can be used).

1. ^{125}I-hFSH is diluted in BBSA-EDTA to 50,000 cpm/ml (approximately 0.25 ng/ml).
2. Rabbit antiserum to hFSH is diluted in BBSA to the usual dilution for RIA of hFSH. Normal rabbit serum is diluted 1:250 with the same buffer. Of the antiserum to be tested, serial dilutions are made up (for example, 1:2.5, 1:5, 1:10, 1:20, and 1:40) using BBSA.
3. Two hundred microliters ^{125}I-hFSH (approximately 50 pg and 10,000 cpm) are incubated

with 200μl antiserum to hFSH at 4°-8° C for 1-3 days. Ten to fifteen tubes are set up. Then 50μl normal rabbit serum dilution (1:250) and 100μl normal human plasma are added to all tubes. Fifty microliters of the antiserum to be tested are added in duplicate or triplicate tubes of each dilution.

4. After incubation for 1 day at 4°-8° C, 500μl of BBSA are added to all tubes.
5. The tubes are centrifuged at 2,500g for 15 minutes.
6. The tubes are decanted, and the precipitated activity is measured in a gamma counter. The precipitated activity is plotted against the dilution of the antiserum tested. A typical result is shown in Fig. 4-2. The antiserum should be used at a dilution where the precipitated activity is relatively independent of its dilution, that is, where the precipitated activity shows a plateau. The antiserum tested in Fig. 4-2 is used in 1:10 dilution.

REMARKS

Precipitating characteristics are generally different in the presence and the absence of human plasma or serum. In double-antibody RIAs it is usually necessary to compensate for this phenomenon. Just before the precipitation step, normal human plasma or serum is added to the standards if they are contained in a buffer diluent. The same volume of diluent is added to the samples to equalize the volumes.

30 / Coupling of antibody to solid phase

Polyacrylamide matrix (Biogel P-200)

PRINCIPLE

The bifunctional reagent glutaraldehyde is reacted with the amido-NH$_2$ groups in polyacrylamide gel. Excess unreacted glutaraldehyde is then removed, and free primary amino groups in the antibody protein are allowed to react with the free aldehyde group of the bound glutaraldehyde.

MATERIALS

1. Biogel P-200 polyacrylamide beads
2. Bovine serum albumin
3. Glutaraldehyde, 50% solution
4. 0.1 M phosphate buffer, pH 6.9

5. 0.1 M phosphate buffer, pH 7.7
6. Immunoglobulin, 10 mg/ml, in 0.1 M phosphate buffer, pH 7.7.

PERFORMANCE

1. Biogel P-200, 0.5 g, is allowed to swell in 0.1 M phosphate buffer (pH 6.9) for 24 hours. The volume is adjusted to 25 ml.
2. Glutaraldehyde, 1.4 ml, 50%, is added to the solution and allowed to react for 48 hours at 37° C in a closed vessel.
3. Then the gel is washed five times with 100 ml of 0.1 M phosphate buffer at pH 6.9 and ten

times with 100 ml of 0.1 M phosphate buffer at pH 7.7.

4. The antibody solution is then added to the activated gel in proportions of about 5 mg immunoglobulin per 0.1 g of dry gel or to 5 ml of the gel suspension.

5. The mixture is reacted for 24-48 hours at 4° C with continuous end-over-end rotation, so that the polyacrylamide beads remain suspended in the solution. (Magnetic stirrers must be used with great care to avoid fragmentation of the gel beads.)

6. Then the gel is washed with 5×50 ml 0.1 M phosphate buffer (pH 7.7) containing 0.1 M glycine. Next the gel is washed with 5×50 ml 0.1 M phosphate buffer containing 0.25% BSA and 0.1% sodium azide.

7. The polyacrylamide-coupled antibody is stored suspended in this buffer at 2°-4° C.

REFERENCE

Weston, P. D., and Avrameas, S.: Proteins coupled to polyacrylamide beads using glutaraldehyde, Biochem. Biophys. Res. Commun. **45:**1574, 1971.

31/Coupling of antibody to solid phase

Sepharose matrix

PRINCIPLE

Cyanogen-bromide-activated Sepharose 4B is reacted with primary amino groups of the immunoglobulin, such as the epsilon amino group in lysine, to produce a Sepharose-coupled antibody complex.

MATERIALS

1. CNBr-activated Sepharose 4B, (Pharmacia, Uppsala, Sweden)
2. Immunoglobulin, approximately 10 mg/ml in 0.1 M NaHCO$_3$
3. 0.1 M NaHCO$_3$ and 0.5 M NaCl
4. 0.001 M HCl
5. 0.1 M acetate (pH 4.0) and 1.0 M NaCl buffer
6. 0.1 M borate (pH 8.0) and 1.0 M NaCl buffer
7. 1 M ethanolamine (pH 8.0)
8. 0.05 M phosphate buffer, pH 7.5, containing 0.25% BSA and 0.1% sodium azide

PERFORMANCE

1. CNBr-activated Sepharose, 1 g, is swollen and washed for 15 minutes on a glass filter with 200 ml of 0.001 M HCl.
2. The immunoglobulin antibody solution (10 mg IgG in 1 ml of 0.1 M NaHCO$_3$) is diluted with 5 ml 0.1 M NaHCO$_3$ containing 0.5 M NaCl. The washed gel is added to this solution in a 15-ml test tube.

3. The solution is rotated end over end for 2 hours at room temperature or 18 hours at 4° C.
4. Uncoupled immunoglobulin is washed away with the coupling buffer (0.1 M NaHCO$_3$ containing 0.5 M NaCl).
5. To neutralize the remaining activated groups of the Sepharose, the solution is reacted with 1 M ethanolamine (pH 8.0) for 1-2 hours.
6. To remove noncovalently adsorbed immunoglobulin, the Sepharose beads are washed with 0.1 M acetate buffer (pH 4.0) containing 1 M NaCl, followed by washing with 0.1 M borate buffer (pH 8.0) with 1 M NaCl. This washing procedure is repeated three times.
7. The Sepharose-coupled antibody is suspended in 0.05 M phosphate buffer (pH 7.5) with 0.25% BSA and 0.1% sodium azide and stored at 2°-4° C.

REFERENCES

Axén, R., Porath, J., and Ernback, S.: Chemical coupling of peptides and proteins to polysaccharides by cyanogen halides, Nature **214:**1302, 1967.

Pharmacia Fine Chemicals A.B.: Affinity chromatography; principles and methods, 1976, Uppsala, Sweden.

Wide, L., Axén, R., and Porath, J.: Radioimmunosorbent assay for proteins; chemical couplings of antibodies to insoluble dextran, Immunochemistry **4:**381, 1967.

32/ Isolation of immunoglobulin from serum by ammonium sulfate precipitation

PRINCIPLE

Immunoglobulin is precipitated by 33% saturated ammonium sulfate.

MATERIALS

1. Ammonium sulfate (NH_4SO_4), saturated solution at 20° C in distilled water
2. 0.1 M sodium bicarbonate ($NaHCO_3$)

PERFORMANCE

1. Add drop by drop 0.5 ml of the saturated NH_4SO_4 to 1.0 ml serum.
2. The solution is mixed gently overnight.
3. Centrifuge for 15 minutes at 2,500g. Decant supernatant.
4. The precipitate is dissolved in 1 ml of 0.1 M $NaHCO_3$ and dialyzed against 2 liters of 0.1 M $NaHCO_3$ for 24 hours.
5. The protein concentration is determined by measuring the absorbance at 280 nm.

33/ Isolation of immunoglobulin from serum by DEAE Sephadex

PRINCIPLE

Reactive cationic functional groups on DEAE Sephadex are used to bind the (predominantly) negatively charged nonimmunoglobulin proteins. The isoelectric point of IgG is sufficiently high so that IgG carries a predominantly positive charge at pH 6.6 and thus passes through the column.

MATERIALS

1. DEAE Sephadex A-50 (Pharmacia Fine Chemicals, Uppsala, Sweden)
2. 0.02 M phosphate buffer, pH 6.6
3. Serum (for example, rabbit serum for production of rabbit IgG antibodies in a double-antibody method)

PERFORMANCE

1. DEAE Sephadex A-50, 5 g, is swollen in 2 liters of 0.02 M phosphate buffer at pH 6.6 overnight. The buffer is then decanted, and another 2 liters of the same buffer are added.

After mixing, the gel is allowed to sediment. The buffer is then decanted, and the same procedure is repeated two times.

2. The gel is transferred to a 25 × 500 mm glass or plastic column in which a gel column 25 × 250 mm is packed.
3. Two hundred milliliters of 0.02 M phosphate buffer (pH 6.6) are passed through the column.
4. Serum, 20 ml, and 20 ml of phosphate buffer are mixed and filtered. The filtrate is added to the column, followed by elution with 0.02 M phosphate buffer (pH 6.6). Ten-milliliter fractions are collected (20-30 fractions). The immunoglobulins pass through the column first, and the concentration of protein in each fraction is determined by measuring absorbance at 280 nm.
5. The purity of various fractions can be verified through agarose gel electrophoresis. The immunoglobulin peak is the first protein peak and usually occurs between fractions 10-20.

34 / Buffers and diluents

Phosphate buffer, 0.05 M, pH 7.5

$Na_2HPO_4 \cdot 2H_2O$, 8.90 g, is dissolved in 500-900 ml distilled water (may need slight heating). After being dissolved, the volume is filled up to 1,000 ml with distilled water (I).

$NaH_2PO_4 \cdot 2H_2O$, 1.95 g, is dissolved in approximately 200 ml distilled water and after being dissolved is filled up to 250 ml (II).

The pH of solution I is adjusted to 7.5 by addition of solution II. The pH meter should previously have been calibrated with a buffer with an exactly known pH.

Phosphate-buffered saline (PBS) (phosphate buffer, 0.01 M, pH 7.0; 0.9% [0.15 M] NaCl; 0.02% sodium merthiolate as preservative)

$Na_2HPO_4 \cdot 2H_2O$, 1.78 g, is dissolved in distilled water (see above) and filled up to 1,000 ml (I).

$NaH_2PO_4 \cdot 2H_2O$, 1.56 g, is dissolved in distilled water and filled to 1,000 ml (II).

The pH of solution I is adjusted to 7.0 by addition of solution II (see above).

NaCl, 9.0 g, and 0.2 g sodium merthiolate are dissolved in about 900 ml of the 0.01 M phosphate buffer. When dissolved, the volume is filled up to 1,000 ml with the same buffer. Check pH and adjust if necessary to 7.0 with 1 M NaOH.

Barbital (barbitone, veronal) buffer, 0.075 M, pH 8.6, with 0.05% sodium azide as preservative

Barbital, 2.07 g, is dissolved by careful heating in 500 ml of distilled water. Sodium barbital, 13.14 g, and 0.5 g sodium azide are dissolved in 400 ml distilled water. The two solutions are mixed, and the volume is adjusted to 1,000 ml with distilled water.

The pH is measured. If necessary, adjust pH to 8.6 with 1 M NaOH.

Glycine buffer, 0.2 M, pH 8.8, with 0.02% merthiolate as preservative

Glycine, 15.0 g, and 0.2 g sodium merthiolate are dissolved in about 900 ml distilled water. After dissolving, the volume is made up to 950 ml. The pH is adjusted to 8.8 by addition of 1 M NaOH. Then the volume is adjusted to 1,000 ml with distilled water.

Tris-HCl buffer, 0.05 M, pH 7.5, with 0.05% sodium azide as preservative

Tris(hydroxymethyl)aminomethane, 6.06 g, is dissolved in 950 ml distilled water. Adjust pH to 7.5 with 1 M HCl by means of a calibrated pH meter.

Sodium azide, 0.5 g, is added. The solution is made up to 1,000 ml with distilled water.

Acetate buffer, 0.1 M, pH 4.0

$C_2H_3NaO_2 \cdot 3H_2O$, 13.61 g, is dissolved in distilled water and then filled up to 1,000 ml. The pH is adjusted to 4.0 with 0.1 M acetic acid.

Bicarbonate buffer, 0.1 M, pH 9.6

$NaHCO_3$, 8.4 g, is dissolved in 900 ml of distilled water. The pH is adjusted to 9.6 with 1 M NaOH. The volume is adjusted to 1,000 ml with distilled water.

Adsorption-preventive agents that may be used in buffers described above

Bovine serum albumin, 0.1%-1.0%; we use 0.25% (2.5 g/liter) BSA in our usual diluents
Human serum albumin, 0.1%-1.0%
Gelatin, 0.1%

35 / Preparation of triiodothyronine (T_3)- and thyroxine (T_4)-free serum

PRINCIPLE

T_3 and T_4 are dissociated from the binding proteins in serum by increasing the pH of the serum to 10.8. Then T_3 and T_4 are removed by passage of the serum through an anion exchange column (QAE Sephadex). The pH of the serum is readjusted to 7.4. The effectiveness of the adsorption is determined by the addition of tracer amounts of ^{125}I-T_3 and ^{131}I-T_4 to the serum.

MATERIALS

1. QAE Sephadex A-25 (Pharmacia, Uppsala, Sweden)
2. 1 M NaOH

3. 1 M HCl
4. ^{131}I-L-thyroxine, specific activity $\geq 50\mu$Ci/μg
5. ^{125}I-L-3,5,3'-triiodothyronine, specific activity $\geq 500\mu$Ci/μg
6. 100 ml normal human serum

PERFORMANCE

1. Fifteen grams QAE Sephadex are swollen in distilled water. The pH is adjusted to 10.8 with NaOH. Two 85 × 25 mm columns are prepared.
2. The pH of 100 ml of serum is adjusted to 10.8 with 1 M NaOH. ^{131}I-T$_4$, 2μCi, and 1μCi ^{125}I-T$_3$ are added to the serum and well mixed. One milliliter of serum is saved for measurement of total added activity.
3. The serum is passed through column 1. The serum remaining in the gel when all of the serum

has passed into the gel is eluted with 20 ml distilled water.
4. The eluate from the first column is then passed through the second column, and the procedure is repeated in exactly the same manner as for column 1. An aliquot of the final eluate from column 2, is taken to determine the amount of ^{131}I-T$_4$ and ^{125}I-T$_3$ activity. The remaining activity should be less than 1% of the original activity.
5. The pH of the T$_3$- and T$_4$-free serum is adjusted to 7.4 with 1 M HCl.

REFERENCE

Burger, A., Sakoloff, C., Stachely, V., Vallotton, M. B., and Ingbar, S. H.: Radioimmunoassay of 3,5,3'-triiodo-l-thyronine with and without a prior extraction step, Acta Endocrinol. (Kbh.) **80:**58, 1975.

36 / Preparation of T$_3$- and T$_4$-free serum by adsorption to activated charcoal

PRINCIPLE

T$_3$ and T$_4$ dissociate from binding proteins in serum and are adsorbed to activated charcoal if the activated charcoal is present in excess. The effectiveness of the adsorption is determined by the addition of tracer amounts of ^{125}I-T$_3$ and ^{131}I-T$_4$ to the serum.

MATERIALS

1. Activated charcoal (Norit decolorizing charcoal)
2. 100 ml normal human serum
3. L-thyroxine (T$_4$) labeled with ^{131}I, specific activity $\geq 50\mu$Ci/μg
4. L-3,5,3'-triiodothyronine, specific activity $\geq 500\mu$Ci/μg

PERFORMANCE

1. To 100 ml serum 2μCi ^{131}I-T$_4$ and 1μCi ^{125}I-T$_3$ are added. A sample is obtained for count-

ing total activity. Fifteen grams of activated charcoal are added.
2. The serum is incubated for 12 hours at 4° C with stirring. Then the charcoal is separated from the serum by centrifugation at 25,000g for 1 hour, with removal of the serum. The serum is centrifuged three more times in the same manner.
3. The remaining ^{131}I-T$_4$ and ^{125}I-T$_3$ activity is measured and should be less than 1% of the original activity.

REFERENCE

Larson, P. R., Dockalova, J., Sipula, D., and Wu, F. M.: Immunoassay of thyroxine in unextracted human serum, J. Clin. Endocrinol. Metab. **37:**177, 1973.

37/Energy calibration of gamma counters

PRINCIPLE

If one knows the correct photopeak energy of a radionuclide and adjusts the gain controls on the gamma spectrometer, it is possible to calibrate the baseline and window settings of a gamma spectrometer in terms of kilo electron-volts (keV) of energy.

MATERIALS

1. Radionuclide sources (preferably ^{125}I, 28 keV; ^{57}Co, 122 keV; ^{131}I, 364 keV, and/or ^{137}Cs, 667 keV); ideally, these sources should give about 10^6 counts per minute when the window is wide open and the baseline is set so that background is less than 1,000 counts per minute (above the noise level)
2. Gamma counter with capability for differential gamma spectroscopy

PERFORMANCE

1. Energy resolution depends on the high voltage applied to the photomultiplier tube. Most modern counters have a recommended high-voltage range for best performance of the photomultiplier tube. This can be used as a starting point for the energy calibration.
2. A small window is set (10 divisions of the 1,000 scale). The baseline is also set to 10. A source of radionuclide is placed in the detector. For example, cobalt 57 may be used for this purpose. Counts are recorded for a short time period, for example, 0.1-0.3 minutes, depending on the count rate (1,000 net cpm). The count rate is recorded as a function of the baseline settings. The baseline is rapidly moved over a spectrum, and a rough plot is made at various baseline settings, such as 10, 50, 100, 150, and 200, and the count rate recorded (it is important to remember that the average energy will be given by the baseline setting plus one half of the window width). If the peak in count rate for ^{57}Co is observed at a scale reading above the expected energy level, the gain must be reduced. However, if the scale reading at which the peak counts are seen is below the energy level, the gain must be increased.
3. The scale is then set with a baseline that is 5 keV below the expected peak of the isotope. For ^{57}Co, this is 122 keV. The window is set at 10 keV. The gain (fine setting) is adjusted upward or downward, and the count rate is noted. Frequently it is possible merely to visually

evaluate the approximate count rate in the window as a function of gain settings. When one has ascertained the approximate range of the gain settings to be used to give the maximum counts in the window, it is usually wise to make a rough plot of gain (x-axis) versus count rate (y-axis). At the point where the count is maximal, the gain setting is noted and recorded. At this gain setting the gamma counter is "peaked in," that is, energy-calibrated.

4. It is usually wise to calibrate the machine using isotopes of several energy levels, such as ^{131}I (364 keV) and ^{137}Cs (667 keV). Although most modern equipment is linear over the range of 0-1,000 divisions on the baseline and window scale, the machine calibration for ^{125}I should be checked to make sure that activity near the photopeak is being counted (see step 6 below). When the scale number of the baseline setting corresponds to the isotope energy, the scale is calibrated for 0-1 meV.
5. On occasion it is necessary to count gamma-emitting radionuclides that have photopeak energies greater than 1.0 meV, such as ^{59}Fe (1.1 and 1.3 meV). As a first step, the calibration may be readily changed by gain adjustments that cut the gain in half (there is a switch on most gamma counters that accomplishes this). This can then be checked by using the same procedure as in step 3 above. In this case, however, the scale reading will correspond to exactly one half of the photopeak energy. For ^{137}Cs, this will be 333. For ^{59}Fe the two peaks should appear at 550 and 650, respectively.
6. Calibration of ^{125}I is usually checked as follows. A counter that has previously been calibrated for 0-1 meV is used, and the baseline is set at 10 and the window at 5 keV. Counts are obtained at baseline settings of 10 to 100 in steps of 5 keV, and a plot of count rate versus energy (baseline setting + 2-5 keV or ½ window) is made. A peak in count rate should be observed near 27 keV. The machine is then calibrated for accurate counting of ^{125}I.
7. ^{129}I ($T_{1/2} = 1.6 \times 10^7$ years) is close enough in energy (29 keV) to ^{125}I to be useful as a convenient means for checking counter performance and proper calibration for ^{125}I counting. The count rate should be identical from day to day. A change in ^{129}I standard count rate means that the machine may need to be recalibrated.

38/Sample method for a laboratory manual

Radioimmunoassay of thyroid-stimulating hormone by a double-antibody technique

PRINCIPLE

Measurement of TSH is accomplished by a competitive RIA using rabbit anti-TSH antibody in the primary step. Since this antiserum cross-reacts with the α-chain of other glycopeptide hormones, human chorionic gonadotropin (hCG) is added to each tube in the assay in order to eliminate this effect. Lacto-peroxidase-labeled ^{125}I-TSH is used as radioligand.

After the primary antibody and the TSH in the samples come into equilibrium, separation of bound from free radioligand is accomplished with a goat anti-rabbit IgG. Some additional normal rabbit serum is added to serve as carrier. After incubation, precipitation of the IgG complex is achieved by centrifugation. Tubes are then counted in an automatic gamma counter. The results in unknown samples are determined by reference to a standard curve.

MATERIALS

1. Buffers
   a. Barbital buffer, 0.075 M, pH 8.6
   b. Barbital-BSA; barbital buffer, 2.5% BSA
   c. Barbital-BSA-EDTA; barbital buffer, 2.5% BSA, 0.25% EDTA
   d. Barbital-BSA with EDTA and hCG. Human chorionic gonadotropin with a purity of 10,000 IU/mg is used; 10.0 mg hCG is dissolved in 50 ml barbital-BSA with EDTA. This solution is stored in 2-ml aliquots in a frozen state (2.0 ml = 4,000 IU). For each assay run, 2.0 ml of this solution is diluted to a final volume of 80 ml with barbital-BSA-EDTA (final concentration of hCG = 50 IU/ml).
2. ^{125}I-TSH prepared by LPO iodination (see Chapter 3). A suitable aliquot of purified ^{125}I-TSH is diluted with barbital-BSA-EDTA-hCG so that 200μl gives about 10,000 cpm. The ^{125}I-TSH may be kept for up to 4 weeks from the day of labeling. The ^{125}I-TSH solution is stored in a frozen state until the day of use. Any prepared dilution should be kept in the refrigerator until immediately before use in the assay.
3. TSH antiserum is obtained from K.A.B.I. Diagnostica, Stockholm. The antiserum is diluted 1:150,000 before use in the assay with barbital-BSA.
4. TSH standard from K.A.B.I. is used (6 IU/mg). The standards are prepared in the ap-

propriate concentration by dilution with barbital-BSA. The following concentrations are utilized: 3.75μU/ml, 7.5μU/ml, 15μU/ml, 30μU/ml, and 60μU/ml. As the 0-standard, barbital-BSA is used. Standards are prepared in 0.5-ml aliquots and are stored in the frozen state until immediately before use.
5. Goat anti-rabbit IgG serum (see Chapter 5 for details of preparation and standardization). A dilution of 1:10 in barbital-BSA is usually adequate for the purpose of this assay.
6. Normal rabbit serum is diluted 1:250 with barbital-BSA (100μl rabbit serum + 25 ml barbital-BSA). This dilution may be kept for up to 2 weeks in the refrigerator. Undiluted serum is stored frozen.
7. "High" and "low" plasma pools. The TSH high and low pools are collected by mixing patient samples with high and low TSH values. When a sufficient volume of each pool has been collected, the pools are mixed well, filtered, aliquoted in small volumes, and stored frozen in 0.3- to 0.5-ml aliquots. These pools are run in order to test the reproducibility at the low and high ends of the plasma curve. Suitable concentrations are approximately $> 4\mu$U/ml in the low pool and 20μU/ml in the high pool.
8. Pool plasma for addition to the standard curve TSH-free plasma is obtained from an individual on a regimen of T_4 suppression. After preparation as previously described, the plasma is divided into 2-ml aliquots and stored in the frozen state.

SAMPLE

2 ml EDTA-plasma

General procedures for collecting samples should be carefully followed.

PERFORMANCE

Reagent solutions and samples should never be kept at room temperature longer than is absolutely necessary. For all pipetting, a semiautomated pipette (for example, Eppendorf-type) is used. All patient samples are run in triplicate.

Day 1

Samples and pools are thawed and stored in a refrigerator (2°-4° C) until immediately before use. A written protocol is made up that identifies standards, pools, and patient samples. Test tubes are numbered sequentially. Ellerman (11 × 55 mm) tubes are used.

Tubes 1-3. These tubes show the total amount of radioactivity added.

Tubes 4-21. These are the standard curve tubes.

Tubes 22-24. After the standard curve tubes come control tubes without antiserum (standard blank). These tubes permit evaluation of nonspecific binding in the standard curve tubes.

Tubes 25-36. The standard curve tubes are followed by the low and high TSH–pool plasma samples in association with sample blanks without antiserum.

Tubes 37-end. The patient samples are all run in triplicate.

Preparation of tubes

1. To the 0-standard tube and the standard blank tubes add 100μl of barbital-BSA.
2. Tubes 5-16 receive 100μl each of the appropriate standard solutions.
3. Tubes 17-*N* receive 100μl of the appropriate pool or patient sample. This includes the sample blanks.
4. To all tubes add 200μl ^{125}I-TSH. Also add 200μl to an empty 11 × 55 mm tube for "total counts." Place a cork in tubes 1-3 and set aside.

5. To all tubes except the blanks add 200μl TSH-antiserum.
6. After mixing all the tubes in a vortex mixer, place the test tube racks into a plastic sack that seals well. The samples are then incubated overnight in the refrigerator at 4° C.

Day 2

1. To all standards and accompanying blanks add 100μl of pool plasma.
2. To all plasma samples (including pools) and accompanying blanks add 100μl barbital-BSA.
3. To all tubes add 50μl goat anti-rabbit antiserum, 1:10 dilution.
4. To all tubes add 50μl normal rabbit serum, 1:250.
5. After thorough mixing of all tubes in a vortex mixer, place the test tube racks into a plastic sack that seals well. Incubate the samples overnight in a refrigerator (4° C).

Day 3

1. To all tubes add 0.5 ml barbital-BSA with an automatic pipette. After careful mixing, centrifuge at 3,000 rpm (2,500g) for 15 minutes.
2. Pour off the supernatant, and place the tubes into 150 × 14 mm counting tubes. Take care that the decanting process is carried out in a uniform manner for each test tube.

39/Sample report for assay performance and data output

Radioimmunoassay of thyroid-stimulating hormone

The assay is set up according to the protocol given in Appendix 38.

Reagents	Dilution	Volume	Date
Antiserum, R 66:2	1:150,000	200μl	6/2
Label, ^{125}I-TSH, 5/24, Fr 4 + hCG	1:1,000	200μl	
Standard samples, plasma (EDTA)			
K.A.B.I. hTSH		100μl	
Double antibody, GAR-G 10	1:10	50μl	6/3
Nonspecific antigen, NRS	1:250	50μl	
Other, 3-26, pool 18; 27-180, diluent		100μl	
Diluent		0.5 ml	6/4

Tube no.	Standard conc./ sample no.	Counter printout			Calculated TSH conc.	
		No.	Time	Counts	Individual sample	Mean of triplicate
1	Total activity	384	120	024348		
2	Total activity	385	120	024174		
3	Total activity	386	120	024398		
4	St$_0$	387	120	012055		
5	St$_0$	388	120	012428		
6	St$_0$	389	120	012346		
7	St 3.75	390	120	011622		
8	St 3.75	391	120	011744		
9	St 3.75	392	120	011824		
10	St 7.5	393	120	011391		
11	St 7.5	394	120	010943		
12	St 7.5	395	120	010764		
13	St 15	396	120	009467		
14	St 15	397	120	009616		
15	St 15	398	120	009831		
16	St 30	399	120	007653		
17	St 30	400	120	007717		
18	St 30	401	120	007925		
19	St 60	402	120	006207		
20	St 60	403	120	006665		
21	St 60	404	120	006115		
22	C$_0$-St	405	120	002405		
23	C$_0$-St	406	120	002406		
24	C$_0$-St	407	120	002404		
25	Pool 88	408	120	008493	23	
26	Pool 88	409	120	008404	24	24
27	Pool 88	410	120	008612	25	
28	Pool 43	411	120	012008	2	
29	Pool 43	412	120	011196	5	3
30	Pool 43	413	120	011784	3	
31	C$_0$–pool 43	414	120	002336		

Continued.

Tube no.	Standard conc./ sample no.	Counter printout			Calculated TSH conc.	
		No.	Time	Counts	Individual sample	Mean of triplicate
32	C_0–pool 43	415	120	001959		
33	C_0–pool 43	416	120	002222		
34	C_0-4444-77	417	120	002108		
35	C_0-4456-77	418	120	002149		
36	C_0-4457-77	419	120	002434		
37	4444-77	420	120	011714	4	
38	4444-77	421	120	011660	4	4
39	4444-77	422	120	011566	4	
40	4456-77	423	120	011049	8	
41	4456-77	424	120	011300	6	7
42	4456-77	425	120	011302	6	
43	4457-77	426	120	009594	15	
44	4457-77	427	120	009397	16	16
45	4457-77	428	120	009387	16	
46	4458-77	429	120	009983	13	
47	4458-77	430	120	009845	14	13
48	4458-77	431	120	010180	12	
49	4459-77	432	120	005450	>60	
50	4459-77	433	120	005283	>60	>60
51	4459-77	434	120	005236	>60	
52	4477-77	435	120	012102	1	
53	4477-77	436	120	012196	1	1
54	4477-77	437	120	012010	2	
55	4478-77	438	120	011406	5	
56	4478-77	439	120	011335	6	5
57	4478-77	440	120	011508	5	
And so on up to 180 tubes						

COMMENTS

Antiserum. R 66:2, rabbit antiserum to hTSH, batch 2

Label. TSH was radioiodinated (lactoperoxidase method) on May 5; fraction 4 from the Sephadex separation is used, diluted 1:1,000 with barbital-BSA-EDTA-hCG.

Double antibody. GAR, goat anti-rabbit, pool 10; NRS, normal rabbit serum.

St_0-St_{60}. Standards containing hTSH in concentrations of $0\mu U$-$60\mu U/ml$.

C_0. Controls without antiserum (substituted by diluent, $200\mu l$). One set is included for the standards C_0St, one set for one pool sample, and three tubes for patient samples (C_0-4444 to C_0-4457); 4444-77 and so forth denote patient sample identification numbers.

Abbreviations used in this text

ACTH adrenocorticotropic hormone (corticotropin)
AFP alpha-fetoprotein
ANS 8-anilino naphthalene sulfonic acid
ATP adenosine triphosphate
B bound
B_0 amount bound in the absence of nonlabeled ligand
BAL dimercaprol
BSA bovine serum albumin
C_0 control without receptor (used as blank), also called "antibody" blank
CEA carcinoembryonic antigen
CNS central nervous system
CRF corticotropin-releasing factor
CSF cerebrospinal fluid
DA double antibody
DASP double antibody solid phase
DFP diisopropyl fluorophosphate
DOC 11-desoxycorticosterone
dps disintegrations per second
ECG electrocardiogram
EDTA ethylenediamenetetraacetic acid
F free
FSH follicle-stimulating hormone
FT_1 free T_4 concentration
GH growth hormone
gon RH gonadotropin-releasing hormone, synonymous with LH-RH or FSH/LH-RH
h human (in association with a hormone abbreviation)
HB_cAg hepatitis B core antigen
HB_sAb hepatitis B antigen–specific antibody
HB_sAg hepatitis B surface antigen
hCG human chorionic gonadotropin
hCS human chorionic somatomammotropin
hPL human placental lactogen
HSA human serum albumin
ICSH interstitial cell–stimulating hormone
IF intrinsic factor
IgE immunoglobulin E
IgG immunoglobulin G
L ligand
LH luteinizing hormone

LH-RH gonadotropin-releasing hormone (*see* gon RH)
L/M liters per mole
LPO lactoperoxidase
LR bound ligand (ligand + receptor)
MSH melanocyte-stimulating hormone
MTHFA methyltetrahydrofolic acid
NRS normal rabbit serum
NSB nonspecific binding
PB phosphate buffer
PBS phosphate-buffered saline
PEG polyethylene glycol
PGA pteroyltriglutamic acid
PIF prolactin inhibitory factor
PRA plasma renin activity
PRC plasma renin concentration
PRS plasma renin substrate
PTH parathyroid hormone
R receptor (unbound sites)
RAIU ^{131}I-thyroid uptake
RIA radioimmunoassay
RT_3U resin T_3 uptake in vitro
T total (usually refers to radioactivity)
T_3 triiodothyronine
T_3 (RIA) total serum T_3 by radioimmunoassay
T_4 thyroxine
T_4 (D) total serum T_4 by competitive protein binding (displacement analysis)
T_4 (RIA) total serum T_4 by radioimmunoassay
T_4-RT_3 index free T_4 index
TBG thyroid-binding (thyroxine-binding) globulin
TBPA thyroid-binding prealbumin
TCA trichloroacetic acid
THFA tetrahydrofolic acid
TLC thin-layer chromatography
TME tyrosine methyl ester
TRF thyrotropin-releasing factor
TRH thyrotropin-releasing hormone
TSH thyroid-stimulating hormone
TSH (RIA) thyrotropin (thyroid-stimulating hormone) by radioimmunoassay

INDEX